Creating Knowledge-Based Healthcare Organizations

Nilmini Wickramasinghe
Cleveland State University, USA

Jatinder N.D. Gupta
University of Alabama in Huntsville, USA

Sushil K. Sharma
Ball State University, USA

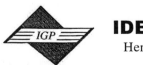
IDEA GROUP PUBLISHING
Hershey • London • Melbourne • Singapore

Acquisitions Editor:	Mehdi Khosrow-Pour
Senior Managing Editor:	Jan Travers
Managing Editor:	Amanda Appicello
Development Editor:	Michele Rossi
Copy Editor:	Bernard J. Kieklak Jr.
Typesetter:	Jennifer Wetzel
Cover Design:	Lisa Tosheff
Printed at:	Yurchak Printing Inc.

Published in the United States of America by
    Idea Group Publishing (an imprint of Idea Group Inc.)
    701 E. Chocolate Avenue, Suite 200
    Hershey PA 17033
    Tel: 717-533-8845
    Fax: 717-533-8661
    E-mail: cust@idea-group.com
    Web site: http://www.idea-group.com

and in the United Kingdom by
    Idea Group Publishing (an imprint of Idea Group Inc.)
    3 Henrietta Street
    Covent Garden
    London WC2E 8LU
    Tel: 44 20 7240 0856
    Fax: 44 20 7379 3313
    Web site: http://www.eurospan.co.uk

Library of Congress Cataloging-in-Publication Data

Creating knowledge-based healthcare organizations / Nilmini Wickramasinghe, editor,
Jatinder N.D. Gupta, editor, Sushil K. Sharma, editor.
    p. ; cm.
  Includes bibliographical references and index.
    ISBN 1-59140-459-2 (hardcover) -- ISBN 1-59140-460-6 (pbk.) -- ISBN 1-59140-461-4 (ebook)
  1. Health facilities--Administration. 2. Health services administration. 3. Evidence-based
medicine. 4. Medical informatics. 5. Health facilities--Information services.
  [DNLM: 1. Health Facilities--organization & administration. 2. Medical Informatics--
organization & administration. 3. Evidence-Based Medicine. 4. Information Management--
organization & administration. 5. Telemedicine--organization & administration. WX 26.5 C912
2005] I. Wickramasinghe, Nilmini. II. Gupta, Jatinder N. D. III. Sharma, Sushil K.
  RA971.C765 2005
  362.1'068--dc22

                       2004003759

British Cataloguing in Publication Data
A Cataloguing in Publication record for this book is available from the British Library.

Creating Knowledge-Based Healthcare Organizations

Table of Contents

Foreword

Elie Geisler, Illinois Institute of Technology, USA

Healthcare organizations are experiencing a quiet revolution. Fueled by economic pressures and a reexamination of the principles of distribution of care, these organizations are also committing to the onslaught of technology. As latecomers, healthcare delivery institutions are faced with the adoption of the prevailing innovations in information technology. The impacts of the Internet and innovations in telecommunications, computing, and the continuing influx of micro-devices are beginning to be felt in healthcare delivery.

The brunt of these effects are found in the confluence of the technology itself with innovations in marketing, management, and the changing perspective of the healthcare consumer. There is a growing trend of increased awareness, empowerment, and changes in the attitudes of healthcare consumers regarding the delivery of healthcare services. The intersection of these forces of change is engendering a tremendous growth in knowledge flowing through the healthcare system. From the bedside to medical school, from the examining room and the medical encounter to the patient and the family's role in the delivery of healthcare services, there are now many new facets to our knowledge about healthcare and its delivery.

The medical profession is confronted with a dramatic rise in medical knowledge. Genetic research, new drugs, and an expanding field of research in areas such as biotechnology and biomedical engineering are creating a strong need to manage this avalanche of knowledge. Medical professionals and particularly medical students are now routinely armed with PDAs and other miniaturized information technology devices that allow them to access this vast array of knowledge. In healthcare delivery, as well as in so many other disciplines and professions, we now produce more knowledge in a day than in hundreds — perhaps thousands — of years of human history. Imagine if we were to produce more automobiles in one day than in the previous 100 years. Our highways and byways would be immediately clogged, and it would be a horrific task to sort out this traffic jam. A similar situation occurs in the growth of knowledge in the healthcare delivery arena.

To sort out the jammed passages of the accumulation of a continuing production of knowledge in healthcare delivery organizations there is a crying need for knowledge management, capable of inserting some order into the increasingly confusing state of affairs. Since healthcare is notoriously slow in adopting such innovations, we are now beginning to see the initial forays of these organizations into the era of knowledge management systems. These are cautious "baby-steps" that the industry is taking, and there is presently very little systematic work that documents such a passage into a new age of managing knowledge.

This book, edited by Professors Wickramasinghe, Gupta and Sharma is a true pioneering effort to open up the field of knowledge management to healthcare organizations and professionals. It's a unique enterprise of the utmost importance. As we witness the transformation of patient care with the advent of wireless hospitals, medical staffs connected to the Internet, and the revolution in the structure and architecture of care and the bedside, it is a perplexing thought that knowledge management in this dynamic area has not yet been adequately studied. This book heralds a new era of the systematic examination of the principles and the practices of knowledge management. It captures the experiences in other, first-adopters industries, and offers potential schemes and methods to better introduce and adopt knowledge management systems in healthcare delivery organizations.

In the final analysis, healthcare delivery is the manipulation of knowledge, and the management of organizations — including healthcare organizations — is the management of knowledge. We are now realizing that unless organizations are capable of effectively administering the knowledge they need to act and to survive, they are destined to failure. This book offers a thoughtful array of topics, ranging from the principles of knowledge management, e-health organizations, knowledge management infrastructure, and how to start and improve knowledge management systems. It's an initial attempt to create awareness of the importance of knowledge management in healthcare delivery. It's also the sounding of a call to other scholars to join in exploring the vital and rapidly growing area of knowledge management in healthcare delivery organizations.

Preface

Healthcare in the 21st Century is facing three very large forces of change; namely, an informed and empowered consumer, the need for e-health adaptability and a shift from focusing on primarily curing diseases to the prevention of diseases. In addition to having to contend with these forces, the cost of delivering quality healthcare is increasing exponentially. While no country spends more per capita than the U.S., most of the 29 countries of the Organization for Economic Cooperation and Development (OECD) have doubled their healthcare expenditures over the last 20 years. Hence, reducing this expenditure as well as offering effective and efficient quality healthcare treatment is becoming a priority globally. New business and technological advances have the potential not only to reduce these costs but also, and equally importantly, to make it possible to achieve high quality, high value and high accessibility to healthcare delivery systems. Thus, the adoption of such advances, specifically knowledge management strategies, processes, techniques and tools into the healthcare industry may not be a panacea for addressing all of today's current healthcare challenges but is certainly an important component for any solution.

The purpose of this book then, is to increase the awareness of the need for embracing knowledge management strategies, processes, techniques and tools throughout various areas of the healthcare sector as well as highlight the benefits such initiatives will provide. The book is divided into four sections described here.

BOOK LAYOUT

Section I, *Knowledge Management in the Healthcare Industry*, includes four chapters.

Chapter I (Sharma, Wickramasinghe and Gupta), *Knowledge Management in Healthcare*, describes the basics of knowledge management and how knowledge management concepts can be applied to the healthcare sector. The authors in their chapter also suggest various approaches that could be used for implementing knowledge management in healthcare organizations.

Chapter II (Desouza), *Knowledge Management in Hospitals*, describes the significance of knowledge management in healthcare organizations. The chapter describes how to develop and foster a knowledge management process model in healthcare organizations. The author also identifies the key barriers for healthcare organizations to cross in order to fully manage knowledge.

Chapter III (Wahle and Groothuis), *How to Handle Knowledge Management in Healthcare: A Description of a Model to Deal with the Current and Ideal Situation*, cites many reasons such as: the introduction of Diagnosis Treatment Combinations (DTCs) in The Netherlands, which makes the learning capacity and competitiveness of the hospital an important factor; the demand for efficiency and effectiveness due to shortages in the job market; the requirement of patients for better quality care and related provision of information, and, the fact that hospitals and/or any other Healthcare Organization (HCO) are becoming more knowledge intensive as principle reasons why healthcare organizations are developing and embracing knowledge management strategies, process techniques and/or tools.

The final chapter in this section, Chapter IV (Rubenstein and Geisler), *How to Start or Improve a KM System in a Hospital or Healthcare Organization*, is based on years of experience in the field and the basic steps required to offer KM solutions in healthcare organizations. The chapter discusses what hospitals and other healthcare organizations need to have in place in order to be successful including, but not limited to, bricks and mortar, human resources, medical technology, financial systems, and other infrastructure items.

Section II, *Approaches, Frameworks and Tools to Create Knowledge-Based Healthcare Organizations*, has nine chapters.

Chapter V (Gargeya and Sorrell) is titled *Moving Toward an e-Hospital*. The authors argue that while some aspects of patient care must continue to be delivered locally, Internet technologies and "e-healthcare experiences" are likely to play an increasing role in the pre-delivery and post-delivery arenas. Their chapter presents an overview of infrastructure issues and technologies that will enable hospitals to "plug into" the evolving e-health continuum.

Chapter VI (Puerzer), *Applying Automatic Data Collection Tools for Real-Time Patient Management*, discusses how hospitals can effectively deal with many of the problems associated with scheduling and overcrowding, and improve the quality of care through the use of automated patient management system. The author argues that knowledge management systems can only be effective if accurate and comprehensive data is accessible to the knowledge management systems.

Chapter VII (Testik, Runger, Kirkman-Liff and Smith), *Data Mining and Knowledge Discovery in Healthcare Organizations: A Decision-Tree Approach*, discusses how healthcare organizations are struggling to find new ways to cut healthcare utilization and costs while improving quality and outcomes. The chapter presents a modern data mining tool, decision trees, which may have a broad range of applications in healthcare organizations.

Chapter VIII (Win and Croll), *Engineering Dependable Health Information Systems*, describes health information systems, in particular automated medical record systems and their role in facilitating effective knowledge management. The chapter outlines key aspects for designing robust and appropriate health information systems, providing some frameworks that can assist in their design and then presenting some case studies that serve to highlight some of the key issues in designing appropriate health information systems.

Chapter IX (Sharma and Wickramasinghe), e-*Health with Knowledge Management: The Areas of Tomorrow*, emphasizes the need for taking a KM perspective when creating or enhancing the efficiency of e-health. In their chapter, the authors describe how the Internet and related new communication technologies enable health professionals to reach large populations with interactive applications, which in turn open enormous opportunities and challenges. The authors argue that e-health solutions should go beyond merely developing and providing technical solutions and must consider social and human factors involved for providing better healthcare.

Chapter X (Wickramasinghe, Sharma and Reddy), *Evidence-Based Medicine: A New Approach in the Practice of Medicine*, describes how evidence-based medicine deals directly with the uncertainties of clinical medicine and has the potential for transforming the education and practice of the next generation of physicians. According to authors, evidence-based medicine will require new skills for the physician, and would need integration of individual clinical expertise with the best available external clinical evidence from systematic research. An integral part of successful evidence-based medicine will be the incorporation of a knowledge management perspective.

Chapter XI (Shadbolt, Wang and Craft), *Moving to an Online Framework for Knowledge-Driven Healthcare*, describes how knowledge is a critical resource in the provision of healthcare guiding improvements regarding clinical decision making, patient care, health outcomes, workforce quality, and organizational behavior and structure. The chapter is focused on knowledge acquisition associated with clinical decision making, patient care and health outcomes. The authors present a framework Protocol Hypothesis Testing (PHT) "a whole-of-health on-line knowledge-based framework," and examine the development of the PHT approach and software application as a case study.

Chapter XII (Engelkemeyer and Muret-Wagstaff), *Using the Malcolm Baldrige National Quality Award Criteria to Enable KM and Create a Systemic Organizational Perspective*, presents how healthcare leaders face an intensifying array of changes and challenges that heighten the need for systematic approaches to knowledge management at the organizational level. This chapter describes the Malcolm Baldrige National Quality Award and its framework, criteria, and scoring system. It also provides insight into pitfalls as well as successful examples of ways that healthcare groups and institutions are becoming learning organizations, successfully employing cycles of learning and effective knowledge management systems in order to enhance performance and better meet the needs of patients and other customers.

Chapter XIII, the final chapter in this section (Fadlalla and Wickramasinghe), is titled *Realizing Knowledge Assets in the Medical Sciences with Data Mining: An Overview*. This chapter provides a survey of the four major data mining techniques and their application to the medical science field in order to realize the full potential of knowledge assets in healthcare. The authors also presented an enhanced framework of the knowledge discovery process to highlight the interrelationships between data, information and knowledge as well as between knowledge creation and the key steps in data mining.

Section III, *Key Issues and Concerns of Various Knowledge Management Implementations: Evidence from Practice*, includes six chapters.

Chapter XIV (Saito, Inoue and Seki), *Organizational Control Mode, Cognitive Activity & Performance Reliability: The Case of a National Hospital in Japan*, presents the findings of a study based in a Japanese context. The authors identify and verify that cognitive activities, work environment and organizational climate/culture are highly related to human performance reliability and that human performance reliability was predicted by organizational control mode, and emphasize that it is important to focus on the implication of latent variables perceived for tacit knowledge as well as articulate knowledge in KM.

Chapter XV (Al-Qirim), *Tele-Medicine: Building Knowledge-Based Tele-Health Capability in New Zealand,* describes the strategic planning of health information systems in New Zealand identifying the major accelerators and impediments of technology adoption and diffusion as well as the role of knowledge management in tele-medicine.

Chapter XVI (Castleman, Swatman and Fowler), *Aligning Multiple Knowledge Perspectives in a Health Services System: A Case Study*, concludes that the most significant impediment to the effective creation and sharing of knowledge is the highly diffused, fragmented and, interlocking organizational structure of the social service administration itself. Their study examines various issues regarding the design of the underlying organizational system for service provision, the level of details required in the service data and the locus of decision-making power among the stakeholders in order to support the higher-level knowledge that is sought.

Chapter XVII (Hughes and Golden), *Knowing How Intranets Enable Knowledge Work: An Exploratory Study in Public Health*, presents findings from longitudinal case studies conducted in two Irish public sector hospitals. This chapter explores the role of intranet technology as an enabling technology for supporting the knowledge worker, knowledge work and various forms of knowledge management in a hospital setting.

Chapter XVIII (Gammack, Desai, Sandhu and Winklhofer), *Knowledge Management in Indian Companies: Benchmarking the Pharmaceutical Industry*, analyzes the KM scenario in the pharmaceutical industry in India. The authors argue that KM must be incorporated into processes, strategies and organizational culture for successful adoption. The study concludes that there is a heavy orientation toward IT-based conceptions of KM, which may be incompatible with the requirements for future success in the pharmaceutical industry globally.

Chapter XIX, the last chapter in this section (Natarajan and Hoffmeister) is titled *"Do No Harm": Can Healthcare Live Up to It.* The chapter describes an important issue, namely, that of the growing percentage of medical errors. The authors highlight the need for the healthcare sector to learn from other industry sectors and embrace techniques to help decrease the number of errors. The authors believe that the embracing of knowledge management by healthcare organizations will serve to decrease medical errors.

Section IV, *Managing Knowledge as an Asset in Healthcare Organizations*, has five chapters.

Chapter XX (Davison), *Temporary Communication Infrastructures for Dynamic KM in the Complex and Innovative Environment of Palliative Care*, describes managing knowledge face-to-face on a human scale. This chapter emphasizes that knowledge creation is a human activity and, therefore, the organizational effort to create and manage knowledge should be based on anthropocentric rather than techno-centric perspectives and the author suggests a personalized approach to knowledge transfer rather than the interaction with a codified knowledge repository.

Chapter XXI (Ahn and Chang), *Managing Healthcare Organizations through the Knowledge Productivity Measurement*, describes how understanding the contribution of knowledge to business performance is important for efficient resource allocations. In this chapter, the author discusses a performance-oriented knowledge management methodology or KP^3 methodology that was applied to the medical domain in Korea and how the contribution of knowledge to the performance was assessed.

Chapter XXII (da Cunha and Paiva), *Knowledge Strategic Management in the Hospital Industry*, analyzes the strategic role of organizational knowledge in the Brazilian hospital industry. Results are presented from a group of eight hospitals, which created a cooperative program related to performance measurement systems (SIPAGEH - Standardized Measurement Systems for Hospital Management). The authors present a three-stage approach to analyze the relationship between strategy and knowledge management based on the cases analyzed.

Chapter XXIII (Mundy and Chadwick), *Secure Knowledge Management for Healthcare Organizations*, argues that as the healthcare industry enters the era of knowledge management it must place security at the foundation of the transition. According to authors, in an age where risks and security threats are rapidly increasing, secure knowledge management is an essential business practice. The chapter presents different approaches to minimize security risks based on the concepts of authentication, authorization, data integrity, availability and confidentiality.

Chapter XXIV (Burdick, Hensing, Kirkman-Liff, Nenaber, Silverman and Simington), *Managing Knowledge to Improve Healthcare Quality in Banner Health*, presents the case study of Banner Health. They argue through their case analysis that the one way to gauge the quality of healthcare is to measure its clinical, financial, and service performance. The chapter suggests that even outstanding performance or outcomes need a review to determine how such results can be consistently achieved.

Acknowledgments

This book would not have been possible without the cooperation and assistance of many people: the authors, reviewers, our colleagues, and the staff at Idea Group Inc. The editors would like to thank Mehdi Khosrow-Pour for inviting us to produce this book, Jan Travers for managing this project, and Michele Rossi as development editor for answering our questions and keeping us on schedule. Many of the authors of chapters in this book also served as reviewers of other chapters, and so we are doubly appreciative of their contributions. We also acknowledge our respective universities for affording us the time to work on this project and our colleagues and students for many stimulating discussions and Fash for all his efforts with formatting draft versions of the manuscript. Finally, the authors naturally wish to acknowledge their families for providing time and supporting them throughout this project.

Nilmini Wickramasinghe, Cleveland State University, USA
Jatinder N.D. Gupta, University of Alabama in Huntsville, USA
Sushil K. Sharma, Ball State University, USA

Section I

Knowledge Management in the Healthcare Industry

Chapter I

Knowledge Management in Healthcare

Sushil K. Sharma, Ball State University, USA

Nilmini Wickramasinghe, Cleveland State University, USA

Jatinder N.D. Gupta, University of Alabama in Huntsville, USA

ABSTRACT

Healthcare organizations are facing many challenges in the 21st Century due to changes taking place in global healthcare systems. Spiraling costs, financial constraints, increased emphasis on accountability and transparency, changes in education, growing complexities of biomedical research, new partnerships in healthcare and great advances in IT suggest that a predominant paradigm shift is occurring. This shift is necessitating a focus on interaction, collaboration and increased sharing of information and knowledge which is in turn leading healthcare organizations to embrace the techniques of Knowledge Management (KM) in order to create and sustain optimal healthcare outcomes. This chapter describes the importance of knowledge management systems for healthcare organizations and provides an overview of knowledge management technologies and tools that may be used by healthcare organizations.

INTRODUCTION

Knowledge Management (KM) is an essential tool in today's emerging healthcare system. Hospitals that seek to deploy KM systems need to understand the human element in the process. Earlier, success factors were only restricted to a few healthcare variables such as patient care and cost, but over the years, technology (both clinical and administrative) has evolved as a differentiating variable, thus redefining the doctrines of competition and the administration of healthcare treatments. For example, in today's healthcare environment we are now treating patients with an emphasis on prevention and managing the patient through good health throughout their life. Such an approach requires significant investment in knowledge assets. One of the key objectives of a KM system is to insulate a hospital's intellectual knowledge from degeneration (Elliot, 2000).

Most hospitals are unaware of their acquired knowledge base. Further, knowledge capital is often lost from a hospital through employee attrition, high turnover rates, cost-saving measures and improper documentation (Chase, 1998). Specific KM tools and metrics help focus the hospital on acquisition, retrieval and storage of knowledge assets both tangible and/or other for activities such as learning, strategic planning and decision making (Oxbrow, 1998). This goes a long way in crafting a coherent and well-designed growth plan for the hospital (Allee, 1997, 1999). KM treats intellectual capital as a managed asset. Improved patient care is directly proportional to a hospital's intellectual assets. The tactical expertise and experience of individual workers should be fully captured and reflected in strategy, policy and practice at all levels of the hospital management and patient care activity (Conklin, 1998). The intangible asset of knowledge of the employee can nurture radical innovation in advance planning, change management, hospital culture and well balanced approaches. Fostering a knowledge-sharing attitude and competency of patient care processes are vital for any KM program in healthcare (Burca, 2000; Matheson, 1995). Hospitals managing and sharing their knowledge assets effectively will have benefits of cycle time reduction, cost reduction, improved return on investment, higher satisfaction index, and better medical and paramedical education levels (Antrobus, 1997; Atkins et al., 2001).

KNOWLEDGE MANAGEMENT

Knowledge Management (KM) is an emerging, interdisciplinary business model dealing with all aspects of knowledge within the context of the firm, including knowledge creation, codification, sharing and how these activities promote learning and innovation (Choo, 1998). Unfortunately there's no universal definition of KM, just as there's no agreement as to what constitutes knowledge in the first place (Beckman, 1999). For this reason, it's best to think of KM in the broadest context:

KM is a discipline that promotes an integrated approach to identifying, managing, and sharing all of an enterprise's information assets, including database, documents, policies and procedures, as well as unarticulated expertise and experience resident in individual workers (Wickramasinghe, 2003). There are many dimensions around which knowledge can be characterized such as storage media, accessibility, typology and hierarchy. Each of these dimensions is explained in this chapter (Brailer, 1999; Broadbent, 1998; Skyrme, 2001, 1999, 1998; Davenport & Prusak, 1997, 1998).

Knowledge Storage Media

There are several media in which knowledge can reside including: the human mind, an organization, a document and/or a computer. Knowledge in the mind is often difficult to access; organizational knowledge is often dispersed and distributed; document knowledge can range from free text to well-structured charts and tables; while computer knowledge can be formalized, sharable and often well structured and well organized. In order to effectively manage KM it is important to pay careful attention to the most useful storage media.

Knowledge Accessibility

Intellectual and knowledge-based assets fall into one of three major categories (Nonaka, 1994; Nonaka & Nishguchi, 2001; Sharma & Wickramasinghe, 2004):

- *Tacit (human mind, organization):* accessible indirectly only with difficulty through knowledge elicitation and observation of behavior.
- *Implicit (human mind, organization):* accessible through querying and discussion, but informal knowledge must first be located and then communicated.
- *Explicit (document, computer):* readily available, as well as documented into formal knowledge sources that are often well organized, often with the help of IT.

In order for effective KM to ensue, it is necessary to understand these categories of knowledge as well as their subtle nuances.

Knowledge Typologies

Typologies are defined, characterized and described in terms of knowledge type-conversion, structural features, elementary properties, purpose and use, and conceptual levels. Knowledge typologies play an integral role in a robust KM system.

Knowledge Hierarchy

A further dimension considers the premise that knowledge can be organized into a hierarchy. Several authors draw distinctions between data, information and knowledge (Allee, 1997; Devenport & Prusack, 1998; Leonard, 1998).

- *Data:* Facts, images and sounds.
- *Information:* Formatted, filtered and summarized data.
- *Knowledge:* Instincts, ideas, rules and procedures that guide action and decisions and are context dependent.

Strictly speaking, KM is a process that identifies and creates knowledge assets. In healthcare, KM optimally utilizes these assets to fulfill the core healthcare objectives. Knowledge assets in hospitals are intangible but they can be defined as knowledge that a medical/paramedical/non-medical person has with respect to patient care, medical needs, operating environment and technologies, something that he or she can utilize in routine medical and healthcare management. KM identifies and maps intellectual assets within the hospital, thereby generating precious knowledge capital for competitive advantage within the medical institution. Since knowledge is dynamically imbedded in organizational and healthcare networks and processes as well as in the staff that use them, hospitals need to have a built-in KM system that "crisscrosses" with its healthcare networks (Jackson, 2000). The result is that employees will then be better informed and continuously updated on the latest tools and best practices. It is important that the techniques adopted to enable KM must take into account some basic factors such as the type of hospital, its culture and its needs to ensure a successful KM system for a healthcare setting (Gokce, 2002; Johnson, 1998; Keeling & Lambert, 2000).

THE NEED FOR KM IN HEALTHCARE

The health sector is large, accounting for between 6% to 12% of GDP across OECD countries. Though the use of healthcare services varies between nations, public expectations of them globally have risen dramatically everywhere since 1950 and the trend is still upwards. Fresh demands arise from the appearance of new drugs and the invention of new technology, from advances in prevention and diagnosis as well as therapy, and from new categories of demand, such as care of the elderly (Eisenberg, 2002). The health sector is complex and includes a range of key actors: patients, providers, practitioners, payers, purchasers, pharmaceutical industry, and professors. The interaction among these actors shapes what counts as relevant knowledge as well as how it is produced, mediated, and used (Conner, 2001). Further, the domain of medical knowledge has expanded to such a degree that a human mind can no longer retain it all. There are now some 20,000 medical journals in the world. A professor of medicine spends on average one day a week to remain abreast of studies in his/her field of interest as well as for his/her research. What can a generalist physician do? How much time can he/she devote to "keeping up"? In France, there are some 7,000 prescription drugs based on some 3,500 active ingredients. A physician has the right to prescribe them all. Can he/she be familiar with all of them? He/she must also be aware of some 300 medical references, some 800 biological tests, more than 1,000 imagery tests, and more than 1,500 surgical interventions. If he/she prescribes six drugs, he/she must also be aware of some 720 potential sources of interaction. The figure reaches 3,328,800 if 10 drugs are prescribed. In addition to the therapeutic value of each molecule, the physician should also know their price and potential effect on specific population groups (diabetics, the obese, children, the elderly, etc. The growth in knowledge has necessarily led to specialization, which too has meant "balkanization" and lack of coordination, especially in hospitals but also in private practice (Halpern, Perry & Narayan, 2001; Dean, 2002). As knowledge is shared, responsibility and decisions about treatment should be shared as well (Eisenberg, 2002). Hospital Information Management (HIM) professionals, like other healthcare personnel, have always sought, used, and valued knowledge about their practice. Managers hire experience because they understand the value of knowledge that has been developed and proven over time. Unfortunately, they are bombarded each day with information in the form of e-mails, voice mails, faxes, reports, memos, and so on — much of which is repetitive or simply not useful. On the other hand, the same professionals spend a great deal of time looking for the information they need by accessing the Web, sending e-mails, making phone calls, and scouring computerized reports. It is in this process that KM can make a difference. Studies have shown that managers get two-thirds of their information from face-to-face meetings or phone conversations. Only one-third comes from documents or other knowledge bases. Unlike material assets, which decrease in value as they are used, the value of knowledge increases with use. For example, new ideas on records storage or retrieval breed other new ideas, and shared knowledge stays with the giver while it enriches the receiver (Jadad, Haynes, Hunt & Browman, 2000). The potential for new ideas arising from the store of knowledge in any healthcare organization is to provide a common entry point for corporate knowledge, such as formularies, clinical road maps, and key financial indicators (Einbinder, Klein & Safran, 1997). Thus what we can see is that the need for KM in healthcare is critical and becomes significant when it begins to focus on the needs of individual users, departmental indicators, and key processes in order to capture and display relevant, useful, and usable knowledge in a customized fashion (Sorrells & Weaver, 1999a, 1999b, 1999c).

APPROACHES TO CAPTURE, STORE AND SHARE KNOWLEDGE

For companies that need to leverage their corporate knowledge, the following four initiatives may help you establish a knowledge sharing system of your own. These initiatives draw upon a predominate, repository model but are also relevant to other models (Morrissey, 1998).

Build the Infrastructure Using Appropriate Technology

Technology enables connectedness to take place in ways that have never before been possible. Harnessing intellectual capital can be expedited through a network-computing infrastructure. Technology has emerged to support each different approach to knowledge management. Document management systems expedite document storage and retrieval. Web-casts allow synchronous communication between experts while discussion groups enable asynchronous interaction. Learning management systems track an employee's progress with continuous learning while data warehousing mines powerful SQL databases, which organize and analyze highly structured information. Paramount to the successful use of these technologies is naturally a flexible, robust IT infrastructure (Sharma & Wickramasinghe, 2004).

Build a Conceptual Infrastructure with Competencies as the Backbone

Technology is important in harnessing intellectual assets, but integrated solutions encompass more than that. You must rethink the conceptual infrastructure of your business. For example, you may need to: ensure intellectual assets reflect your vision and values; articulate the theoretical framework for your processes; establish a taxonomy or categorization scheme to organize your information; create cross references that reflect relationships between entries; or index your information using attributes or meta-tags. The notion of competence plays a critical role in knowledge indexing and sharing. Karl Erik Sveiby, noted Swedish expert on managing and measuring knowledge-based assets, observes, "The concept of competence, which embraces factual knowledge, skills, experience, value judgments and social networks is the best way to describe knowledge in the business context." Once competencies or target proficiencies are defined, they become the backbone, which connects users to useful, relevant knowledge.

Create a Repository of Reusable Components and Other Resources

Before the Industrial Revolution, products were handcrafted; each piece was unique and couldn't be reused. The genius of the Industrial Revolution centered on making reusable parts and components became standardized and interchangeable. The

Information Revolution is similar. Instead of crafting a unique solution each time, knowledge sharing creates a warehouse of "stored parts" — e.g., standardized and interchangeable components which can be reused and adapted: skills, best practices, models and frameworks, approaches and techniques, tools, concepts, specific experiences, presentation aids, white papers, etc. Adding to this, resources such as directories of experts indexed by their field can help you gain access to knowledge outside of your core competencies.

Set High Standards for Quality and Usability

Ensure that your information complies with high quality standards because it is the foundation upon which to build a knowledge-centric healthcare organization. In addition, it is important to make sure that the system meets the users' needs, which may involve reworking or restructuring information. Leonard Caldwell observed: "Critical information must first be reorganized so that information is presented in a way that mirrors users' needs and parallels a thought process occurring within a job function or task." Establishing consistent patterns helps end-users find information quickly. Online coaching can provide users with tips and techniques on how to modify, customize, or tailor information. Leveraging organizational knowledge is not an option — it is an imperative if one is to flourish in the marketplace. It can lead into a new phase of quality and innovation. It will reduce cycle time and gives a competitive advantage as a company. The synergy will also contribute to growth as individuals. Companies who have the foresight to manage their knowledge capital now will have an advantage in the future (Herbig, Bussing & Ewert, 2001).

KM TOOLS AND TECHNOLOGIES

The paraphernalia of the information revolution — computers, communications networks, compact discs, imaging systems and so on — are now widely expected to make a vital contribution to helping doctors and other medical professionals do their work better (Gokce, 2002). New information technologies include:

- Electronic patient records, which are more up to date, easier to access, and more complete than paper ones;
- Standardized medical terminologies and languages, both within and across natural language communities;
- Methods and tools to support faster dissemination of information via the Internet that leads to new scientific understanding of diseases and their treatment;
- More timely and reliable methods and tools to support better communication and coordination among members of healthcare teams;
- A creative approach to KM can result in improved efficiency, higher productivity and increased revenues in practically any business function.

The technical goal of KM initiatives is to give the organization the ability to mine its own knowledge assets, which could include creating such tools as a centralized search capability, automatic indexing and categorization, content analysis and preparation, data analysis, and customizable features integrated in a digital dashboard. Process improvement is a precursor to providing a knowledge-centered environment. Before an organization can foster collaboration and knowledge sharing, the organization must possess an understanding of information flows and of the overall knowledge infrastructure. There is no such thing as the perfect KM product. Instead, different tool sets can be integrated with the organization's legacy systems (Heathfield & Louw, 1999). Technical issues that KM projects must address include:

- Setting up electronic delivery strategies for information
- Identifying information sources and services
- Building decision support tools and data-mining templates
- Establishing enterprise-wide business rules
- Implementing process improvement techniques

Knowledge Mapping

Knowledge management is rapidly becoming a critical success factor for competitive organizations. Carrying out knowledge management effectively in an industrial environment requires support from a repertoire of methods, techniques and tools, in particular knowledge engineering technology adapted for knowledge management. Knowledge mapping creates high-level knowledge models in a transparent graphical form. Using knowledge maps, management can get an overview of available and missing knowledge in core business areas and make appropriate knowledge management decisions. Knowledge mapping is a good example of a useful knowledge management activity with existing knowledge acquisition and modeling techniques at its foundations (Strawser, 2000). Knowledge mapping is a technique rather than a product. A knowledge map could be used as a visual example of how information is passed from one part of an organization or group to another and is usually a good place to start understanding what types of intellectual assets the organization has at its disposal. Most organizations that have implemented KM applications provide a context and framework for the way knowledge is gained. KM is usually an integral part of continuous quality improvement or total quality management projects. Several consultants offer knowledge-mapping methodologies (Heathfield & Louw, 1999).

Process-Based Knowledge Map

A process-based knowledge map is essentially a map or diagram that visually displays knowledge within the context of a business process. In other words, the map shows how knowledge should be used within the processes and sources of this knowledge. The overview of the business process is prepared before the knowledge and the sources are mapped to this process. Any type of knowledge that drives the process or results from execution of the process can be mapped. This could include tacit knowledge (knowledge that resides in people such as know-how, experience, and intuition) and explicit knowledge (codified knowledge that is found in documents); customer knowledge; knowledge in processes; etc.

Intelligent Agents

In the early days of online information retrieval systems, individuals met with search intermediaries who were trained to use the online systems. The intermediaries were often knowledgeable about the information seeker's area of interest. Today, technology in the form of personal computers and the Internet provides users with the means to access the online databases from their own offices. However, distributed sources of online information, e.g., the World Wide Web (WWW), compound the problem of information searching. Both novice and experienced users still need support with the search process and the integration of information. To address this problem, agents have been developed for information management applications. The goal of intelligent search agents is to allow end-users to search effectively, be it either a single database of bibliographic records or a network of distributed, heterogeneous, hypertext documents. The approaches range from desktop agents specialized for a single user to networks of agents used to collect data from distributed information sources. Intelligent agents use a combination of profiling techniques, search tools, and recognition algorithms to "push" information to the decision maker on a regular basis. Because intelligent agents use a standard Web analogy, users can quickly set up "net casts" of internal information to automatically receive knowledge bases when they become available. For example, a physician can request that lab results be forwarded to his or her individual dashboard as soon as the lab has completed the procedure. One cautionary note: using push technologies can result in an information flood if filters are not configured to reduce unwanted or unnecessary data (Strawser, 2000).

Web Browsers

Web browsers such as Microsoft's Internet Explorer are practical because of their cost and relative ease of use, and they have become the preferred presentation layer for accessing knowledge bases. The productivity potential inherent in browsers is similar to that of wireless phones. The freer the knowledge worker is of place, time, medium, and device, the less time is spent on the process of messaging, and the more time is available for results. The less time spent on process, the shorter the knowledge cycle, which can be a significant productivity advantage (Strawser, 2000).

KM Applications

Most new KM applications consist of two major elements (often integrated into one interface): a means for employees looking for specialized knowledge to hook up with other people in the organization with the same knowledge (usually via a web application), in other words, an easy way for employees to tap into tacit knowledge resources (people); and a means for employees looking for specialized knowledge to search relevant documents/data (also usually via a web application), in other words, an easy way for employees to tap into explicit knowledge. KM applications are usually designed to support a particular information set in an organization, such as length-of-stay margin management, physician profitability, or accounts receivable recovery. Some consulting firms offer a base set of templates as a core application, focusing on desktop applications, whereas others have developed information sets that provide encyclopedic knowledge of a particular healthcare segment, such as physician issues (Strawser, 2000).

Workflow Applications

In the software world, and in particular in the imaging subset of that world, the need arose to send a particular (bit-mapped) document to a particular workstation or users on a network. This simple routing and distribution was called "workflow." It was quickly learned that these work items could be "tracked," which allowed the accumulation of data

Table 1: Data Banks, Knowledge Banks and KM Software

Data banks	(Involving text and images as well as figures) which act as medicine's memory to be used for research (clinical, pharmaceutical, epidemiological, etc.)
Knowledge banks	(Bibliographies, sites for exchanges among professionals, etc.), which make it possible to have access at any moment to the state of the art and can help in making medical decision (diagnosis or treatment)
Software	To help with diagnosis and prescribing which does not replace the physician but acts to extend their knowledge

about not only where an item had been but also on what happened to it along the way. Who worked on it, how long it was there, the status it had leaving a point, and where it went next was starting to look much more like the manufacturing model. If data was also accumulated about the workers in this operation (how many did they complete, to what status, how long did it take for each) the model was complete. Workflow applications, such as Lotus Notes or Outlook 2000, also play an important role in a KM implementation. For example, a KM solution based on Office 2000 could serve as a nurse triage application, integrating automatic call distribution and transaction-processing systems, in concert with a knowledge base of typical responses to patient questions and symptoms (Strawser, 2000). These described technologies and tools can be exploited to create data banks, knowledge banks and a KM software as shown in *Table 1*, which will be a great help for providing better solutions for healthcare.

These data banks can be readily accessed through a network (Internet or intranet) if the user has at his/her disposal a workstation, software, and passwords that give access to these networks and their different sites. The system should be made flexible so that it can be adaptable in time and space, and can be customized: each physician can, when he/she wishes, consult one of the banks or receive specific information on the fields which he/she has chosen in advance. Access need not be limited to physicians alone, but can also be made available to health professionals and the public, and the latter could adapt behavior to help prevent the onset of illness. Of course, these data banks have to be organized, updated continuously and meet users' expectations by allowing them to ask questions and to engage in discussions among themselves, so that it is always possible to evaluate the quality of the information consulted (Fitchett, 1998). The knowledge bank can make it possible to consult experts located elsewhere and to transmit images and other elements of a patient's file to a colleague to obtain an opinion, a practice currently known as "tele-medicine" (Hansen & Nohria, 1999). Software can help to offer software diagnostic and prescription aids to extend this knowledge (Confessore, 1997; Wyatt, 2000; Timpson, 1998).

CONCLUSIONS

Until recently, most of the knowledge experience and learning about KM had been accessible to only a few practitioners. However, during the past three years an explosion of interest, research, and applications in KM has occurred. There is some concern among the practitioners that KM might suffer a fate similar to business reengineering, artificial intelligence, and total quality management. That is, interest in the discipline must last long enough to iron out the bugs while simultaneously delivering significant business value. The irony is that just when the discipline works well, potential users often have lost interest in the fad, point to the inevitable early failures, and thus miss out on the real benefits. Unless the very ambitious and interesting KM initiatives in healthcare evolve differently, even if they work in a technical sense, they will not work in the economic sense and the healthcare system will continue to be what it is today: an immense apparatus for reimbursing healthcare costs. However, there will still be a health/social services network and a medical profession that is familiar with the tools and power of the Internet. The experience will not be totally negative, even if it is likely to reach goals that are different from those set at the outset. Although considerable progress has been achieved in KM across a broad front, much work remains to fully deliver the business value that KM promises. Ultimately, in order to realize the enormous potential value from KM, organizations must motivate and enable creating, organizing and sharing knowledge.

This chapter has served to highlight the need for healthcare in general to embrace the strategies, protocols, tools, techniques and technologies of knowledge management in order to contend with key challenges pertaining to access, quality and value of healthcare delivery. The following chapters in the book will highlight specific areas within the healthcare industry and key issues regarding knowledge management that are pertinent. This will serve to develop a detailed understating of the essential requirements for creating knowledge-based healthcare organizations.

REFERENCES

Allee, V. (1997). *The Knowledge Evolution: Building Organizational Intelligence.* London: Butterworth-Heinemann.

Allee, V. (1999). Knowledge Management: Moving the Care Model from a "Snapshot" to a "Story." *Health Forum Journal.* Retrieved from the World Wide Web: http://www.healthforum.com/hfpubs/asp/ArticleDisplay.asp?PubID=7&Article ID=1305&Keyword=knowledge.

Antrobus, S. (1997). Developing the nurse as a knowledge worker in health - learning the artistry of practice. *Journal of Advanced Nursing*, 25 (4), 823-829.

Atkins, J., Cooper, L., Hughes, E., Kingston, P. & Mayne, A. (2001, January). The healing power of KM. *Knowledge Management*, 1.

Beckman, T. J. (1999). The current state of knowledge management. In J. Liebowitz (Ed.), *Knowledge Management Handbook*. New York: CRC Press.

Brailer, D. J. (1999, January). Management of knowledge in the modern health care delivery system. *Joint Commission Journal on Quality Improvement*, 25 (1), 1999.

Broadbent, M. (1998). The phenomenon of knowledge management: What does it mean to the information profession? *Information Outlook*, 2 (5), 23-36.

Burca, S. (2000). The learning healthcare organization. *International Journal for Quality in Healthcare*, 12 (6), 457-458.

Chase, R. L. (1998). Knowledge navigators. *Information Outlook*, 2(9), 18.

Choo, C. W. (1998). *The Knowing Organization: How Organizations Use Information to Construct Meaning, Create Knowledge, and Make Decisions.* New York: Oxford University Press.

Confessore, S. J. (1997). Building a learning organization: communities of practice, self-directed learning and continuing medical education. *Journal of Continuing Education in the Health Professions,* 17(1), 5-11.

Conklin (1996). Capturing organizational memory. In R. M. Baecker (Ed.), *Groupware and Computer-Supported Cooperative Work* (pp. 561-565). San Mateo, CA: Morgan Kaufmann.

Conner, M. (2001). Developing network-based services in the NHS. *International Journal of Health Care Quality Assurance including Leadership in Health Services,* 14(6-7), 237-244.

Davenport, T. H. & Prusak, L. (1997). *Information Ecology: Mastering the Information and Knowledge Environment.* New York: Oxford University Press.

Davenport, T. H. & Prusak, L. (1998). *Working Knowledge: How Organizations Manage What They Know.* Boston, MA: Harvard Business School Press.

Dean, B. (2002). Learning from prescribing errors. *Quality and Safety in Healthcare,* 11(3), 258-260.

Einbinder, J. S., Klein, D. A. & Safran, C. S. (1997). Making effective referrals: A knowledge management approach. *Proceedings AMIA Annual Fall Synposium,* (pp. 330-334).

Eisenberg, H. (2002). Transforming Hospitals into Knowledge Management Centres [presentation]. Retrieved from the World Wide Web: http://www.syntrek.com/kmppt/.

Elliot, S. (2000). Sharing knowledge & best practices: The hows and whys of tapping your organization's hidden reservoirs of knowledge. *Health Forum Journal.* Retrieved from the World Wide Web: http://www.healthforum.com/hfpubs/asp/ArticleDisplay.asp?PubID=7&ArticleID=1343&Keyword=knowledge.

Fitchett, J. (1998). Managing your organization's key asset: Knowledge. *Health Forum Journal.* Retrieved from the World Wide Web: http://www.healthforum.com/hfpubs/asp/ArticleDisplay.asp?PubID=7&ArticleID=12869&Keyword=knowledge.

Gokce, C. (2002, July/August). Knowledge management in the NHS. *Managing Information,* 9 (6).

Halpern, S., Perry, S. C. & Narayan, S. (2001, January/February). Developing clinical practice environments supporting the knowledge work of nurses. *Computers in Nursing,* 19 (1), 17-23.

Hansen, M. T. & Nohria, N. (1999). Thomas Tierney. What's your strategy for managing knowledge? *Harvard Business Review,* 77(2), 106-116.

Heathfield, H. & Louw, G. (1999, June). New challenges for clinical informatics: Knowledge management tools. *Health Informatics Journal,* 5(2), 67-73.

Herbig, B., Bussing A. & Ewert, T. (2001). The role of tacit knowledge in the work context of nursing. *Journal of Advanced Nursing,* 34 (5), 687-695.

Jackson, J. R. (2000). The urgent call for knowledge management in medicine. *The Physician Executive,* 26 (1), 28-31.

Jadad, A. R., Haynes, B. Hunt, D. & Browman, G. P. (2000). The Internet and evidence-based decision-making: A needed synergy for efficient knowledge management in health care. *CMAJ,* 162 (3), 362-365.

Johnson, D. E. L. (1998, July). Knowledge management is new competitive edge. *Health Care Strategic Management,* 16 (7), 2-3.

Joyce, L. (2000). Translating knowledge into good practice. *Professional Nurse,* 16 (3), 960-963.

Keeling, C. & Lambert, S. (2000). Knowledge management in the NHS: Positioning the healthcare librarian at the knowledge intersection. *Health Library Review,* 17 (3), 136-143.

Kenner, C. (2002). *Knowledge Management and Nursing Education.* Retrieved from the World Wide Web: http://eknowledgecenter.com/articles/1011/1011.htm.

Krogh, G., Ichijo, K. & Nonaka, I. (2000). *Enabling Knowledge Creation: How to Unlock the Mystery of Tacit Knowledge and Release the Power of Innovation.* New York: Oxford University Press.

Leonard, D. (1998). *Wellsprings of Knowledge: Building and Sustaining the Sources of Innovation.* Boston, MA: Harvard Business School Press.

Matheson, N. W. (1995). Things to come: Postmodern digital knowledge management and medical informatics. *Journal of the American Medical Informatics Association,* 2 (2), 73-8.

Morrissey, J. (1998). Principles of knowledge management. *Modern Healthcare,* 28 (7), 42.

Nonaka, I. (1994). A dynamic theory of organizational knowledge creation. *Organizational Science,* 5, 14-37.

Nonaka, I. & Nishiguchi, T. (2001). *Knowledge Emergence.* Oxford: Oxford University Press.

Nutkis, D. S. (1997, November). Webcasting: Knowledge management coming to health care providers. *Surgical Services Management,* 3 (11), 18-21.

Nutley, S. M. & Davies, H. T. O. (2001). Developing organizational learning in the NHS. *Medical Education,* 35, 35-42.

O'Conner, G. T. et al. (1996). A regional intervention to improve the hospital mortality associated with coronary artery bypass graft surgery. *Journal of the American Medical Association,* 6 (4), 55-73.

Odden, J. R. (1998). Developing web-based knowledge management systems for healthcare call centers. *Journal of Healthcare Information Management,* 12 (2), 87-95.

OECD. (2000). *Knowledge Management in the Learning Society, OECD.* Retrieved from the World Wide Web: www.brint.com/km.

Open Clinical. (2000). *The Medical Knowledge Crisis and Its Solution Though Knowledge Management [draft white paper].* Retrieved October 25, 2000 from the World Wide Web: http://www.openclinical.org/docs/whitepaper.pdf.

Oxbrow, N. & Abell, A. (1998). Putting knowledge to work: What skills and competencies are required? In *Knowledge Management: A New Competitive Asset.* Washington, DC: SLA State-of-the-Art Institute, 25.

Pfeffer, J. & Sutton, R. I. (2000). *The Knowing-Doing Gap: How Smart Companies Turn Knowledge into Action.*

Sharma, S. & Wickramasinghe, N. (2004). A framework for building a learning organization in the 21ˢᵗ Century. (forthcoming). *International Journal of Innovation and
Learning.*

Skyrme, D. J. (1998, March). Knowledge Management: Solutions: The Role of Technology. *ACM SIGGROUP Bulletin,* Special Issue on Knowledge Management at
Work.

Skyrme, D. J. (2001). *Capitalizing on Knowledge: From e-Business to k-Business.*
Butterworth-Heinemann.

Skyrme, D. J. & Amidon, D. M. (1999). The knowledge agenda. In J. D. Cortada & J. A.
Woods (Eds.), *The Knowledge Management Yearbook* (pp. 108-125). Butterworth-
Heinemann.

Sorrells, J. J. (1999). The role of the chief nurse executive in the knowledge-intense
organization of the future. *Nursing Administration Quarterly,* 23 (3), 17-25.

Sorrells, J. J. & Weaver, D. (1999a, July/August). Knowledge workers and knowledge-
intense organizations, Part 1: A promising framework for nursing and healthcare.
Journal of Nursing Administration, 29 (7/8), 12-18.

Sorrells, J. J. & Weaver, D. (1999b, September). Knowledge workers and knowledge-
intense organizations, Part 2: Designing and managing for productivity. *Journal
of Nursing Administration,* 29 (9), 19-25.

Sorrells, J. J. & Weaver, D. (1999c). Knowledge workers and Knowledge-intense organizations, Part 3: Implications for preparing healthcare professionals. *Journal of
Nursing Administration,* 29 (10), 14-21.

Strawser, C. L. (2000). Building effective knowledge management solutions. *Journal of
Healthcare Information Management,* 14 (1), 73-80. Retrieved from the World
Wide Web: http://www.himss.org/asp/ContentRedirector.asp?ContentID=948.

Timpson, J. (1998). The NHS as a learning organization: Aspirations beyond the rainbow?
Journal of Nursing Management, 6 (5), 273-274.

Wickramasinghe, N. (2003). Practising what we preach: Are knowledge management
systems in practice really knowledge management systems? *Business Process
Management Journal,* 9 (3), 295-316.

Wyatt, J. C. (2000). Clinical questions and information needs. *Journal of the Royal
Society of Medicine,* 93 (4), 168-171.

Chapter II

Knowledge Management in Hospitals

Kevin C. Desouza, University of Illinois at Chicago, USA

ABSTRACT

The medical field in recent years has been facing increasing pressures for lower cost and increased quality of healthcare. These two pressures are forcing dramatic changes throughout the industry. Managing knowledge in healthcare enterprises is hence crucial for optimal achievement of lowered cost of services with higher quality. The following chapter focuses on developing and fostering a knowledge management process model. We then look at key barriers for healthcare organizations to cross in order to fully manage knowledge.

INTRODUCTION

The healthcare industry is information intensive and recent trends in the industry have shown that this fact is being acknowledged (Morrissey, 1995; Desouza, 2001). For instance, doctors use about two million pieces of information to manage their patients (Pauker, Gorry, Kassirer & Schwartz, 1976; Smith, 1996). About a third of doctor's time is spent recording and combining information and a third of the costs of a healthcare provider are spent on personal and professional communication (Hersch & Lunin, 1995). There are new scientific findings and discoveries taking place every day. It is estimated that medical knowledge increases fourfold during a professional's lifetime (Heathfield & Louw, 1999), which inevitably means that one cannot practice high quality medicine without constantly updating his or her knowledge. The pressures toward specialization in healthcare are also strong. Unfortunately, the result is that clinicians know more and more about less and less. Hence it becomes difficult for them to manage the many patients whose conditions require skills that cross traditional specialties. To add to this, doctors also face greater demands from their patients. With the recent advances of e-health portals, patients actively search for medical knowledge. Such consumers are increasingly interested in treatment quality issues and are also more aware of the different treatment choices and care possibilities.

Managing knowledge in healthcare enterprises is hence crucial for optimal achievement of lowered cost of services with higher quality. The fact that the medical sector makes up a large proportion of a country's budget and gross domestic product (GDP), any improvements to help lower cost will lead to significant benefits. For instance, in 1998 the healthcare expenditure in the US was $1.160 billion, which represented 13.6% of the GDP (Sheng, 2000). In this chapter, we look at the knowledge management process and its intricacies in healthcare enterprises.

KNOWLEDGE MANAGEMENT PROCESS

Knowledge management from a process perspective is concerned with the creation, dissemination, and utilization of knowledge in the organization. Therefore, a well-structured process needs to be in place to manage knowledge successfully. The process can be divided into the following steps: beginning with knowledge creation or elicitation, followed by its capture or storage, then transfer or dissemination, and lastly its exploitation. We now elaborate on the various stages of the process:

Creation and Elicitation

Knowledge needs to be created and solicited from sources in order to serve as inputs to the knowledge management process. For the first scenario where knowledge has to be created, we begin at the root — data. Relevant data needs to be gathered from various sources such as transaction, sales, billing, and collection systems. Once relevant data is gathered, it needs to be processed to generate meaningful information. Transaction processing systems take care of this task in most businesses today. Just like data, information from various sources needs to be gathered. An important consideration to be aware of is that information can come from external sources in addition to internal sources. Government and industry publications, market surveys, laws and regulations, etc., all make up the external sources. Information once gathered needs to be integrated. Once all necessary information is at our disposal, we can begin analyzing it for patterns, associations, and trends — generating knowledge. The task of knowledge creation can be delegated to dedicated personnel, such as marketing or financial analysts. An

Figure 1: Knowledge Management Process

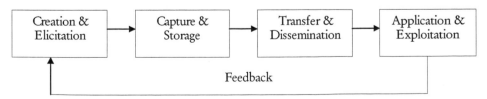

alternative would be to employ artificial intelligence-based computing techniques for the task such as genetic algorithms, artificial neural networks, and intelligent agents (Desouza, 2002a). Data mining and knowledge discovery in data bases (KDD) relate to the process of extracting valid, previously unknown and potentially useful patterns and information from raw data in large data bases. The analogy of mining suggests the sifting through of large amounts of low grade ore (data) to find something valuable. It is a multi-step, iterative inductive process. It includes such tasks as: problem analysis, data extraction, data preparation and cleaning, data reduction, rule development, output analysis and review. Because data mining involves retrospective analyses of data, experimental design is outside the scope of data mining. Generally, data mining and KDD are treated as synonyms and refer to the whole process in moving from data to knowledge. The objective of data mining is to extract valuable information from data with the ultimate objective of knowledge discovery.

Knowledge also resides in the minds of employees in the form of know-how. Much of the knowledge residing with employees is in tacit form. To enable for sharing across the organization, this knowledge needs to be transferred to explicit format. According to Nonaka and Takeuchi (1995), for tacit knowledge to be made explicit there is heavy reliance on figurative language and symbolism. An inviting organizational atmosphere is central for knowledge solicitation. Individuals must be willing to share their know-how with colleagues without fear of personal value loss and low job security. Knowledge management is about sharing. Employees are more likely to communicate freely in an informal atmosphere with peers than when mandated by management. Desouza (2003b) studied knowledge exchange in game rooms of a high-technology company and found significant project-based knowledge exchanged.

Capture and Storage

To enable distribution and storage, knowledge gathered must be codified in a machine-readable format. Codification of knowledge calls for transfer of explicit knowledge in the form of paper reports or manuals into electronic documents, and tacit knowledge into explicit form first and then to electronic representations. These documents need to have search capabilities to enable ease of knowledge retrieval. The codification strategy is based on the idea that the knowledge can be codified, stored and reused. This means that the knowledge is extracted from the person who developed it, is made independent of that person and reused for various purposes. This approach allows many people to search for and retrieve knowledge without having to contact the person who originally developed it. Codification of knowledge, while being beneficial for distribution purposes, does have associated costs. For instance, it is easier to transfer strategic know-how outside the organization for scrupulous purposes. It is also expensive to codify knowledge and create repositories. We may also witness information overload in which large directories of codified knowledge may never be used due to the overwhelming nature of the information. Codified knowledge has to be gathered from various sources and be made centrally available to all organizational members. Use of centralized repositories facilitates easy and quick retrieval of knowledge, eliminates duplication of efforts at the departmental or organizational levels and hence saves cost. Data warehouses are being employed extensively for storing organizational knowledge (Desouza, 2002a).

Transfer and Dissemination

One of the biggest barriers to organizational knowledge usage is a blocked channel between knowledge provider and seeker. Blockages arise from causes such as temporal location or the lack of incentives for knowledge sharing. Ruggles' (1998) study of 431 US and European companies shows that "creating networks of knowledge workers" and "mapping internal knowledge" are the two top missions for effective knowledge management.

Proper access and retrieval mechanisms need to be in place to facilitate easy access to knowledge repositories. Today almost all knowledge repositories are being web-enabled to provide for the widest dissemination via the Internet or intranets. Group Support Systems are also being employed to facilitate knowledge sharing, with two of the most prominent being IBM's Lotus Notes and Microsoft's Exchange. Security of data sources and user friendliness are important considerations that need to be considered while providing access to knowledge repositories. Use of passwords and secure servers is important when providing access to knowledge of a sensitive nature. Access mechanisms also need to be user-friendly in order to encourage use of knowledge repositories.

Exchange of explicit knowledge is relatively easy via electronic communities. However, exchange of tacit knowledge is easier when we have a shared context, co-location, and common language (verbal or non-verbal cues), as it enables high levels of understanding among organizational members (Brown & Duguid, 1991). Nonaka and Takeuchi (1995) identify the processes of socialization and externalization as means of transferring tacit knowledge. Socialization keeps the knowledge tacit during the transfer, whereas externalization changes the tacit knowledge into more explicit knowledge. Examples of socialization include on-the-job training and apprenticeships. Externalization includes the use of metaphors and analogies to trigger dialogue among individuals. Some of the knowledge is, however, lost in the transfer. To foster such knowledge sharing, organizations should allow for video and desktop conferencing as viable alternatives for knowledge dissemination.

Exploitation and Application

Employee usage of knowledge repositories for purposes of organizational performance is a key measure of the system's success. Knowledge will never turn into innovation unless people learn from it and learn to apply it. The enhanced ability to collect and process data or to communicate electronically does not — on its own — necessarily lead to improved human communication or action (Walsham, 2001). Recently the notion of communities of practice to foster knowledge sharing and exploitation has received widespread attention. Brown and Duguid (1991) argued that a key task for organizations is thus to detect and support existing or emergent communities. Much of knowledge exploitation and application happens in team settings and workgroups in organizations, hence support must be provided. Davis and Botkin (1994) summarize the six traits of a knowledge-based business as follows:

1.   The more *they* (customers) use knowledge-based offerings, the smarter *they* get.
2.   The more *you* use knowledge-based offerings, the smarter *you* get.
3.   Knowledge-based products and services adjust to changing circumstances.
4.   Knowledge-based businesses can customize their offerings.

5. Knowledge-based products and services have relatively short life cycles.
6. Knowledge-based businesses react to customers in real time.

KNOWLEDGE MANAGEMENT IN HOSPITALS

We now apply the generic discussion of knowledge, knowledge management, and the process in the context of healthcare enterprises. For purposes of this chapter, we focus our attention on hospitals, although much of the discussion can be applied to other healthcare enterprises, such as pharmaceutical companies, insurance providers, etc.

Knowledge in Hospitals

In healthcare, we have the presence of both explicit and tacit forms of knowledge. Explicit knowledge is available in medical journals, research reports, and industry publications. Explicit knowledge can be classified under: internal and external. Internal are those that are relevant to the practice of medicine, such as medical journals and research reports. External are legal, governmental, and other publications that do not directly affect patient treatment methodology but govern general medical practices. Three dimensions in health information outlined by Sorthon, Braithewaite and Lorenzi (1997) include management information, professional information, and patient information. Overlap and commonalties are identified, but fundamental differences exist in the types of information required for each dimension, the way the information is used, and the way standards are maintained. The achievement of a comprehensive and integrated data structure that can serve the multiple needs of each of these three dimensions is the ultimate goal in most healthcare information system development. Tacit knowledge is found in the minds of highly specialized practitioners, such as neurosurgeons or cardiac arrest specialists. Much of tacit knowledge resides in the minds of individuals. Seldom does efficient knowledge sharing take place. One exception to this is where practitioners exchange know-how at industry or academic conferences. This, however, happens on an all-too-infrequent basis.

Knowledge Management in Hospitals

In the following section we step through the various stages of the knowledge management process.

Knowledge Creation and Elicitation

Creation and elicitation of knowledge can be handled in one of two modes: controlled or free form. In the controlled scenario, we can have an individual department responsible for overseeing knowledge gathering from the various functional areas. This department can be in lieu of the current medical records department in most hospitals, which are responsible for centrally storing patient information. We can also have a variation in which control is divested to each department. In this method, each department will be responsible for coordinating knowledge-sharing efforts from their constituents. For instance, a person in the pharmaceutical department will be responsible for

Figure 2: Staged Look at Knowledge Management

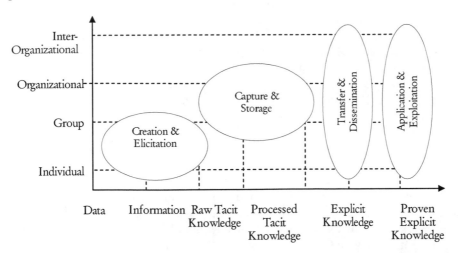

gathering all knowledge on drugs administered to patients. In the second approach, i.e., free form, each individual is responsible for contributing to the organization's knowledge resource. A strong locus of control is absent. Individuals as end users of organizational resources share equal burden to contribute into the asset. A variation of the free-form strategy can be one in which each group, rather than individuals, are responsible for knowledge creation and sharing. An example would be a group of neurosurgeons that research new knowledge on surgical practices. Each of the above-mentioned strategies has associated pros and cons. For instance, with a controlled strategy, we need to have dedicated individuals responsible for knowledge creation and elicitation from group members. In the free-form strategy, while we do not have the overhead of a dedicated person, we lose a structured knowledge-creation process. Choosing a given strategy is a function of the hospital's resources. Along with soliciting internal knowledge, a hospital should also acquire relevant knowledge from external entities such as government, regulatory bodies, and research organizations. Gathering of external knowledge is crucial for hospitals due to the high nature of external pressures and their involvement in day-to-day operations.

As portrayed in *Figure 2*, knowledge creation and elicitation takes place at the individual and group level. Much of the elements gathered at this stage might be raw data, which after processing, becomes information. Information is then applied on experiences, learned associations, and training of employees to generate knowledge. This knowledge remains in tacit form until it is called upon for sharing with peers. Tacit knowledge stored with employees is raw to a large degree, as it is has not been checked for quality or validated against standards.

The other option in the healthcare industry is to generate knowledge through discovery. Data mining and other statistical techniques can be used to sift through large sets of data, and discover hidden patterns, trends, and associations. For instance, in the medical domain all resources are not only very expensive but also scarce. Optimal planning and usage of them is, hence, not a luxury but a requirement. To illustrate this let us take the case of simple blood units. Annually well over 12 million units of blood are transferred to patients (Clare et al., 1995; Goodnough, Soegiarso, Birkmeyer & Welch, 1993) with a cost-per-unit ranging from $48 to $110 with a national average of $78 (Sheng, 2000; Forbes et al., 1991; Hasley, Lave & Kapoor, 1994). Ordering of excess units of blood for operations is the primary cause of waste and corresponding increases in transfusion costs (Jaffray, King & Gillon, 1991). Blood ordered that is not used takes it out of supply for at least 48 hours (Murphy et al., 1995). Even though blood can be returned, it needs to be tested and routed which costs on average $33. In recent years, supply of blood has been decreasing in recent years due to an aging population and increased complexity of screening procedures (Welch, Meehan & Goodnough, 1992). Given these circumstances, any improvements in blood-need prediction can realize significant benefits. Data mining techniques such as artificial neural networks have been employed to sift through large medical databases and generate predictive models which can better forecast blood transfusion requirements. Kraft, Desouza and Androwich (2002a, 2002b, 2003a, 2003b) examine the discovery of knowledge for patient length-of-stay prediction in the Veterans Administration Hospitals. Once such knowledge is generated, it can be made available to external sources.

Knowledge Capture and Storage

Once gathered, knowledge needs to be captured and stored to allow for dissemination and transfer. Two strategies are common for capture and storage: codification and personalization. The codification strategy is based on the idea that knowledge can be codified, stored and reused. This means that the knowledge is extracted from the person who developed it, is made independent of that person and reused for various purposes. This approach allows many people to search for and retrieve knowledge without having to contact the person who originally developed it (Hansen et al., 1999). Organizations that apply the personalization strategy focus on dialogue between individuals, not knowledge objects in a database. To make the personalization strategies work, organizations invest heavily in building networks or communities of people. Knowledge is shared not only face-to-face, but also by e-mail, over the phone and via videoconferences. In the medical domain, the codification strategy is often emphasized, because clinical knowledge is fundamentally the same from doctor to doctor. For instance, the treatment of an ankle sprain is the same in London as in New York or Tokyo. Hence it is easy for clinical knowledge to be captured via codification and to be reused throughout the organization.

Knowledge capture has been one of the most cumbersome tasks for hospitals. Until rather recently much of the patient knowledge was stored in the form of paper reports and charts. Moreover, the knowledge was dispersed throughout the hospital without any order or structure. Knowledge was also recorded in different formats, which made summarization and storage difficult.

Recently we have seen advancements in the technology of Electronic Medical Records (EMRs). EMRs are an attempt to translate information from paper records into a computerized format. Research is also underway for EMRs to include online imagery and video feeds. At the present time they contain patients' histories, family histories, risk factors, vital signs, test results, etc. (Committee on Maintaining Privacy and Security in Healthcare Applications of the National Information Infrastructure, 1997). EMRs offer several advantages over paper-based records, such as ease of capture and storage. Once in electronic format, the documents seldom need to be put through additional transformations prior to their storage.

Tacit knowledge also needs to be captured and stored at this stage. This takes place in multiple stages. First, individuals must share their tacit know-how with members of a group. During this period, discussions and dialogue take place in which members of a group validate raw tacit knowledge and new perspectives are sought. Once validated, tacit knowledge is then made explicit through capture in electronic documents such as reports, meeting minutes, etc., and is then stored in the knowledge repositories. Use of data warehouses is common for knowledge storage. Most data warehouses do have web-enabled front-ends to allow for optimal access.

Knowledge Transfer and Dissemination

Knowledge in the hospital once stored centrally needs to be made available for access by the various organizational members. In this manner knowledge assets are leveraged via diffusion throughout the organization. One of the biggest considerations here is security. Only authorized personnel should be able to view authorized knowledge. Techniques such as the use of multiple levels of passwords and other security mechanisms are common. However, organizational security measures also need to be in place. Once the authorized users get hold of the knowledge, care should be taken while using such knowledge, to avoid unscrupulous practices. Moreover, employees need to be encouraged to follow basic security practices, such as changing passwords on a frequent basis, destroying sensitive information once used, etc. Ensuring security is a multi-step process. First, the individual attempting to access information needs to be authenticated. This can be handled through use of passwords, pins, etc. Once authenticated, proper access controls need to be in place. These ensure that a user views only information for which he or she has permission. Moreover, physical security should also be ensured for computer equipment such as servers and printers to prevent unauthorized access and theft.

Disseminating healthcare information and knowledge to members outside the organization also needs to be handled with care. Primarily physicians, clinics, and hospitals that provide optimal care to the patients use health information. Secondary users include insurance companies, managed care providers, pharmaceutical companies, marketing firms, academic researchers, etc. Currently no universal standard is in place to govern exchange of healthcare knowledge among industry partners. Hence, free flow of healthcare knowledge can be assumed to a large degree. From a security perspective, encryption technologies should be used while exchanging knowledge over digital networks. Various forms are available such as public and private key encryptions, digital certificates, virtual private networks, etc. These ensure that only the desired recipient has access to the knowledge. An important consideration while exchanging knowledge with external entities is to ensure that patient identifying information is removed or disguised. One common mechanism is to scramble sensitive information such as social security numbers, last and first names. Another consideration is to ensure proper use by partners. Knowledge transferred outside the organization (i.e., the hospital) can be considered to be of highest quality as it is validated multiple times prior to transmittal.

Medical data needs to be readily accessible and should be used instantaneously (Schaff, Wasserman, Englebrecht & Scholz, 1987). The importance of knowledge management cannot be stressed enough. One aspect of medical knowledge is that different people need different views of the data. Let us take the case of a nurse, for instance. He or she may not be concerned with the intricacies of the patient's condition, while the surgeon performing the operation will. A pharmacist may only need to know the history of medicine usage and any allergic reactions, in comparison to a radiologist who cares about which area needs to be x-rayed. Hence, the knowledge management system must be flexible to provide different data views to the various users. The use of intelligent agents can play an important role here through customization of user views. Each specialist can deploy customized intelligent agents to go into the knowledge repository and pull out information that concerns them, thus avoiding the information overload syndrome. This will help the various specialists attend to problems more efficiently instead of being drowned with a lot of unnecessary data. Another dimension of knowledge management is the burden put on specialists. A neurosurgeon is paid twice as much, if not more, than a nurse. Hence, we should utilize their skills carefully to get the most productivity. Expert systems play a crucial role here in codifying expertise/ knowledge. When a patient comes for treatment, preliminary test and diagnosis should be handled at the front level. Expert systems help by providing a consultation environment whereby nurses and other support staff can diagnose illness and handle basic care, instead of involving senior-level doctors and specialists. This allows for the patients that need the care of experts to receive it and also improves employee morale through less stress.

Knowledge Application and Exploitation

The last stage, and the most important, is the application and exploitation of knowledge resources. Only when knowledge stored is used for clinical decision-making does the asset provide value. As illustrated in *Figure 3*, knowledge application and exploitation should take place at all levels from the individual to inter-organizational efforts. We draw a distinction here between application and exploitation. Applications are predefined routines for which knowledge needs are well defined and can be programmed. For instance, basic diagnosis when a patient first enters the hospitals, these efforts include calculation on blood pressure, pulse rates, etc. Knowledge needed at this level is well defined and to a large extent is repetitive. On the other hand, exploitation calls for using knowledge resources on an ad-hoc basis for random decision-making scenarios. For instance, if a hospital wants to devise an optimal nurse scheduling plan, use of current scheduling routines, plus knowledge on each individual's skill sets can be exploited for devising the optimal schedule. Decisions like these, once handled, seldom repeat themselves on a frequent basis.

With knowledge management being made easy and effective, quality of service can only increase. A nurse, when performing preliminary tests on a patient, can provide them with better information on health issues through consultation with an expert system. Primary care doctors normally refer patients for hospital care. Some of the primary care doctors may work for the hospital (Network) and the rest are independent of the hospital (Out-of-Network). Today there are a lot of inefficiencies associated with referring patients to hospitals. If a patient is referred, he or she has to contact the hospital personnel who then first take in all patient information and then schedule an appointment. The normal wait time can be any where from one to four weeks depending on seriousness. With the Internet revolution today, all patients, doctors, and hospitals can improve the process tremendously through the deployment of dedicated intelligent agents. Each doctor can be provided with a log-on and password to the hospital's web site. Upon entry to the web site, the doctor can use search agents to browse through appointment schedules, availability of medical resources, etc. These agents can then schedule appointments directly and electronically receive all documentation needed. Hospitals within a certain location can set up independent networks monitored by agents whereby exchange of medical knowledge and resources can take place. Patients can use search agents to browse through hospital web sites, request prescriptions, learn about medical treatments, view frequently asked questions, etc. Intelligent agents can also be trained to learn patient characteristics. Once this takes place, they can be deployed to monitor various medical web sites and send relevant information to the patient in the form of e-mails. Expert systems can be deployed to help the user navigate through the various knowledge bases through recommendations. If a user chooses the main category of "common cold," the expert system can ask for symptoms, suggest medications, etc. Patients can then use these notifications to improve the quality of their health. Intelligent agents also help in improving quality of service through providing only relevant decision-making information. Personnel can then act quickly and reduce time lags. An added benefit of a successful knowledge management system is less burden and stress on personnel. Hospitals are characterized for being highly stressful and always "on pins and needles" when it comes to employees. Through artificial intelligence, much of the routine details can be automated. This reduces the burden on personnel. Also, specialists and highly valued personnel can concentrate efforts on selected matters, the rest can be handled by junior level staff and intelligent systems. This makes for a more welcoming atmosphere.

IMPENDING BARRIERS TO KNOWLEDGE MANAGEMENT

The medical field has to overcome a few hurdles in order to realize the potential benefits of open connectivity for knowledge sharing among the partners of the supply chain and internal personnel such as doctors, surgeons, nurses, etc. We now highlight three of the most prominent issues:

Unified Medical Vocabulary

The first barrier is the development of a unified medical vocabulary. Without a unified vocabulary, knowledge sharing becomes close to impossible. There is diversity of vocabulary used by medical professionals, which is a problem for information retrieval (Lindberg, Humphreys & McCray, 1993). There are also differences in terminology used by various biomedical specialties, researchers, academics, and variations in information accessing systems, etc. (Houston, 2000). To make matters more complex, expertise among users of medical information also varies significantly. A researcher in neuroscience may use precise terminology from the field, whereas a general practitioner may not. Medical information also must be classified differently based on tasks. Researchers may need information summarized according to categories, while a practitioner or doctor may need patient-specific details that are accurate (Forman, 1995).

To help bridge some of the gap in terminology, we have two main medical thesauri in use. Medical Subject Headings (MeSH) and Unified Medical Language System (UMLS) are meta-thesauri developed by the National Library of Medicine (NLM) (Desouza, 2001). UMLS was developed in 1986 and has four main components: meta-thesaurus, specialist lexicon, semantic net, and information sources map. The meta-thesaurus is the largest and most complex component incorporating 589,000 names for 235,000 concepts from more than 30 vocabularies, thesauri, etc. (Lindberg et al., 1993). Approaches to organizing terms include human indexing and keyword search, statistical and semantic approaches. Human indexing is ineffective as different experts use varying concepts to classify documents, plus it is time-consuming for large volumes of data. The probability of two people using the same term to classify a document is less than 20% (Furnas, Landauer, Gomez & Dumais, 1987). Also different users use different terms when searching for documents. Artificial Intelligence-based techniques are making headway in the field of information retrieval. Houston et al. (2000) used a Hopfield network to help in designing retrieval mechanism for the CANCERLIT study. The issue of standardization of terminology continues to be a great debate. The Healthcare Financing Association (HCFA) is adopting some Electronic Data Interchange (EDI) standards to bring conformity to data (Moynihan, 1996). We can expect more standards to be released in the next few years to enable sharing of data.

Security and Privacy Concerns

With sharing of data comes the inherent risk of manipulation and security issues. Security of patients' data and preventing it from entering the wrong hands are big concerns in the field (Pretzer, 1996). Strict controls need to be put in place before open connectivity can take place. Patients' data are truly personal and any manipulation or unauthorized dissemination has grave consequences. Sharing of patient-identifiable data between members of the healthcare supply chain members is receiving serious scrutiny currently. Government and other regulatory bodies will need to set up proper laws to help administer data transmission and security (Palmer et al., 1986). The recent Health Insurance Portability and Accountability (HIPPA) Act can be seen as one of many governmental interventions into the healthcare industry for the protection of consumer privacy rights. Enterprises will have to go to the basics of ethics and operate carefully.

Organizational Culture

In every organization we can see the application of the 20/80 rule. Knowledge providers make up 20% of the workforce, as they possess experiences and insights that are beneficial to the organization. The remaining 80% are consumers of this knowledge (Desouza, 2002a). The providers are often reluctant to share and transfer knowledge as they fear doing so will make them less powerful or less valuable to the organization (Desouza, 2003a, 2003b). Between departments we also find knowledge barriers, in which one group may not want to share insights collected with the other. To help alleviate some of these issues, management should strive to provide incentives and rewards for knowledge-sharing practices. A highly successful approach is to tie a portion of one's compensation to group and company performance, thus motivating employees to share knowledge to ensure better overall company performance. Additionally, Foucault (1977) noted the inseparability of knowledge and power, in the sense that what we know affects how influential we are, and vice versa our status affects whether what we know is considered important. Hence, to alleviate this concern, an enterprise-wide initiative should be carried out making any knowledge repository accessible to all employees without regard to which department or group generated it.

A key dimension of organizational culture is leadership. A study conducted by Andersen and APQC revealed that one crucial reason why organizations are unable to effectively leverage knowledge is because of a lack of commitment of top leadership to sharing organizational knowledge or there are too few role models who exhibit the desired behavior (Hiebeler, 1996). Studies have shown that knowledge management responsibilities normally fall with middle managers, as they have to prove its worth to top-level executives. This is a good and bad thing. It is a good thing because normally middle-level managers act as liaisons between employees and top-level management, hence they are best suited to lead the revolution due to their experience with both frontline, as well as higher-level authorities. On the other hand it is negative, as top-level management does not consider it important to devote higher-level personnel for the task. This is changing, however. Some large companies are beginning to create the position of chief knowledge officer, which in time will become a necessity for all organizations. A successful knowledge officer must have a broad understanding of the company's operation and be able to energize the organization to embrace the knowledge revolution (Desouza & Raider, 2003). Some of the responsibilities must include setting up knowledge management strategies and tactics, gaining senior management support, fostering organizational learning, and hiring required personnel.

It is quite conceivable that healthcare enterprises will start creating the positions of chief knowledge officers and knowledge champions. Top management involvement and support for knowledge management initiatives cannot be underestimated. This is of pivotal importance in hospitals, as their key competitive asset is medical knowledge.

CONCLUSIONS

Some researchers and practitioners have expressed concern about knowledge management being a mere fad (Desouza, 2003b). To deliver promised values, knowledge management must address strategic issues and provide for competitive advantages in enterprises. McDermott (1999) noted that companies soon find that solely relying on the use of information technology to leverage organizational knowledge seldom works. The following chapter has introduced knowledge management and its process. We have also applied it to healthcare enterprises focusing on hospitals. Finally, we justified the knowledge management process by looking through two main strategic frameworks.

Knowledge management initiatives are well underway in most healthcare enterprises, and we can expect the number and significance of such efforts to increase over the next few years. Areas of future and continued research include: automated search and retrieval techniques for healthcare information, intelligent patient monitoring systems, and optimal knowledge representation semantics.

REFERENCES

Brown, J. S. & Duguid, P. (1991). Organizational learning and communities of practice: Towards a unified view of working learning and innovation. *Organization Science, 2*(1), 40-57.

Clare, M., Sargent, D., Moxley, R. & Forthman, T. (1995). Reducing health care delivery costs using clinical paths: A case study on improving hospital profitability. *Journal of Health Care Finance, 21*(3), 48-58.

Committee on Maintaining Privacy and Security in Health Care Applications of the National Information Infrastructure. (1997). *For the record: Protecting Electronic health information.* Washington, DC: National Academy of Sciences.

Davis, S. & Botkin, J. (1994). The coming of knowledge-based business. *Harvard Business Review*, 165-70.

Desouza, K. C. (2001). Artificial intelligence for health care management. *Proceedings of the First International Conference on Management of Health care and Medical Technology.* Enschede, The Netherlands.

Desouza, K. C. (2002a). *Managing knowledge with artificial intelligence: An introduction with guidelines for non-Specialists.* Westport, CT: Quorum Books.

Desouza, K. C. (2002b). Knowledge management in hospitals: A process oriented view and staged look at managerial issues. *International Journal of Health Care Technology Management, 4*(6).

Desouza, K. C. (2003a). Barriers to effective use of knowledge management systems in software engineering. *Communications of the ACM, 46*(1), 99-101.

Desouza, K. C. (2003b). Facilitating tacit knowledge exchange. *Communications of the ACM, 46*(6), 85-88.

Desouza, K. C. & Raider, J. J. (2003). Cutting corners: CKO & knowledge management, *Business Process Management Journal.* (Forthcoming).

Forbes, J. M. et al. (1991). Blood transfusion costs: A multicenter study. *Transfusion, 31*(4), 318-323.

Forman, P. N. (1995). Information needs of physicians. *Journal of the American Society of Information Sciences, 46*(10), 729-736.

Foucault, M. (1977). Two lectures. In C. Gordon (Ed.), *Power/Knowledge: Selected Interviews and Other Writings.* New York: Pantheon Books.

Furnas, G. W., Landauer, T. K., Gomez, L. M. & Dumais, S. T. (1987). The vocabulary problem in human-system communication. *Communication of the ACM, 30*(11), 964-971.

Goodnough, L. T., Soegiarso, R. W., Birkmeyer, J. D. & Welch, H. G. (1993). Economic impact of inappropriate blood transfusions in coronary artery bypass graft surgery. *The American Journal of Medicine, 94*(5), 509-514.

Hansen, M. T., Nohria, N. & Tierney, T. (1999). What's your strategy for managing knowledge? *Harvard Business Review, 77*(2), 106-116.

Hasley, P. B., Lave, J. R. & Kapoor, W. N. (1994). The necessary and the unnecessary transfusion: A critical review of reported appropriateness rates and criteria for red cell transfusions. *Transfusion, 34*(2), 110-115.

Heathfield, H. & Louw, G. (1999). New challenges for clinical informatics: Knowledge management tools. *Health Informatics Journal, 5*, 67-73.

Hersch W. R. & Lunin L. F. (1995). Perspectives on medical informatics: Information technology in health care — Introduction and overview. *Journal of American Social Infrastructure Science*, 46, 726-727.

Hiebeler, R. (1996). Benchmarking knowledge management. *Strategy and Leadership*, *24*(2).

Houston, A. L. et al. (2000). Exploring the use of concept spaces to improve medical information retrieval. *Decision Support Systems, 30*(2), 171-186.

Jaffray, B., King, P. M. & Gillon, J. (1991). Efficiency of blood use and prospects of autologous transfusion in general surgery. *Annals of the Royal College of Surgeons of England, 73*(4), 235-238.

Kraft, M., Desouza, K. C. & Androwich, I. (2002a). Knowledge discovery in clinical databases: issues and process. In M. Khosrow-Pour (Ed.), *Issues & Trends of Information Technology Management in Contemporary Organizations - 2002 Information Resource Management Association Conference* (Vol. 1, pp. 168-171). Hershey, PA: Idea Group Publishing.

Kraft, M., Desouza, K. C. & Androwich, I. (2002b). Length of stay predictions for spinal cord injury patients using neural networks and nursing diagnoses data: methodological issues, results and applicability. *Proceedings of the Second International Conference on Management of Health Care and Medical Technology*, Chicago, Illinois, July 28-30, 2002.

Kraft, M., Desouza, K. C. & Androwich, I. (2003a). Data mining in health care information systems: Case study of a veterans administration spinal cord injury population. *Proceedings of the Thirty-Sixth Hawaii International Conference on System Sciences (HICSS-36)*, Los Alamos, CA: IEEE Press, Big Island, Hawaii, January 6-9, 2003.

Kraft, M., Desouza, K. C. & Androwich, I. (2003b). Health care information: From administrative to practice databases, In G. Grant (Ed.), *ERP & Data Warehousing: Issues and Challenges*. Hershey, PA: Idea Group Publications.

Lindberg, D. A. B., Humphreys, B. L. & McCray, A. T. (1993). The unified medical language system. *Methods of Information in Medicine, 32*, 281-291.

McDermott, R. (1999). Why information technology inspired but cannot deliver knowledge management. *California Management Review, 41*(4), 103-117.

Morrissey, J. (1995). Managed care steers information systems. *Modern Health Care, 25*(8).

Moynihan, J. J. (1996). A milestone for paperless claims processing. *Health Care Financial Management, 50*(1), 68-69.

Murphy, W. G. et al. (1995). Blood use for surgical patients: A study of Scottish hospitals transfusion practices. *Journal of Royal College of Surgeons of Edinburgh, 40*(1), 10-13.

Nonaka, I. & Takeuchi, H. (1995). *The Knowledge-creating Company*. New York: Oxford University Press.

Palmer, R. H., Kane, J. G., Churchill, W. H., Goldman, L. & Komaroff, A. L. (1986). Cost and quality in the use of blood bank services for normal deliveries, cesarean sections, and hysterectomies. *Journal of the American Medical Association, 256*(2), 219-223.

Pauker, S. D., Gorry, G., Kassirer, J. & Schwartz, W. (1976). Towards the simulation of clinical cognition: Taking a present illness by computer. *American Journal on Medicine, 65,* 981-996.

Pretzer, M. (1996). Why should you have a health lawyer's convention? *Medical Economics, 73*(16), 160-168.

Ruggles, R. (1998). The state of the notion: Knowledge management in practice. *California Management Review, 40*(3), 80-89.

Schaff, R., Wasserman, G., Englebrecht, R. & Scholz, W. (1987). Medical treatment assistance with an interactive drug information system. *Medical Expert Systems Using Personal Computers,* 45-51.

Sheng, O. R. (2000). Decision support for health care in a new information age. *Decision Support Systems, 30*(2), 101-103.

Smith, R. (1996). What clinical information do doctors need? *British Medical Journal, 313,* 1062-1068.

Sorthon, F., Braithwaite, J. & Lorenzi, N. (n.d.). Strategic constraints in health informatics: Are expectations realistic? *International Journal of Health Planning and Management, 12,* 3-13.

Walsham, G. (2001). *Making a World of Difference: IT in a Global Context.* Chichester, UK: Wiley.

Welch, H. G., Meehan, K. R. & Goodnough, L. T. (1992). Prudent strategies for elective red blood cell transfusions. *Annals of Internal Medicine, 116*(5), 393-402.

ENDNOTE

[1]   A previous version of this article was published in: Desouza, K. C. (2002). Knowledge management in hospitals: A process oriented view and staged look at managerial issues. *International Journal of Healthcare Technology and Management,* 4(6). I would like thank Yukika Awazu for her assistance with this research project.

Chapter III

How to Handle Knowledge Management in Healthcare:
A Description of a Model to Deal with the Current and Ideal Situation

A.E. Wahle, Cap Gemini Ernst & Young B.V., The Netherlands

W.A. Groothuis, Cap Gemini Ernst & Young B.V., The Netherlands

ABSTRACT

There are many arguments why healthcare organizations need knowledge management. In The Netherlands, there are some things going on, like a new defrayment and remuneration system for the hospitals, the increasing aging population, the focus on quality, efficiency and effectiveness and the existence of more, very specialized disciplines, that there is a need for knowledge management. This chapter describes a model that can be used to chart the current situation regarding knowledge management. The model is based upon the primary and supported processes, a division in types of knowledge and a knowledge cycle. The use of the model is demonstrated by a case description. Conclusions which are drawn from the recap of the case description showing that the model can be useful but some things must be taking into account, such as the size of a case and its boundaries.

INTRODUCTION

There are many arguments why healthcare organizations (HCO's) need knowledge management. The argument for HCO's to develop knowledge management lies in:

• the hospital, or any other HCO, is a knowledge intensive organization;
• there is a big demand for optimizing the support and primary processes;
• the demand for efficiency and effectiveness due to shortages on the job market;
• the requirement of the patient for better quality care and related provision of information;
• the introduction of Diagnosis Treatment Combinations (DTCs) in The Netherlands which makes the learning capacity and competitiveness of the hospital an important factor.

HCO's make use of multiple knowledge areas, such as those of medicine and policy making (Lucardie, Ribbens & Singeling, 1998). These multiple knowledge areas and the existence alongside one another of a large number of interdependent disciplines each with their own professional autonomy makes a healthcare organization a knowledge intensive organization. Furthermore, there is a tendency toward more superspecialism. Especially medical doctors specialize towards small but very specialized areas, and as a result they have very unique knowledge. And this very unique knowledge has to be secured, disseminated and utilized.

In The Netherlands, through an increasingly aging population, the demand for care grows. At the moment the care sector has to cope with a shortage of staff. Improving the present capacity is mainly an issue of the last couple of years. Particularly due to the existence alongside one another of interdependent disciplines, the shortage in one professional group can also be felt directly by other professional groups. The shortage of (good) personnel is a challenge to knowledge management. The available knowledge must be secured and disseminated.

In The Netherlands the focus has in particular been on improving the quality, efficiency and effectiveness of care. Certainly in the last decade the Dutch government has paid a lot of attention to quality in the care sector. In particular, it has attempted to ensure the quality of care through legislation (Van Dijen, 1999). Much of this legislation relates to quality control and improving the position of the client/patient. With respect to the latter position, the Dutch Consumer Association (Consumentenbond) carried out a large-scale survey in 2002 into the quality of hospital care based expressly on patient opinion (Consumer Association, 2002). The conclusions and recommendations of the Consumer Association report offer starting points for using knowledge management in (hospital) care. In particular the provision of information for the patient about the period after discharge, or after care, is often found to fall short. Improvements can also be made in the information transfer between the various professional groups.

The introduction of a new defrayment and remuneration system in the Dutch hospitals stresses the need to develop, disseminate and utilize knowledge. After all, due to the introduction of market forces into the Dutch healthcare system an institution is more dependent on its own knowledge and skills to stay a step ahead of (or at least level with) the competition. The current system is a system of job-based budgeting of hospitals and the lump sum funding of medical specialists. This system will be replaced by a new defrayment and remuneration system for hospitals and medical specialists. It is a system based on the Diagnosis and Treatment Combinations (DTCs).

Added Value of KM

When using knowledge management a number of objectives can be pursued (Konter, 2002). In our view the most important objectives that also show the added value of knowledge management are:

1. to make (better) informed decisions
2. uniform action through the entire organization
3. learning organization which continually improves one and two above
4. as a result achievement of:
    (a) common vision of policy and objectives
    (b) quality improvement
    (c) efficiency increase
    (d) cost saving
    (e) greater competitiveness
5. patient empowerment

Everyone makes decisions, from medical specialist to staff manager. By becoming aware of the available knowledge (knowledge management), one is in a better position to make informed decisions. This can involve using decision support systems as well as many other types of solution (see section "Knowledge Activities"). By making informed decisions, one can also increase the quality of patient care (Friedman, Gatti, Elstein, Franz, Murphy & Wolf, 2001).

It can bring an efficiency increase when everyone in the organization acts uniformly, i.e., everyone has access to protocols, guidelines and procedures and also follows them. Uniform action also implies a shared view of the organizations policy and objectives.

If protocols, guidelines and procedures have been drawn up in accordance with the latest (medical) state of the art, this leads to an improvement in patient care. In various publications (Everdingen, 1993; O. Y., 1999) it has been demonstrated that using protocols, guidelines and procedures reduces the inter- and intra-care provider variance and the number of errors in care provision.

When staff is given the opportunity to follow a continuous learning process, the organization as a whole has a greater learning capacity and competitiveness. The introduction of a new defrayment and remuneration system in the Dutch hospitals stresses the need to develop, disseminate and utilize knowledge. The success of a self-learning organization depends very much on the culture and behavior of the staff. Change management will therefore be an important aspect in the implementation and the continuous process of knowledge management (see also "Knowledge Activities").

Another important aspect of the learning capacity of an organization concerns the ability to learn from one another's mistakes. Good incident and accident records are important here, as well as a culture in which incidents and accidents are actually reported (van Everdingen, 1993). The number of reports says something about the quality of the prevention policy. However paradoxical that sounds, the more reports, the better the quality.

By sharing knowledge about diseases with (future) patients, for example through certified websites and databanks, a degree of self-care is encouraged. This means that with good patient information one can achieve a lower care consumption, but also when a patient reaches the consulting room, he is better informed and can ask more specific questions.

It can be argued that knowledge management, in addition to making informed decisions, will result in an improvement due to a uniform procedure, an increased learning capacity, a reduction in costs due to greater efficiency and improved communication with the patient, as well as an improvement in the overall quality of the care provided. The various objectives are interrelated and interdependent. Quality standards can, for example, be built into the decision support systems, enabling the system to take quality standards into account when giving advice to the user. The system can also take into account legislation and regulations, which contributes to an improved quality. By acting uniformly in accordance with prescribed procedures, the quality is also improved. Another point that improves quality is that everyone can have the information they want and so can make informed decisions.

KM and Quality Improvement Projects

Describing the added value of KM, we have described the ideal situation. Many HCOs do one of the mentioned activities and call it a quality improvement project. KM and quality management often have the same purpose, namely to improve the processes and outcome involved. However, the added value of active knowledge management is to see all these activities/processes in cohesion with each other while quality management tends to look at individual processes/activities.

An ideal situation can only be approached by getting insight in the current situation. To do this, we have described below a model with which the current situation can be mapped and the (knowledge management) activities are presented in cohesion with each other.

METHODS

Before we deal with the model, first we make clear our way of thinking about knowledge management. We feel obliged to do this for a better understanding of the structure and way of reasoning used in the model.

Definition of Knowledge Management

When talking about knowledge management, many aspects are covered. Still, well-functioning knowledge organizations can be characterized by:
*   the coherent promotion of common knowledge;
*   the screening/filtering of only the knowledge that is necessary (less is more);
*   the stretching of knowledge, communication and capturing.

With knowledge management it is like looking through a magnifying glass at information management. For example, a structured look is taken of how the current and ideal provision of information, for example of the professional groups and patients, is organized.

We define knowledge management as the management of the knowledge cycle. The knowledge cycle consists of *developing, disseminating and utilizing knowledge* (Oldenkamp, 2001, 2002; Brailer, 1999). Development consists of both the gathering and creating of knowledge. Disseminate means structuring, making explicit, distributing and explaining. Utilize refers to finding and (re-)deploying knowledge.

Several other authors have introduced similar cycles or "knowledge value chains" (Van der Spek & Spijkervet, 1996; Weggeman, 1997). We have opted for the definition as described above because of its simplicity and because in our view the cycle and its management includes all aspects referred to by the other authors. On the basis of the "develop, disseminate and utilize" knowledge cycle, the section titled "Case" discusses this.

Knowledge

Knowledge management, as we have said, is the management of a cyclical process centered on knowledge. But what do we understand by knowledge? It can be defined as the capacity to act competently. In acting, we necessarily make use of information. Further information puts us in a position to act more competently (Oldenkamp, 2001)

We can distinguish different kinds of knowledge. A common, and much used, division is one into procedural, declarative, social and contextual knowledge (Oldenkamp, 2001; Boers & Kruithof, 1998; Boersma & Stegwee, 1996). We find the following terminology more suitable:

* *know what* (declarative) – factual knowledge. This knowledge often forms the basis for the "know how" type of knowledge;
* *know how* (procedural) – knowledge of procedures. To deal with routine matters, established procedures are often available, which capture factual and background knowledge;
* *know who* (social) – who knows what or meta-knowledge. You do not have a monopoly on wisdom, so you need to call upon others with the specific knowledge you need;
* *know why* (contextual) – background knowledge. This knowledge is required when new procedural knowledge is drawn up and when lines of reasoning have to be explained.

The "know what" and "know how" types of knowledge are also seen as the two most important types of knowledge for management and control of the organization (Boersma & Stegwee, 1996).

We have chosen the above division because in our opinion it fits in with the terminology and the experience of the professional groups in the healthcare sector. For example, doctors and nurses use mainly factual knowledge, but also use background knowledge and experience. By calling in colleagues, they are calling upon who-knows-what knowledge or meta-knowledge and everyone in his or her work comes up against certain guidelines, procedures, etc. The medical specialist follows a particular procedure for an operation, the nurses follow procedure when dressing wounds and a receptionist follows procedure when identifying the patient.

The use of a division into types of knowledge has often been found useful in structuring the knowledge present (Oldenkamp, 2001).

A Model for the Care Sector

In the care sector a distinction is often made between primary and support processes. The primary processes are geared to (para)medical and nursing care. Support processes are geared to the direct support of the primary processes and the deployment of people and resources.

Table 1 sets out the processes in more detail. The support processes are broken down into care-support and general support processes. The aim is not for completeness here as different care institutions can have slightly different classifications or names for the processes. The main lines do, however, correspond.

In combination with the knowledge cycle and the breakdown into types of knowledge, a framework is drawn up. For each process, for each type of knowledge and for each phase of the knowledge cycle, it is indicated which activities are being used in the current situation. *Figure 1* shows the model. It shows the ideal situation because all parts are being filled.

The model can be filled in with even more detail, depending on the organization's requirement. The setup of the model is three-dimensional so that it can be looked at from three points of view of the knowledge processes. For example, what kind of process is used knowledge being used in, what sort of knowledge are we talking about and which phase of the knowledge cycle is the knowledge pointing at. In this manner a three-dimensional reproduction of the current situation can be acquired. In "Cases" we make clear how we can do this.

Knowledge Activities

In this section, brief examples of possible activities for applying knowledge management in an organization are given. These examples will be outlined to make clear

Table 1: Breakdown of Processes

Primary processes	1. Central registration 2. Outpatient consultation 3. Patient admission 4. Nursing and care 5. Outpatient treatment 6. Clinical treatment
Care-support processes	1. Medication 2. Diagnostic procedures[1] 3. Other care support
General support processes	1. Staff provision 2. Finance 3. Provision of information 4. Management 5. Facilities 6. (Education)

Figure 1: Model for the Care Sector

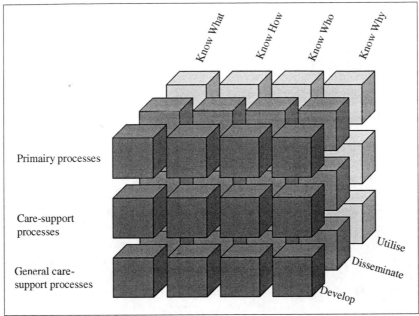

what kind of activities are ranged under knowledge management. The framework of "A Model for the Care Sector" can be filled in with these activities, allowing one to see at a stroke where the activities are concentrated and to see them in cohesion with each other.

Per phase of the knowledge cycle, a few activities are listed, accompanied by a brief description. For each activity, the type of knowledge is indicated in brackets.

Develop

Developing knowledge involves gathering or creating knowledge. An example of gathering knowledge is recruiting new staff.[2] New staff often have an unprejudiced view of existing — and often habitual — procedures and as a result they bring a measure of renewal, in addition to the knowledge and skill in a particular specialist area that they have made their own (*know what, know why*).

The buying of books[3] can also be seen as gathering knowledge. For example, the (medical) library purchases specialist literature or the organization buys handbooks for interns/trainee specialist registrars and specialists to support them in their work (*know what, know why*).

By giving staff the opportunity to subscribe to specialist journals or other media — and to have these costs reimbursed — the development of knowledge is stimulated (*know what, know why*).

The development (or the creation) of knowledge is also carried out, for example, by continuing vocational training or via external training, courses, congresses or seminars. It is possible to work on knowledge development through continuing vocational training in the traditional lecturer-student form, as well as via online-training courses.[4] Online-training courses have the advantage that they can be followed independently of time and place (*know what, know why*).

Registration systems are a separate example. Filling the registration systems with data so that the data can be subsequently analyzed, can be seen as the development of knowledge. Only when this is done, can we talk of disseminating and then utilizing the knowledge stored in the record systems.

Disseminate

Thanks to the facilities that ICT offers, copying and distributing knowledge takes hardly any time at all. However, the possible (ICT) solutions are very diverse. A well-known example is the knowledge bank, of which a protocol system[5] is an example. This is the type of knowledge bank that is often found nowadays in hospitals. More and more hospitals also make their guidelines for treatment available for patients, though in understandable language[6] (*know how, know what, know why*). This knowledge is made available through information pillars in the hospital or via websites containing a variety of information on treatment. Hospitals themselves also often refer to reliable sources on the Internet (*know how, know what, know why*).

In discussing the development phase, the registration system was already mentioned as a system for developing knowledge in the first instance. A specific example is a system for registering incidents and accidents. Making these records as complete and accurate as possible gives the organization an opportunity to learn from mistakes and so to increase the knowledge in certain areas as a result of which a quality jump and efficiency gain is achieved.[7] Another example of a registration system for learning from mistakes is a system faults.

For disseminating knowledge, patient discussions or clinical lessons are an excellent form. By organizing regular meetings on certain clinical pictures or unique patients, knowledge can be disseminated (*know what, know why*).

Marketplaces, communities, discussion groups and forums are places, often on the Internet, where staff can exchange knowledge with one another (*know what, know why*). This is certainly not necessarily an internal or institutional matter, as they are more often aimed at groups such as heart patients or users of a particular software package. These places can moreover be regarded as a system for knowledge development.

Utilize

The investment of time, money and energy in the previous two phases is paid back in the last phase, i.e., knowledge utilization. By better utilizing the available knowledge, comparable work can be carried out (qualitatively) better, faster or perhaps cheaper. However, the success of this phase largely depends on the behavior of the staff and the culture of sharing knowledge. Does the staff think that they can learn something from others and do they also want to? This does of course happen in the first two phases of the knowledge cycle, for before the knowledge can be utilized, it is first necessary to develop and disseminate it.

A decision support system (DSS) is a well-known example of knowledge utilization. With the help of decision support systems, informed decisions can be made. Decision support systems are mainly important where many variables have to be weighed up against one another to arrive at a decision.[8] This mainly occurs in the diagnostic process of the specialist (*know what*).

Other examples of a decision support system are an physician order entry system (POES) for achieving better decisions and savings on medication.[9] In particular, general practitioners in The Netherlands make increasing use of POESs that are often already incorporated in their GP information systems.

Another example of utilizing knowledge is making use of literature. The modern physician is expected to base his decisions on the best and most recent evidence from the medical science literature (Rijssenbeek, 2001; Offringa, 2001). However, as Offringa (2001) notes, 40,000 medical science journals are published annually with more than one million articles. This means for an internist that he would have to read between 17 and 22 articles per day to keep up with the publication rate. For a general practitioner, this number is even higher. Medical information is easily available without restriction via MEDLINE. The Cochrane Collaboration is an organization that has taken upon itself "preparing, maintaining and promoting the accessibility of systematic reviews of the effects of healthcare interventions" (www.cochrane.nl). There are Cochrane Centers all over the world. By using the Cochrane Library, a doctor is able to obtain up-to-date information on the state of research regarding the efficacy of medical treatment (*know what, know why*).

In guidelines for medical practice, knowledge is stored or obtained through vocational training or external training or literature. By using a guideline this particular knowledge is utilized (*know how*).

Setting up a competence matrix can also facilitate the utilization of knowledge. With the help of such a competence matrix (who-knows-what), one can search for specific knowledge that is already present with a colleague (*know who*).

CASE

In this section the model will be put into practice by a case description and recap. This case will show our three-dimensional approach of the model.

Description

Mrs. W. is send by the midwife to the gynecologist because of an incomplete breech presentation of her baby. Mrs. W. is in her 34th week of pregnancy. With the help of echography, the gynecologist looks at precisely how the baby is presenting and also carries out an external examination. He discusses with Mrs. W. and her partner exactly what is happening — the baby is lying with its buttocks in the birth canal and with its head and legs upward — and what the policy will be for the coming weeks. This is in accordance with the guidelines drawn up for this specific condition by the scientific association (www.nvog.nl). Mrs. W. must come back the following week. The gynecologist expects that the baby can still turn itself.

The next week, Mrs. W. and her husband come back to see the gynecologist. An extensive echograph is scheduled and in addition to checking the presentation, a number of length measurements are taken of the baby and the pelvic passage. A co-assistant will accompany them. He tells them that if pelvic narrowing is suspected, there is an increased risk of fetal mortality/morbidity in case of vaginal birth. However, there is no question of this. The baby is also of normal length. Mrs. W's abdomen does not, however, offer the baby much room. The gynecologist decides to wait another week so that the baby can still turn itself, but considers that chance small. He also wants to wait as long as possible for any external turning. This is a guideline the gynecologists have implemented in their practice. There is a significant chance when external turning will be done, the delivery of the baby can start. When this is happening, the baby has to be mature/developed enough.

In the 36th week of her pregnancy, Mrs. W. comes back again. Again the gynecologist looks with the help of echography at how the baby is lying. The baby is still lying in an incomplete breech presentation. The doctor discusses the options with the couple. He does not want to turn the baby externally because of the limited room in the abdomen, the placenta that is under the navel and Mrs. W's very contractile abdomen. The two options for the delivery, which cannot be left for long, are a breech delivery and a planned caesarean section. He refers the couple to the website of the scientific association for some background information in order to make their choice. In the waiting room is a big notice on the wall drawing attention to the website as being reliable information.

Once home, Mrs. W. and her husband study the information on the website and discuss the risks, advantages and disadvantages of one option or the other. They decide on a c-section.

When they notify the gynecologist of this decision, he agrees with their choice. He tells them that he recently took part in a clinical lesson of a nurse from the gynecology/obstetrics ward where the results of a randomized "multi-centre trial" have been presented in which for more than 2,000 women with a fetus in breech presentations and with a pregnancy term of 37 weeks, a policy aimed at a vaginal delivery was compared with one aimed at a planned c-section. Perinatal mortality, neonatal mortality and serious neonatal morbidity were significantly lower in the group with a policy aimed at a planned c-section. Between the two groups, there was no significant difference in maternal mortality and serious maternal morbidity in the short term (www.nvog.nl). The gynecologist did not tell the couple this at the previous meeting so as not to influence their choice. As they leave, he gives them a brochure containing information on the how and what for a c-section.

The c-section is planned for two weeks later, in the 39th week of the pregnancy. However, a week after her last appointment with the gynecologist, Mrs. W. starts spontaneous contractions and a healthy baby boy is born after a c-section, without complications for either mother or son.

Recap

The recap is divided into three parts according to the model described earlier. The case will be analyzed by looking at the processes in which it takes place, what kind of knowledge is being used and to which phase of the knowledge cycle the case refers.

The knowledge activities are taking place in the primary and care-support processes. The patient has an outpatient consultation several times (primary process), whereby diagnostic procedures (care-support process), e.g., an echograph, are carried out. It is possible to break down the primary and care-support process to be more detailed in what specific part of the process the case is taking place. For instance, the knowledge is being transferred from the gynecologist to the patient while performing the consultation. Writing it down in the patient record is disseminating the information. Performing the consultation and writing down the information (i.e., knowledge to decide what kind of guideline to use) are subprocesses of outpatient consultation.

We can also point out the diagnostic procedure, e.g., an echograph, at a sub-level, namely radio-diagnostics. We can even go one level deeper, for example, by performing an echograph. During performance, the gynecologist gives the co-assistant, who has to learn this profession, information about what he is doing and why: he disseminates his knowledge.

The case points itself especially at two phases (disseminate and utilize) of the knowledge cycle. The clinical lesson of the nurse, which the gynecologist took part in, and the website where the patient was referring to for reliable background information are knowledge activities which fall under the disseminating phase. The gynecologist, when explaining the "what" and "why" as he was doing an extensive echograph, disseminates his knowledge to the co-assistant. By using the guidelines for incomplete breech presentation and external turning, the gynecologist utilizes the knowledge, which is stored in these guidelines.

The case uses three kinds of knowledge: know what, know how and know why. The information on the web site contains factual and background knowledge. When the gynecologist quotes a remarkable survey, the patient and her husband are given more background knowledge. During his performance of the extensive echograph, he gives the co-assistant factual knowledge. The brochure contains know how, i.e., procedural knowledge.

Figure 2 shows the results of charting the case in the 3D model described where all the different activities are presented in cohesion with each other.

The case is an example of several objectives that can be pursued by using knowledge management, namely uniform treatment (all gynecologists follow the same

Figure 2: Results of the Case

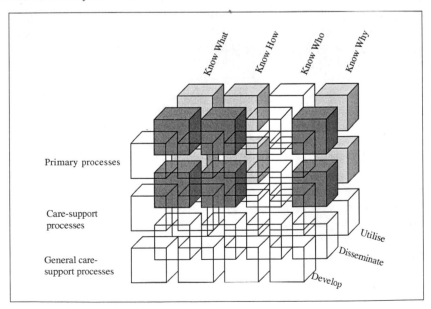

guidelines), making informed decisions (clinical lesson and the choice the couple had to make) and patient empowerment (informing the patient by referring to a reliable web site and brochures).

CONCLUSIONS

In this chapter a model is presented that can be used to chart the current situation regarding knowledge management. A fully filled model represents the ideal situation, whereby all activities are in cohesion with each other. In the beginning of the chapter, we described the ideal situation. How the model can be used to chart the current situation is then described.

By applying the model to our case in section 3 the following conclusions can be drawn:

• The model appears to be suitable for positioning the case in terms of process types, cycle and types of knowledge involved. The question is, however, whether this picture is also obtained when a whole organization is examined. It is therefore recommended to use a more detailed breakdown of the primary and support processes so that more distinction is made within the processes;

• During the recap of the case, all the different activities were brought together in cohesion. This resulted in a useful overview, in addition to the separated descriptions of the activities one by one;

• Also, during the recap of the case, it was difficult to draw a boundary — what is the scope of a process and what is not. In practice this boundary will be difficult to indicate as a hospital is not independent and the processes extend outside the walls of the hospital. The process approach is a good starting point;

• The distinction between the types of processes gives a clear picture of where in the organization the knowledge processes are affected. The question is, however, whether the distinctions can be maintained in daily practice, as the processes tend to be so strongly intertwined. Take, for example, the diagnostic process which forms a considerable part of the out/in-patient treatment of the patient;

• To fill in the model, a person who knows much about knowledge management is needed.

When dealing with KM-projects, it is recommended to start with the processes where "quick wins" are to be expected. This will motivate the people involved to adapt to and work with the necessary change for a better KM process. It is expected that the outcome of active knowledge management, when the results become clearly noticeable, will have a positive effect on staff motivation and staff/patient satisfaction.

To conclude, knowledge management can certainly contribute to optimizing primary and support processes. The case in this chapter has shown that the objectives to be achieved with knowledge management are no utopian dream. By pursuing these objectives, one is not only working on the efficiency and learning capacity of the organization, but also on improving the quality of care which are, and should be, supplemental to each other.

REFERENCES

General

Consumentenbond [Consumer Association, Hospital Comparison Group]. (2002). Ziekenhuisvergelijkingssysteem.

Everdingen, J. J. E. van (red.). (1993). Smetten op de witte jas [Stains on the white coat].

Lagendijk, P. J. B, Schuring, R. W. & Spil, T. A. M. (2001). Elektronisch Voorschrijf Systeem, van kwaal tot medicijn [Electronic Prescription Service, from complaint to medicine].

Raad voor de Volksgezondheid en Zorg. (2002). E-health in zicht [National Health Care Council, E-health in sight].

Van Dijen, M.E.M. (1999, September). Adviesgroep Gezondheidszorg, Kwaliteitsmanagement, alternatieven voor de gezondheidszorg [Health Care advisory group, Quality management, alternatives for health care], Ernst & Young Consulting.

General Knowledge Management

Boers, A. & Kruithof, E. (1998). Procesbenadering [Process approach], reeks IT Professional & Onderneming, Kluwer Bedrijfsinformatie.

Boersma, S. K. Th. & Stegwee, R. A. (1996). Exploring the issues in knowledge management. Information Resources Management Association International Conference.

Brailer, D. J. (1999, January). Management of knowledge in the modern health care delivery system. *Journal on Quality Improvement*, 1(25), 6-19.

Konter, M. D. (2002, September). Kennismanagement bij ziekenhuizen (een onderzoek naar de behoefte aan en toegevoegde waarde van kennismanagement bij ziekenhuizen) [Knowledge management in hospitals (a survey into the need for added value in knowledge management in hospitals)], afstudeerscriptie/master's thesis, University of Twente.

Lucardie, L., Ribbens, H. & Singeling, H. (1998). Transformatie van kennisintensieve naar kennisgebaseerde organisaties: het ziekenhuis als voorbeeld [Transformation from knowledge-intensive to knowledge-based organisations: the hospital as an example]. *Informatie & zorg: kwartaaluitgave VMBI*, 103-108.

Oldenkamp, J. H.. (2001). Succesvol overdragen van kennis [Succesful knowledge transfer], Utrecht: Lemma.

Oldenkamp, J. H. (2002). Professioneel leren [Professional learning], Utrecht: Lemma.

O. Y. (1999, September). Kennismanagement in de zorg [knowledge management in health care], *Informatie & zorg: kwartaaluitgave VMBI*, 3, 97-102.

Rijssenbeek, A. (2001). Kennismanagement in de zorg [Knowledge management in the care sector]. MIC-congres 2001, Noordwijk.

Van der Spek, R. & Spijkervet, A. L. (1996). Kennismanagement: intelligent omgaan met kennis [Knowledge management handling knowledge intelligent]. Utrecht, Kenniscentrum CIBIT.

Weggema, M.C.D.P. (1997). Kennismanagement: inrichting en besturing van kennisintensieve organisaties [Knowledge management: set-up and control of knowledge-intensive organisations]. Schiedam: Scriptum.

Applications: Protocols and Guidelines

Richtlijn 07 Stuitligging, Nederlandse Vereniging voor Obstetrie en Gynaecologie [Guideline 07 Breach presentation, Dutch Association for Obstetrics and Gynaecology]. Retrieved December 30, 2002 from the World Wide Web: www.nvog.nl.

www.rdgg.nl (n.d.). Retrieved November 30, 2002.

Applications: Decision Support Systems

Friedman, C., Gatti, G., Elstein, A., Franz, T., Murphy, G. & Wolf, F. (2001). Are clinicians correct when they believe they are correct? Implications for medical decision support. Medinfo 2001, Amsterdam.

Offringa, M. (2001). Workshop: Gebruik van snel toegankelijke, voorbewerkte informatie bij klinische beslissingen in het Evidence Based Medicine tijdperk [Use of rapidly accessible, pre-processed information in clinical decisions in the Evidence Based Medicine age], MIC-congres 2001, Noordwijk.

www.cochrane.nl (n.d.). Retrieved November 10, 2002 from the World Wide Web.

ENDNOTES

[1]   Diagnostic procedures also include diagraphs and procedures in the clinical chemistry laboratory (clinical chemistry and hematology, parasitology and microbiology).

[2]   This can be done on an individual basis, but by mergers and take-overs new knowledge is also gathered in the form of new staff.

[3]   This does not necessarily immediately lead to the spreading and utilisation of knowledge. The acquired material must be brought to the attention of staff where there may be a potential need.

[4]   From the report "E-health in zicht" (E-health in sight) (Raad voor de Volksgezohdheid en Zorg, 2002) it appears that 84% of Dutch doctors would like to receive continuing vocational training via the Internet.

[5]   Guidelines are also often included in a protocol system.

[6]   A good example of this is the treatment of breast cancer in the Reinier de Graaf Groep (in Dutch) where various paths can be followed, depending on the treatment that is necessary for this diagnosis (www.rdgg.nl).

[7]   In The Netherlands the care institutions have MIP (*Melding Incidenten Procedure* - incident reporting procedure)-/FONA (*Fouten, Ongevallen en Near Accidents* — errors, accidents and near accidents) committees. Accidents and errors (for example, falls or medication errors) are reported via a form and dealt with by the committee or, in the most serious case, by the management. It does, however, appear that via the reporting committees an insufficient idea is obtained of the number and nature of the incidents. The number of reports does in fact say something about the quality of the prevention policy in institutions. It sounds paradoxical, but the more reports that are made, the better the quality (Everdingen, 1993). This does of course depend on the reporting culture in an institution.

8   Investigation shows that people can weigh up a maximum of seven related variables to come to the right conclusion. Often the assessment is influenced by things such as tiredness, mood, prejudice, etc. And knowledge and experience of other experts is not available.

9   According to a recent publication, the use of POESs is not what was expected (Lagendijk, Schuring & Spil, 2001). There is no appreciable saving among general practitioners because they already prescribe economically and sensibly and are not the greatest generators of medication costs. Being able to make better justified decisions for therapy is however considered an advantage.

Chapter IV

How to Start or Improve a KM System in a Hospital or Healthcare Organization

A.H. Rubenstein, IASTA Inc., USA

E. Geisler, Illinois Institute of Technology, USA

ABSTRACT

One of the key factors that distinguishes enterprises of the 21st Century is the emphasis on knowledge and information. Knowledge management is an important means by which organizations can better manage information, and more importantly, knowledge. Unlike other techniques, knowledge management is not always easy to define, because it encompasses a range of concepts, management tasks, technologies, and practices, all of which come under the umbrella of the knowledge management. This chapter deals with two aspects of knowledge management systems: (a) why KM systems are needed, and (b) how to get started on designing and rolling out a new or improved KM system. The inferences are drawn from the direct experiences the authors have had during their academic and consulting activities in many health sector organizations.

INTRODUCTION

Hospitals and other healthcare organization need bricks and mortar, human resources, medical technology, financial systems, and other infrastructure items. In addition, they need effective ways of capturing, preserving, transforming, retrieving, and applying *knowledge* about past experiences and subsequent "lessons learned" to *current* and *future* needs. These are commonly called *Knowledge Management (KM)* systems.

Here are some brief definitions:

1. *KM* is the management of intellectual capital (IC) in the interests of the enterprise.
2. *IC* includes knowledge, information, lessons learned, and other data held for use over time.
3. Intellectual nuggets (*nuggets*) are the units that carry knowledge, lessons learned, etc.
4. *Super-nuggets* are items tied specifically to express or implied needs of the organization.
5. The most valuable structure of a nugget (N) is a compound statement which has an "If x, ...then y" format: If you do this in a certain way, ... then you can achieve or avoid the following consequence(s).
6. Some nuggets are, in fact, *causal statements*, but many others only suggest strong *correlations* or *influence* of actions on outcomes (consequences).

QUESTIONS SURROUNDING KM SYSTEMS

Why does a hospital or healthcare organization need a new or improved KM system?

- To bridge knowledge "*silos*" in specialties and support functions.
- To learn from its own experiences and experiences of other organizations.
- To avoid repeating or duplicating major or even disastrous mistakes in, for example:
  - disease management;
  - infection control;
  - misuse or abuse of instruments;
  - duplication of expensive equipment.
- To support training at all levels.
- To support weaker or resource-poor units with experience from stronger or resource rich units.
- To share "tricks of the trade."
- To help avoid pitfalls in:
  - organizational design;
  - staffing;
  - work flow.
- To exchange methods of:
  - productivity improvement;
  - cost savings;
  - patient services.

Does everyone need a KM system?

- In general, *yes*, to help: organize, preserve, retrieve, and use lessons learned and other nuggets about his/her job, and the internal and external environment.
- However, there are vast differences among individuals and individual information needs and style — some people still pine for the all-but-obsolete card catalog in the public library. Others have gone "all electronic" and will never look back.

- There are also differences in the relevance and value of past experience or the experience of others.
- Although it is hard to imagine or accept, people in responsible positions may be completely ignoring lessons from the past.
- It is important that the organizational KM system is able to accommodate a wide range of individual differences and bring lessons learned across organizational lines.

Many areas of professional and staff practice have *common elements* where experience can be fruitfully codified and exchanged. Such commonalities can transcend narrow medical, healthcare, and administrative specialties. KM systems can also help transcend temporal and spatial distances in the organization and between organizations. Two such areas are: managing medical technology and medical and staff errors.

Managing Medical Technology

Application areas include computerized patient records, telemedicine, and improved utilization and management of equipment. These all provide opportunities for sharing knowledge and experience, but the pace of such sharing lags far behind the leading edge in industry and the evolving state of the art. Progress is slow toward achieving ease of use, standardization, and connectivity between databases and different record systems. A key challenge is to incorporate existing and new knowledge systems into integrated and comprehensive systems that can be used effectively and cooperatively by caregivers, administrators, payors, and regulators.

Medical Errors

Dealing with medical errors systematically requires improved codification, increased sharing, e.g., the "mortality and morbidity" sessions conducted in hospitals, but generally not recorded and disseminated.

How to Get Started

- Who should initiate a new or redesigned KM system — the role of "champions."
- The design and rollout teams — size, skills, experience, knowledge of the organization.
- How to keep it simple.
- How to get started in a modest way — not across the whole organization at once.
- Possible modest field experiments to test ideas and components of the system.

The champion should be a sponsor at a high enough level to provide credibility as well as material support — e.g., a CEO, other top manager, an operating division manager. The team should include three to six people with: (1) technical understanding of information and communication systems, (2) credibility and experience within the organization, and (3) good people skills.

How to Keep it Simple
- Don't start with a "greenfields" approach.
- Utilize existing components where feasible. All healthcare organizations have many existing information systems that might be adapted.
- Get something useful going quickly.
- Do not ignore possibly useful legacy systems.
- Design the size and "shape" to fit the existing organization — not an ideal one.
- Don't start on too broad a front.
- Select a functional or operating area with high success potential for KM.
- Design a fast prototype that can be readily rolled out to demonstrate the KM principle.

How to Get Started
- Identify information/knowledge needs and styles of key individuals and groups of potential users.
- Examine the current, if any, versions of KM in use or being developed.
- Develop metrics for assessing:
  - The operation of the KM system:
  - The impacts — immediate or direct, intermediate, and ultimate.
- Design and test a systematic procedure for the extraction and refinement of knowledge "nuggets."
- Design and test a monitoring and assessment procedure for system usage and effectiveness.

Some methodologies we have used for designing systems from the viewpoint of the users include:
1. Personal communication charting and communication flow matrix.
2. Individual information-seeking propensity profile.
3. Critical incident method — Effective and ineffective use of the system.
4. Black hole analysis — Where do key pieces of information disappear to?
5. Gatekeeper analysis — Who are the key intermediaries in searching for information?
6. Knowledge transfer and application mapping — What happened to a nugget or super-nugget in terms of application?
7. Individual and group risk-taking propensities.
8. Blame-placing behavior.
9. Bureaucratic analysis and the role of organizational politics.
10. Indicators for statistically out-of-control behaviors.
11. As to KM technology, adequate technology is in hand or on the way. The key problems in designing, installing, using, and management of KM systems are primarily human (user behavior) and organizational (politics, culture, and communication).

SOURCES

Davenport, T. & Prusak, L. (1997). *Working Knowledge: How Organizations Manage What They Know.* Boston, MA: Harvard Business School Press.

Dixon, N. (2000). Common *Knowledge: How Companies Thrive by Sharing What They Know.* Boston, MA: Harvard Business School Press.

Geisler, E. (1999). Mapping the Knowledge-Base of Management of Medical Technology. *International Journal of Healthcare Technology and Management,* 1(1), 3-10.

Geisler, E., Krabbendam, K. & Schuring, R. (2003). *Technology, Healthcare and Management in the Hospital of the Future.* Westport, CT: Greenwood Publishing Group.

Martin, W. (2000). Approaches to the Measurement of the Impact of Knowledge Management Programs. *Journal of Information Science,* 26(1), 21-27.

Nonaka, I. & Nishiguchi, T. (eds.) (2001). *Knowledge Emergence: Social, Technical and Evolutionary Dimensions of Knowledge.* New York: Oxford University Press.

Rapport, M. (2001). Unfolding Knowledge. *Knowledge Management,* 4(7), 44-49.

Rubenstein, A. H. (1989). *Managing Technology in the Decentralized Firm.* New York: John Wiley & Sons.

Rubenstein, A. H. (2001). Knowledge-Management Systems: Effective Rollout and Operation to Meet User Needs. *Annual Review of Communications, International Engineering Consortium,* 54, 1-9.

Rubenstein, A. H. & Geisler, E. (1992). Intelligent Support Systems: An Analysis of User Needs. *Siemens Review,* 6, 32-36.

Rubenstein, A. H. & Geisler, E. (2003). *Installing and Managing Workable Management Systems.* Westport, CT: Praeger.

Rubenstein, A. H. & Schwaertzel, H. (eds.) (1992). *Intelligent Workstations for Professionals.* New York: Springer Verlag.

Section II

Approaches, Frameworks and Tools to Create Knowledge-Based Healthcare Organizations

Chapter V

Moving Toward an e-Hospital

Vidyaranya B. Gargeya, The University of North Carolina at Greensboro, USA

Deborah I. Sorrell, High Point Regional Health System, USA

ABSTRACT

Healthcare organizations, like other information intensive organizations, cannot ignore the rapid progression to a digital network economy. While some aspects of patient care must continue to be delivered locally, Internet technologies and "e-healthcare experiences" are likely to play an increasing role in the pre-delivery and post-delivery arenas. Creating the infrastructure to quickly take advantage of this paradigm shift, while adding value to the local delivery system is paramount to the long-term success of healthcare organizations. To achieve the level of data integration necessary to move to an e-hospital, the complicated web of patient data must flow automatically and instantaneously between information systems within and external to the organization. This chapter presents an overview of infrastructure issues and technologies that will enable hospitals to "plug into" the evolving e-health continuum.

INTRODUCTION

The typical hospital information system application architecture can be separated into systems that support: (1) patient care, (2) administrative and regulatory processes, and (3) decision-making and quality improvement (Mon and Nunn, 1999). At the foundation of these broad categories are the network architecture, the hardware components, and the connectivity software and data architectures that unite the e-hospital within and without the evolving digital network. Noting that e-healthcare is a vehicle of change, Lin and Umoh (2002) stated that the e-healthcare system would not only be a win-win concept for the providers and the patients, but also for other stakeholders in the system. Over the last few years, dozens of articles and a few books have been written on the benefits of e-healthcare (Kelly and Unsal, 2002; Siau, Hong, and Southard, 2002;

Walter and Tung, 2002; Goldstein, 2000). The e-hospital is only one, yet important, element of the e-healthcare system. This chapter takes stock of the state-of-the-art and examines critical infrastructure elements central to the realization of an e-hospital, a critical component of the e-health continuum. This would help the leading-edge practitioners in validating their work and provide practitioners moving towards an e-hospital environment some tips for their journey. There is also some food for thought for academics in terms of research agenda for the future.

The automation of the transactions surrounding a patient visit to the hospital and the transformation of the diagnostic, treatment, and other patient-centric observations into digital data is a prerequisite for e-health. Although most of the current e-health hype focuses on the pre-delivery and post-delivery aspects of healthcare, the core application systems and the niche applications that support the menagerie of hospital provider specialists surrounding the delivery of care to hospital patients will be explored in this chapter. Next, the technologies and standards that seem to be shaping the healthcare digital network will be given. The technologies and open standards that placed the Internet revolution into perpetual motion will allow hospitals to reap the same gains in productivity and quality being realized in other industries. Healthcare decision-makers must select products, vendors, and applications that incorporate Internet technologies for the e-hospital to be realized. Perhaps the most fundamental and essential building blocks of the e-hospital are the hardware components and the rich network connectivity media that allow humans and computers to communicate. The user-friendliness, reliability, and availability of the tools that patients and healthcare providers use to complete healthcare transactions and to manage and access health-related knowledge are paramount. A sampling of the variety of communication devices and the necessary physical and technological infrastructures will be offered, along with key issues. Finally, the challenges posed to the end-users in an e-hospital environment will be presented in this chapter. The hospital is part of a larger system. Perhaps the greatest challenge to the realization of e-health both inside and outside of the hospital walls is the psychological and socio-economical issues that will determine the overall benefits of a digital healthcare delivery system.

APPLICATION ARCHITECTURE SUPPORTING THE ENTERPRISE BUSINESS PROCESSES

This will be discussed in terms of patient admission process, communication of patient admission data, supporting diagnostic and therapeutic sciences, and the point-of-care data entry.

Patient Admission Process

Hospital administration and registration systems are used to "register" patients into the hospital. It is the first point where the potential for drastic reductions in per-transaction costs could be realized via e-commerce. It is estimated that in the US it costs $8 per claim for providers to carry out the check-in, verifying eligibility, and billing. In aggregate, some $250 billion is spent annually on medical claims paperwork in the United

States. Online, Internet-based transactions could drop that figure nearly tenfold. In addition, the processing time could be cut from months to seconds (DeJesus, 2000). Conversion to online healthcare has been mandated by the US federal government program, the Health Insurance Portability and Accountability Act (HIPAA). Admission and registration staffs need a personal computer (PC) with Internet access and ample hardware configuration to run a browser with 128 encryption. Integration of the verification and eligibility system data with the admission and registration systems completely automates the process. Systems have long been in place for obtaining eligibility information for Medicare and Medicaid patients electronically. Internet eligibility and claims processing is a natural progression. The "Y2K" effort forced equipment updates resulting in the replacement of outdated terminals. The profit potential in this area has sparked the attention of several companies, each with their own strategy for being the provider of Web transactions. Key players in this market are Healtheon/WebMD and Pointshare.

A powerful first point-of-contact (point-of-sale) approach for the hospital is the use of embedded-chip smart cards. These cards are capable of holding compact patient medical record and biometrics identifiers. This would enable quick, automated registration and admitting, as well as information for health and health insurance purposes such as eligibility, referral, and pharmacy approval. Humetrix.com and the MedicAlert Foundation plan a product rollout of a smart card that holds emergency pattern record information and allows card holders to access their personal medical records online automatically by dialing up a web site. Smart card use is already more widespread in some European countries than it is in the US. The degree of computerization in the US would allow healthcare to capitalize on the technology. Smart cards (which will be given to the patients) will satisfy one of the basic security requirements under HIPAA by creating a security apparatus around automated patient information and documenting any accessing of confidential information with use of the audit trails automatically generated in smart card systems. Infrastructure set-up costs for the deployment of smart cards is steep. The cards cost approximately $2 to produce and card readers run between $50 and $100 right now. Prices are expected to decline but the cultural acceptance may take longer (Hagland, 2000).

The lure of instantaneously adjudicated medical claims has its downsides. Providers must change the way they do business, payers lose their float and patients would lose the two to three month lag in being faced with their share of the medical costs. The population in general remains risk-averse when it comes to using any new technology that would threaten the privacy of their healthcare information. The real-time exchange of funds could make healthcare providers, payers and patients dubious about using the web to administer transactions. However, the dramatic reduction in transaction cost may be the final determinant for acceptance.

Communication of Patient Admission Data

The data associated with the admission of a patient is of a relatively generic nature. Made up of standard patient demographic data, insurance particulars, and the patient's location (department, room number, and bed), the information associated with the event of admitting a patient is of interest to most if not all of the other information systems used in the hospital. In an e-hospital, this patient information is communicated with all other applications in the hospital. Hospitals organize themselves around specialized diagnos-

Figure 1: e-Hospital Information Systems Architecture

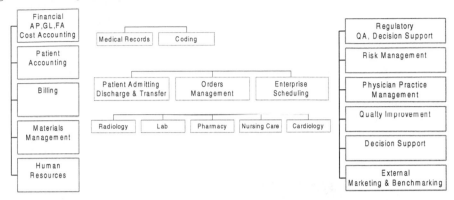

Adapted from Mon and Nunn (1999)

tic methods, focused medical interventions, and various therapeutic care strategies. This business architecture is supported by the application architecture required to implement the enterprise processes (Gordon, 1999). *Figure 1* shows the layers of system architecture. Note that the core clinical information systems for delivering patient care are shown at the center with administration systems and administrative decision support systems around the periphery.

Supporting Diagnostic and Therapeutic Sciences

According to Becich (2000), it is estimated that 50% to 70% of the major decisions that affect patients are based on information available from clinical pathology (laboratory tests) and anatomical pathology (tissue samples). If the other diagnostic areas such as radiology, cardiovascular diagnostic procedures, and nuclear medicine are also included, then the value of immediately accessible results of diagnostic patient tests to decision-makers is obvious. The popular adage "deliver information anywhere, anytime, any place, from any source" holds great potential value in healthcare, and particularly in an e-hospital.

The key diagnostic areas (of clinical and anatomical pathology) are far ahead of the patient point-of-care areas with respect to process automation and digital data capture. Clinical laboratories have been "computerized" for several decades: radiology, cardiovascular laboratories, nuclear medicine, and other areas are close behind. The classical x-ray film processing has been replaced with "film-less" imaging processes that produce digital images in many hospitals worldwide. A rich variety of patient data collected via sophisticated medical diagnostic sciences is available in a digital format waiting for collection, storage, and display on the web. Hospital pharmacies are highly automated from automated drug dispensing devices to robotic workstations used to package and barcode patient medication.

Medical errors, however, occur at an alarming rate despite the digital readiness and automation of patient care supporting processes. The Institute of Medicine (IOM) reported, on the basis of a 1999 study conducted in New York, that as many as 98,000 people die annually in the US as a result of medical errors. A similar study in Colorado and Utah revealed that at least 44,000 people die from medical mistakes in US hospitals each year. In addition to the loss of life, mistakes cost money. In the US alone, hospital mistakes cost an estimated $8.5 to $14.5 billion per year (Stammer, 2000). Leveraging information technology is imperative, and many experts believe that quality improvement begins with the physician and automation of point-of-care functions such as physician order entry and e-prescribing (paperless communication of patient drug orders from a physician using the Internet and aligned technologies). The Food and Drug Administration (2004) has targeted the reduction of preventable medical errors as a top priority for 2004 in its paper, *Protecting and Advancing Consumer Health and Safety*. Bar coding of drugs and biologics, e-prescribing and real time data mining tools capable of searching electronic medical records to improve tracking of adverse events are three bulleted information technology initiatives.

Point-of-Care Data Entry

Automation of point-of-care data is one of the greatest challenges for the e-hospital. The technical hurdles are being overcome but the resistance to change by healthcare providers remains strong. Paper documentation continues to dominate the majority of hospital settings. For example, the physician writes orders for diagnostic tests, pharmaceuticals, diet, and nursing care. These written orders are typically "typed" into an orders management system by hospital clerical staff. Procedures (e.g., surgeries, laboratory tests, or x-rays) can be scheduled in an enterprise scheduling system to better allocate many types of resources. Integration between the admitting and orders systems makes the process more efficient and accurate. These orders are communicated to the appropriate clinical system (e.g., radiology or laboratory) electronically if interfaced or integrated with the order management system. Otherwise, the orders must be "retyped" in the clinical system from a printer audit trail. Once an order is placed in a clinical system, the process of performing the ordered diagnostic test or delivering the specified medication or service begins. If the physician could consistently digitize these "paper instructions," the improvements in the accuracy, the timeliness, and the appropriateness of patient care would be staggering. In addition, the patient vital sign data (e.g., blood pressure, fluid input and output, temperatures) are written on the patient's chart. Technology already exists to convert physician voice dictations to digital text (typically the patient's admitting history and physical and the discharge plan and diagnosis). Hand-held devices and wireless technologies are realistic enabling tools. Point-of-care automation and digital data capture promises dramatic increases in patient care effectiveness and efficiency. However, simply putting the technological infrastructure in place without assuring the acceptance and uniform adoption of the technology by all of the healthcare providers will produce only marginal results. The defining leap in productivity will be realized when the enabling technical tools are used uniformly across the patient's visit.

CONNECTIVITY TECHNOLOGIES AND COMMUNICATION STANDARDS

Several core technologies form the glue that links the specialized and often very disparate e-hospital software applications together. They form the basis for connectivity both inside and outside the hospital. *Figure 2* illustrates a sampling of technologies and communication standards (Synder-Halpern, 1999).

The World Wide Web and the Internet have shown that linking and communicating digitally can be easy. The standard Internet protocols (for example, HTTP, TCP/IP) quickly became the universal wire protocol for distributed systems communication. Led by the Object Management Group (OMG), object or component technologies offer a way of providing a standard external interface to link very different applications together by "wrapping" or modularizing in a common way to exchange messages (data) between the components. OMG's CORBA (Common Object Request Broker Architecture) interoperability platform was recently adopted by the International Organization for Standards (ISO) as an international standard (Object Management Group, 2000a). CORBA is an architecture and is a set of specifications that enables distributed object computing over virtually any network or combination of interconnected networks, especially the Internet. The CORBA component framework is language-neutral and is supported on a wide variety of platforms. The Object Request Broker (ORB) is at the heart of the framework and the Internet Inter-ORB Protocol (IIOP) is used to achieve communication between objects (Object Management Group, 2000b). Microsoft has its own proprietary, distributed object architecture holdout. DCOM, distributed component object model, has been an integral part of all Windows systems since the introduction of Windows '95. A gateway approach can be used to allow interoperability between CORBA and COM/DCOM.

Figure 2: Connectivity Software and Data Architecture

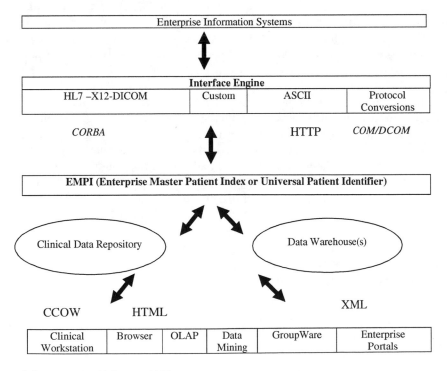

Adapted from Synder-Halpern (1999)

HTML (Hypertext Markup Language) and XML (eXtensible Markup Language) provide flexible data-packaging mechanisms to further facilitate open communication, just as open communication and interoperability distributed architecture standards have enabled the Internet backbone. XML can be used to create common information formats to allow data to be shared between programs. XML is a meta-language that allows communication partners to define industry vocabularies.

Health Level Seven (HL7) is the American National Standards Institute's (ANSI) approved group that develops standards for healthcare. HL7 is the name of the non-profit organization as well as one of many healthcare standards the organization develops and supports. HL7 recently proposed what it believes to be the first XML-based standard for healthcare: the Clinical Document Architecture (CDA). The CDA provides an exchange model for the clinical documents that comprise a patient's medical record. The CDA leverages the use of XML, making documents machine-readable for easy electronic processing and human-readability so they can be easily used when anywhere needed. XML-aware browsers or wireless applications, such as cell phones, can display CDA documents. Nokia showed a demo of this functionality at the 2000 Healthcare Information and Management Systems Society conference (HIMSS 2000) HL7 demonstration. This is just the start of the incorporation of XML-based e-healthcare technologies in development by HL7 (Health Level Seven, 2000a).

Dunbar (1990) reported that a consortium of 51 hospitals came on board with the HL7 standards effort. With the adoption of HL7 communication standard, Zale Lipshy University Hospital, a 160-bed private teaching hospital in Dallas, improved its flexibility in its operations with staffers accessing any type of information at a moment's notice (Eckerson, 1990). The laboratory at the University of Nebraska Medical Center (UNMC) became one of the first laboratories in the country to adopt a laboratory automation system, the Lab-Inter-Link system. The system uses robotic technology, HL7 interfacing to the Sunquest Laboratory Information System, and a rules-based database to automatically route and track specimens throughout the laboratory (Weis, 1996). This system has enabled UNMC to cut down the errors, reduce labor costs, and increase efficiencies.

Digital Imaging and Communications in Medicine (DICOM) is an organization devoted to setting standards to ensure that medical imaging devices can exchange data. Similarly, the National Council for Prescription Drug Programs, NCPDP, mission is to create and promote data-exchange standards for the pharmacy and healthcare industries. X12 is the standard mandated by HIPAA for the communication of healthcare claims transactions. The number of standards organizations surrounding the healthcare industry is staggering and continues to grow as does the organizations devoted to distributed computing. For interface needs that are not facilitated by distributed object technologies, message-oriented middleware software applications (such as interface engines) are used (Marietti, 2000). Dunbar (1993) reported that Bayfront Medical Center in St. Petersburg, Florida, improved its flexibility in communication through the use of client/server technologies. Similarly, Ortman (2001) noted that Aventail, network management service provider for Mt. Sinai NYU Health in New York, reduced costs by appropriate use of intranet/internet/middleware technologies.

At the end-user level, the Clinical Context Object Workgroup (CCOW) is a technical committee within HL7. The group focuses on the collaboration among visual (GUI-based) applications on a clinical workstation. It works to use software component technologies and reduce the re-engineering costs in order to bring its benefits to the industry as rapidly as possible. It publishes standards for the visual integration of cooperative interaction among independently authored healthcare applications at the point of use (Health Level Seven, 2000b).

In June 2003, the Public-Private Collaboration, Connecting for Health, announced consensus on an initial set of healthcare data standards. The data standards and protocols include: HL7 v2.x data interchange standard, the HL7 Reference Information Model, the DICOM standard for imaging, the National Council for Prescription Drug Program, NCPDP, SCRIPT prescription drug information standard, the LOINC vocabulary for laboratory tests, the Institute of Electrical and Electronic Engineers (IEEE), Central European Nations (CEN) International Standards Organization (ISO) [IEEE/CEN/ISO] 1073 medical device communication standard, the American Standards Committee (ASC) X12 administrative transaction standard, HL7 Data Types, Clinical Document Architecture (CDA) and the HL7 Clinical Context Management Specification (CCOW). This list sets a vender supporting standards requirement base line that e-hospital decision-makers should include for information technology procurement decisions (Markle Foundation, 2003).

THE e-HOSPITAL NETWORK

An absolutely essential component for the system to work is the network. It is possibly the most critical element of the entire system as well. The network infrastructure varies from hospital to hospital, but certain characteristics of the network will remain the same across the hospital. The network in e-hospitals needs to be not only robust, but also has to comply with regulations imposed by HIPAA, both in terms of transmission protocols and security standards. In addition, innovations in network technology facilitate better and more efficient patient care through such things as mobile devices connected via wireless networks and Internet and Intranet technologies.

Network Infrastructure

A significant obstacle for hospitals to achieving the quality of the network required in creating the e-hospital environment is the existing network infrastructure. Most hospital's IT infrastructures have been built in a piecemeal fashion (Gillespie, 1999). Consequently, it would not be uncommon for a hospital to have multiple networks using multiple protocols. This creates the situation where certain information is online but can't be accessed by certain people because the network they are on won't "talk to" (or communicate with) the network on which the desired information resides. Also, in the past, legacy networks were not built to handle the volume of workstations and the bandwidth demands in today's environment. Attempting to just add devices to the existing network as the IT infrastructure grows could bring the whole system to a grinding halt. This was the case with Saint Raphael hospital in New Haven, Connecticut. They spent $10 million on a computer-based patient records system that proved to be first-rate. However, as the CIO of that organization explained: "[The network backbone] was so unreliable that the whole system became more of a liability than an asset" (Gillespie, 1999). These legacy networks were also not equipped to deal with the issues introduced by the Internet, particularly security needs. To get up to speed with the e-hospital, considerable attention has to be paid to many existing networks.

In the e-hospital environment, the network needs to meet high standards. To get an idea of those standards, listed below are high-level requirements for one hospital's network (University of Rochester Medical Center, 2000). The University of Rochester Medical Center (URMC) described its vision of an appropriate network design as one that must:

- Be ubiquitous, reliable, scalable, manageable, and secure;
- Be capable of supporting voice and multimedia data transmission, including applications such as tele-medicine and teleconferencing;
- Utilize industry standard protocols and topologies;
- Be capable of supporting the diverse network requirements associated with patient care, research, education, and administration; and
- Be cost effective in both implementation and operation.

The URMC's Network Infrastructure Planning/Review Group lists several aspects of the network infrastructure that will be necessary to meet these requirements. Though the network infrastructure varies from hospital to hospital, it is helpful to look at the specifics of a good network infrastructure for the e-hospital as described by the URMC's Network Infrastructure Planning/Review Group. That group specifies that the network should support a minimum speed of 155Mbs. Reliability and stability will be assured through the use of fault tolerant electronics and redundancy. They divide security into two different areas: physical and logical. The physical security requirements will be met by using fiber cabling in the backbone and putting all electronic components in locked closets. Using point-to-point switched connections and screening devices such as firewalls will meet logical security requirements. Other core components of the URMC's network will include authentication servers, security services, remote access, and e-mail gateways (University of Rochester Medical Center, 2000).

Privacy and Security

A reliable, fully integrated, constantly accessible e-hospital assures minimal success without the public's and healthcare system's trust for the privacy and security of health information. The Health Insurance Portability and Accountability Act (HIPAA) final Security Rule prompted the establishment of the NIST/URAC/WEDi Health Care Security Workgroup in late 2002. The Workgroup's mission is to facilitate communication and consensus on the best practices for information security in healthcare and to promote the implementation of a uniform approach to security practices and assessments. The founding organizations include the National Institute of Standards and Technology (NIST), URAC, an independent, nonprofit leader in promoting healthcare quality via its accreditation and certification programs and WEDI, the Workgroup for Electronic Data Interchange. The Secretary of Health and Human Services is directed per the HIPAA legislation to consult WEDi regarding the implementation of the administrative simplification requirements (NIST/URAC/WEDi, 2004). These organizations offer a wealth of information for more detailed discussions on both HIPAA and privacy and security.

In a nutshell, HIPAA deals with the privacy, confidentiality and security of patient health information. In the context of HIPAA, privacy focuses on who should have access, what constitutes the patients rights to confidentiality, and definition of inappropriate access to health records. From O'Reilly, 1972, privacy is defined as a "security principle that protects individuals from the collection, storage and dissemination of information about themselves and the possible compromises resulting from unauthorized release of that information" (Russell and Gangemi, 1992). Confidentiality establishes how paper records or the information systems that store the records are protected from inappropriate access so that it is not made available or disclosed to unauthorized individuals, entities or processes (e.g., kept private). Security is the means used to ensure both privacy and confidentiality.

The HIPAA Security Rule breaks the requirements into six categories: administrative procedures, physical safeguards, security configuration management, technical security services, technical security mechanism and electronic signature. The e-hospital network infrastructure encompasses the hardware and software used to shuffle electronic data to and from the systems that store the data regardless of the physical location of the device used to access and create the data or the physical location of the data storage system. In today's market, that can mean moving data to and from anywhere in the world. In other words, e-hospital network infrastructures and security services must move to the same level of electronically integrated service delivery that is currently provided by other industries such as the financial services industry.

Emerging Trends

Since physicians and healthcare providers are constantly on the move, another emerging standard is the usage of mobile, wireless devices connected to the network. For example, therapists in a South Carolina hospital have effectively used a wireless Local Area Network (LAN) to improve productivity and enhance patient care. According to the director of this department, they "lost 10 hours a day in therapists pushing paperwork" (Goedert, 1999). Now the medical supplies cart is equipped with a laptop with a wireless connection to the network instead of a clipboard. The therapists can retrieve treatment orders and enter clinical data into the system as well as view previous test results and treatment information about a patient. This system also enables the hospital to keep families better informed as to a patient's progress. Another example is the use of palm computers in a Phoenix, Arizona, emergency room. With these palm computers, Emergency Room (ER) physicians can access, via a wireless link, expert systems that walk them through a series of questions when diagnosing such things as heart attacks, using the most current knowledge available (Mitchell, 1999).

Examples of innovative uses of both old and new technologies abound but the realization of the true "e-hospital" remains elusive. The dream is becoming closer to a reality. For the first time, a President of the United States has backed the use of information technology to provide a unified system of computerized records as a tool not only to prevent medical errors but also reduce costs (U.S. White House press, 2004). This, along with the legislation and funding this endorsement spawns, will elevate both awareness and focus of the healthcare industry on information technology. The industry should see the maturity and increased implementation of Electronic Medical Record, EMR, solutions, deployment of more wireless handheld tablet devices and other similar ease of use and convenience innovations, further digitization and integration of all patient related data into various data repositories and further standardization of security services in keeping with the general security industry (e.g., single sign on solutions, stronger secure data messaging such as S-MIME, stronger authentication strategies such as smart cards and biometrics, uniform adoption of standard network protocols and infrastructure topologies).

THE END-USER

The user interface, the tools that physicians, other healthcare specialists, and customers use to work with digital data, is a critical component of the e-hospital network. The simplicity, reliability, and ease of use of the devices, or mechanisms used to access, review, and respond to information, are the ultimate determinants of success. The variety of the tools available is in itself an explosive industry. While the traditional PC with its "windows" desktop metaphors remains common, browser-based GUIs (graphical user interfaces) and full-blown clinical workstations are becoming more common. Enterprise-wide or individually customized portals are a direction many software vendors are headed.   Perhaps the most convenient are the wireless varieties. The use of laptops, handheld PCs, PDAs and mobile phones is skyrocketing. Information users demand to be mobile. *Figure 3* shows an overview of the evolving e-hospital. This figure has been developed based on the earlier work of Forman and Saint John (2000). This picture of total digital communication, commerce, and interaction is technically possible and is being embraced around the globe. It brings with it the possibility of true freedom of information and the promise of improved health and well-being. It also carries a burden of responsibility for adopters: that access and ability to use the digital network will be uniform so as to level the standard of healthcare for all citizens.

Gartner Group has recently published a white paper on the "digital divide" phenomenon (Gartner Group, 2000). Gartner's CEO Michael Fleisher also recently made a presentation on the subject before US Congress (Fleisher, 2000). The studies by the Gartner group found that socioeconomic status (SES) as defined by one's household incomes and educational level is a good predictor of one's likelihood to have access to the Internet and all the benefits that such access brings. The paradox fueling this gap can be summarized as: unlimited access to knowledge is available, but to get it you must have the means. Possessing the knowledge is what propels one upward to acquire the means.

The "digital divide" and the implications it has for the e-hospital, particularly in the post-hospital discharge stage and the pre-admission phase, cannot be ignored. It is a common misconception that the "digital divide" is a divide between the "haves" and the "have-nots" — those who can afford computers and an Internet connection and those who can't. However, as with many social issues, the problem is more complicated than this. Many efforts are being made to provide access to the Internet for those who do not have it. For example, in addition to stand-alone literacy centers in areas of need, more than 11,000 public libraries and 1,100 accredited community colleges offer access to the Internet. Where it gets more complicated is with content barriers. A study done by The Children's Partnership estimates that at least 50 million Americans are not able to benefit from the Internet because of one or more content-related barriers. The content barriers listed in this study are lack of local information, literacy, language, and lack of cultural diversity. Lack of local information has to do with the fact that it is less likely that there will be content on the Internet directly related to the communities where access is limited. The cultural barrier results from the lack of content directly related to and expressive of

Figure 3: e-Hospital Infrastructure Components

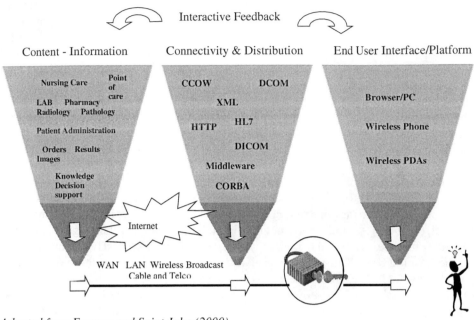

Adapted from Forman and Saint John (2000)

various ethnic groups. This is a formidable barrier because "distinctive cultural practices and beliefs among ethnically diverse Americans influence the ways in which these groups participate in everything from their children's education to use of health services to civic activities like voting" (Children's Partnership, 2000, Section II). Does this mean that with a wide disparity in the availability of computer access amongst the general populace, e-hospital services may not be available for or may not be used by certain segments of society? A survey done by harrisinteractive.com (of Harris market research and polling) revealed that 86% of Internet users (in the year 2000) said that they were scanning the web for healthcare and disease-specific information as compared to 71% of Internet users in the year 1999 (McCarthy, 2000). This suggests that e-hospital services may be a viable alternative to more Internet users. Time will tell how the overall barriers to usage of the Internet will affect the quality of healthcare provided to affected populations. In light of these barriers to accessing and utilizing e-hospital services, laws, policies, procedures, and practices must be sensitive to this potential disparity. During the e-Health Summit hosted at the University of California at Berkley in March of 2000, a group of business, academic, and government leaders met to discuss the "health digital divide." These discussions seem to indicate that closing the digital divide gap as it pertains to healthcare will be harder than closing it for the Internet Economy. According to Molly Coye, former director of the California Department of Health Services, one reason for this is that "we're dealing with two huge cultures, health and government. These are the two systems that have invested the least and are the most ignorant about what technology can do" (Woody, 2000). However, governments and healthcare providers must seize the opportunity to use the potential of e-health (in the form of the e-hospital) for extending care and providing medical knowledge to all people.

CONCLUSIONS

As e-healthcare evolves, the e-hospital will be an important part of the continuum. To fully realize the potential of the e-hospital: (1) the transactions surrounding a patient's hospital visit need to be automated, (2) diagnostic, treatment, and other patient-centric observations need to be digitized, and (3) a robust, secure, and standardized network needs to be in place to handle the transmission of all of this data. This chapter has explored the various systems that are part of a hospital's IT infrastructure and the changes and additions to that infrastructure that will be necessary to achieve the goal of the e-hospital. In addition, some emerging trends and innovations in information technology that are improving the quality and efficiency of the e-hospital were discussed. Finally, the human factor pertaining to the prevalence of IT in the hospital system, especially relating to the effect on hospital staff and the health "digital divide," is considered.

There is still a lot of work to be done in understanding the move towards an e-hospital. One of the paradigms that need to be looked into in greater depth is how the e-hospital, technologies, and infrastructure, fit into the overall healthcare service chain. Many of these issues presented in the chapter relate to activities directly associated with what the hospital does after the patient visit has been initiated and before the patient leaves the hospital. The role of the e-hospital in preventive care (prior to the hospital visit by the patient) and post-hospital visitation has to be explored in greater detail. Qualitative and quantitative cost-benefit analyses of the e-hospital should be carried out so that the long-term effectiveness and efficiency of such an environment is ensured. Implementation issues for putting the e-hospital in place should be addressed. Finally, performance measures (in terms of quality, reliability, delivery, flexibility, cost, etc.) for an e-hospital should be researched and put in place for the hospital of tomorrow. Many of the technologies described in the chapter have been in existence for more than a decade. It is imperative that research be carried out for gauging the effectiveness and efficiency and, in turn, productivity of these technologies in the e-hospital environment.

REFERENCES

Becich, M. (2000, October). Pathology informatics in the new millennium. *Advance for Administrators of the Laboratory,* 68.

Blair, J. S. (2000). *An Overview of Healthcare Information Standards.* Retrieved October 29, 200 from the World Wide Web: http://www.cpri.org/resource/docs/overview.html.

Children's Partnership. (2000). *Low-Income and Underserved Americans: The Digital Divide's New Frontier, A Publication of the Children's Partnership.* Retrieved October 29, 2000 from the World Wide Web: http://childrenspartnership.org/pub/low_income/index.html.

DeJesus, E. X. (2000, June). Claims processing speeds up. *Healthcare Informatics,* 45-50.

Dunbar, C. (1990). Sam Schultz and the University Hospital Consortium. *Computers in Healthcare,* 11(5), 18-24.

Dunbar, C. (1993). Medical Center in Florida Enjoys Client/Server Benefits but Stresses Documentation. *Computers in Healthcare,* 14(9), 22.

Eckerson, W. (1990). Hospital Hopes HL7-Based Net Will Ensure Versatility. *Network World*, 7(34), 19-20.

Fleisher, M. D. (2000). *FirstGov.gov: Is It a Good Idea*. Testimony before a hearing of the Subcommittee on Government Management, Information, and Technology, September 12, 2000. Retrieved January 16, 2001 from the World Wide Web: http://www.house.gov/reform/gmit/hearings/001002.FirstGov/001002mf.htm.

Forman, P. & Saint John, R. W. (2000, November). Creating Convergence. *Scientific American*, 283(5), 50-56.

Gartner Group. (2000). *Gartner's Digital Divide Report: 50 Percent of U.S. Households now have Internet Access*. Gartner Group Press Release, October 2, 2000. Retrieved January 16, 2001 from the World Wide Web: http://gartner3.gartnerweb.com/public/stataic/aboutgg/pressrel/pr20001002a.html.

Gillespie, G. (1999, September). Laying a New Foundation. *Health Data Management*.

Goedert, J. (1999, August). Going Wireless to Boost Productivity. *Health Data Management*.

Goldstein, D. E. (2000). *E-Healthcare: Harnessing the Power of Internet e-Commerce and e-Care*. Frederick, MD: Aspen Publishers.

Gordon, D. (1999). *Merging Multiple Institutions: Information Architecture Problems and Solutions*. AMIA '99 Annual Symposium. Retrieved October 29, 2000 from the World Wide Web: http://www.amia.org/pubs/symposia/D005435.htm.

Hagland, M. (2000, October). Smart Cards Knock at Healthcare's Door. *Healthcare Informatics*, 77-82.

Health Level Seven. (2000a). HL7 to Release First XML-based Standard for Healthcare. Health Level Seven, Inc. Press Release, 3300 Washtenaw Ave., Suite 227, Ann Arbor, MI 48104-4261, October 4, 2000.

Health Level Seven. (2000b). Retrieved January 16, 2001 from the World Wide Web: www.hl7.org.

Kelly, E. P. & Unsal, F. (2002). Health Information Privacy and E-Healthcare. *International Journal of Health Technology & Management*, 4(1/2), 41-52.

Lin, B. & Umoh, D. (2002). e-Healthcare: A Vehicle of Change. *American Business Review*, 20(1), 27-32.

Marietti, C. (2000, June). Middleware: Enabling the '2' in B2B. *Healthcare Informatics*, 30-31.

MARKLE Foundation's CONNECTING FOR HEALTH Press Release (2003, June 5). Connecting For Health Unites Over 100 Organizations To Bring American Healthcare System into Information Age. Retrieved February 20, 2004 from the World Wide Web: http://www.connectingforhealth.org/news/pressrelease_060503.html.

McCarthy, R. (2000). E-health, your Workforce and You. *Business & Health*, 18(10), 46.

Mitchell, M. (1999, September). Working Smart Maximizing the Payoff from IT. St. Joseph's Hospital's Heart Attack Risk Assessment. *CIO Magazine*. Retrieved Octoober 29, 2000 from the World Wide Web: http://www.cio.com/archive/090199_smart.html.

Mon, D. T. & Nunn, S. (1999, February). Understanding CPR Architecture: An HIM Professional's Guide. *Journal of AHIMA*, American Health Information Management Association. Retrieved April 20, 2000 from the World Wide Web: http://www.ahima.org/journal/features/feature.9902.1.html.

Morrissey, J. (2000, April). Internet dominates Providers' Line of Sight. *Modern Healthcare*, 72.

NIST/URAC/WEDi Health Care Security Workgroup White paper, NIST/URAC/WEDi (2004). Retrieved February 20, 2004 from the World Wide Web: http://www.wedi.org/cmsUploads/pdfUpload/WhitePaper/pub/2004-02-09NUWWP.pdf.

Object Management Group. (2000a). *OMG news release: CORBA Interoperability approved as ISO Standard.* Retrieved October 29, 2000 from the World Wide Web: http://www.omg.org/news releases/pr2000/2000-10-25.htm.

Object Management Group. (2000b). *E-Business: Success On A Sound Software Architecture.* Retrieved October 29, 2000 from the World Wide Web: http://www.omg.org/attachments/pdf/OMG.pdf.

Ortman, N. (2001). Healthcare Intranets are Healthy Investments that Pay for Themselves. *Managed Healthcare Executive*, 11(8), 42-45.

Russell, D. & Gangemi, Sr., G. T. (1992). *Computer Security Basics.* O'Reilly & Associates, Inc.

Siau, K., Hong S. & Southard, P. (2002). e-Healthcare Strategies and Implementation. *International Journal of Healthcare Technology & Management*, 4(1/2), 118-131.

Stammer, L. (2000, October). Seeking Safety. *Healthcare Informatics*, 65-72.

Synder-Halpern, R. (1999, September/October). A Model-Based Context Assessment Approach for the Informatics Nurse Specialist Consultant. *Computers in Nursing*, 17(5), 221-228.

Tieman, J. (2000, October). Rules Change Business Basics. *Modern Healthcare*, Supplement (Eye on Info), 12.

University of Rochester Medical Center. (2000). Final Report of the Network Infrastructure Planning/Review Group of the IAIMS at the University of Rochester Medical Center. Retrieved January 16, 2001 from the World Wide Web: http://www.urmc.rochester.edu/iaims/planning/committees/network/fnlrpt2.html.

U.S. Food and Drug Administration (2004). Protecting and Advancing Consumer Health and Safety. Retrieved February 20, 2004 from World Wide Web: http://www.fda.gov/oc/whitepapers/consumers.html.

U.S. White House press release, "The President's Address to the Nation" (2004, January 24). Retrieved February 20, 2004 from the World Wide Web: http://www.whitehouse.gov/news/releases/2004/01/20040124.html.

Walter, Z. & Tung, Y. A. (2002). e-Healthcare System Design: A Consumer Preference Approach. *International Journal of Healthcare Technology & Management*, 4(1/2), 53-87.

Weis, D. (1996). UNMC Laboratory System Cuts Errors and Labor Costs. *Health Management Technology*, 17(11), 35-36.

Woody, T. (2000, March). Bridging the Digital Divide. *The Standard.* Retrieved October 29, 2000 from the World Wide Web: http://news.idg.net/crd__145980.html.

ENDNOTE

[1]   The authors wish to thank Mr. Kevin E. Thompson for his contributions in developing the preliminary draft of a paper, based on which this chapter has been written.

Chapter VI

Applying Automatic Data Collection Tools for Real-Time Patient Management

Richard J. Puerzer, Hofstra University, USA

ABSTRACT

The management of patients in healthcare facilities, such as outpatient clinics and hospital emergency departments, is a significant hospital management problem. In an effort to deal with the volume of patients who visit an emergency department, hospitals often haphazardly add more resources to their emergency department, such as hiring more personnel or adding more treatment rooms, without proper analysis of the impact of the additional resources on the system. These solutions can be quite expensive and yet their effect on improving problems in the system is often negligible. Knowledge management can make these challenges tractable and lead to more effective solutions. For example, through the application of an automated patient management system that collects and utilizes information concerning the status of patients, the flow of patients can be better managed. Hospitals can effectively deal with many of the problems associated with scheduling and overcrowding, and improve the quality of care provided by their institution. To accurately capture and provide access to the volume of precise information required to effectively manage a healthcare facility, an extensive information acquisition system must be created. The information collected can then be used for both real-time and long-term management decisions. These ideas are discussed and elaborated upon in this chapter.

INTRODUCTION

The purpose of this chapter will be to investigate the problems involved in managing patient flows and to describe the application of automatic data collection tools that will optimize the use of resources through knowledge management. Improvements in knowledge management through the collection and utilization of information and, subsequently, in the control and management of the emergency department, will result in increased productivity and cost effectiveness of emergency department resources, better flow of patients through the department, and improved quality of patient care.

This chapter will describe, as a case study, the development of tools capable of addressing the issues involved with patient management. The case study will describe the development of an information systems framework for the creation of a patient flow management system. It will then describe the use of this framework in the creation of an experimental patient tracking and control system that was developed utilizing automatic data collection tools with a computer-based interface to track the flow of patients throughout a model hospital emergency department. The experimental system utilizes a graphical interface to aid emergency department staff in the control and management of patients. In addition, the system has built-in monitoring and analysis tools. Control is accomplished by increasing the use of information and by providing more information feedback to emergency department staff.

The goal of the chapter will be to further the understanding of the use of technology for the improvement of the quality of patient care, specifically through the use of automated data collection technology and control systems for the management of patients and patient information. Advances in these technologies for real-time decision making allow for optimization of resource allocation and, ultimately, the care of patients. On a larger scale, these technologies thus represent advancement in the knowledge management of healthcare systems and enterprises.

PATIENT OVERCROWDING PROBLEM

The overcrowding of patients in hospital emergency departments and outpatient clinics throughout the United States is a serious problem that often results in increased facilities and/or personnel. Research shows that the patient overcrowding problem affects hospitals of all types throughout the United States. One survey (Ranseen, 1991) states that 38% of United States households include someone who has visited a hospital emergency department for a minor illness or non-life-threatening emergency in the last two years. Another study (Kellerman & Lynn, 1991) shows that three of four institutions have reported that their rate of emergency department usage has increased in the past few years. That same study reported that during one reference month, 40% of reporting hospitals diverted ambulances to other hospitals part of the time, and one-third were required to transfer patients to other hospitals due to overcrowding. The introduction of managed care is supposed to have an effect on the usage of emergency departments. However, Shortell and Reinhardt (1992) report that, "while managed care is being touted as an effective approach to both cost control and quality improvement, there is relatively little research to document the extent to which these savings and quality improvements have been realized."

All types of healthcare institutions are affected by this problem. When investigating whether the overcrowding problem affected only public hospitals, Kellerman and Lynn (1991) found that private hospitals have reported mean occupancy rates just as high as those reported by public hospitals. They suggest that the increasing population in the United States, changes in technology associated with healthcare, and changes in the demands made on healthcare systems, will continue in the foreseeable future. These studies serve as evidence of both the breadth and significance of the patient overcrowding problem.

A major effect of overcrowding and patient gridlock is the creation of problems in patient management. These problems include long waiting periods for patients between healthcare procedures and processes. Patients also face long waits when they require the use of any ancillary resources such as laboratory tests or imaging procedures. Long waits have a subsequent negative effect on the care and treatment of patients and the quality of care provided. The previously mentioned survey of emergency department directors by Kellerman and Lynn (1991) found that 65% of those responding reported that patient overcrowding was having a moderate-to-severe negative impact on their quality of patient care.

There is a great deal of variation in the care required by the patients who come to the emergency department and clinics, depending on the type and severity of the patient's illness or injury. Some patients need little or no actual medical attention, while others require a great deal of treatment and resources over a period of several hours. Many patients seen in the emergency department are eventually admitted to the hospital. The emergency department must first stabilize, treat, and monitor these patients. Thus, the emergency department staff is performing multiple roles in the care and treatment of many patients. This position of patient treatment provider and patient transition facilitator in the healthcare system results in the emergency department being a critical point of care. This creates a dual problem for the emergency department because it is prone to overcrowding problems caused by the hospital when a large percentage of hospital beds are full and by high arrival rates of new patients.

This overcrowding problem increases costs and dangerously compromises the abilities of already strained emergency departments (Andrulis et al., 1991). One consequence of overcrowding is that when patients must wait for long periods of time, many become extremely annoyed or leave the emergency department before they receive treatment. Baker et al. (1991) found that when the average waiting time increases, the population of patients who leave without being seen increases in both in size and in the severity of illness. In addition, they found that these patients who leave do not differ from those who stay for treatment in terms of age, race, or insurance status. This phenomenon causes another management problem. Any delay in the care of a patient creates a delay in the care of other patients, which also contributes to patient overcrowding. An example of this is when a patient exits the emergency department before the completion of the care process. In such a case, emergency department staff cannot be certain that the patient has left. They must assure that the patient has not been moved or become "lost." This obviously requires time. This is time that could be better utilized.

Studies have also shown that the patients who leave the emergency department are not doing so because their illnesses are trivial or nonexistent. Kellerman (1991) found that many patients are leaving because they are, in fact, too sick to wait and are too uncomfortable in the waiting room. One case study (Bindman et al., 1991) reported that 27% of the patients who left without treatment returned to an emergency department.

These studies refute the claim that it is simply those who require little or no medical attention who leave without treatment. Therefore, it cannot be predicted who will leave the emergency department and, thus, management cannot make any assumptions when a patient is missing. On an economic level, most, if not all, of the patients who leave the emergency department can be thought of as unsatisfied customers as well as lost revenue. However, an overcrowded emergency department means not only the loss of revenue and the perception of poor quality of care by many of the patients, but also means that the health of some patients may be put in jeopardy. Anything that endangers the health of patients is obviously an unacceptable condition.

EFFECTS OF OVERCROWDING ON QUALITY OF PATIENT CARE

In today's healthcare environment there is a growing emphasis on the quality of patient care. Gedde and Gupta (1992) stated that the successful healthcare provider of the future will be the provider who adopts those concepts that contain or reduce costs while, at the same time, improve quality. Hospital overcrowding significantly impacts the quality of patient care. It is not surprising then, that a study by Hagland (1991) found that the majority of the quality complaints by patients who had been cared for in the emergency department were concerned with the amount of time spent in the emergency department as opposed to complaints regarding the clinical care provided. Unnecessary delays in patient admission, long delays in receiving medical attention, large queues and/or long delays for testing and diagnostic procedures, and periodic temporary "loss" of patients in the system contribute to non-value-added time in the hospital. In the increasingly competitive healthcare environment, problems with the patients' perception of quality of care must be addressed.

Because these quality issues are predominately concerned with time, hospital management may address them as they work with the related problems associated with overcrowding. However, in attempting to improve quality through these methods, hospital management should be cognizant of McCabe's (1992) statement that warns: "quality is not an end in itself, but the strategic method that the hospital uses to effectively and efficiently perform its mission." Through the use of a knowledge management approach and knowledge management tools, the problems associated with overcrowding can be ameliorated and a continuous effort can be made to improve the quality of patient treatment. Implementation and maintenance of such an approach will allow for a method for improving patient care delivery systems, maintaining these improvements, and providing the means for further improvement.

FACILITATING KM THROUGH AUTOMATIC DATA COLLECTION

Automatic data collection tools such as bar codes and readers, magnetic stripe cards, and radio identification tools, have in recent years been utilized for innovative purposes in a variety of healthcare applications. For example, bar code collection tools are used by an eye bank to track time-critical donor tissue. Winters (1990) reported that automatic data collection tools, specifically bar code technologies, were being used by a hospital for the general purpose of improving patient care quality. In particular, bar codes have been used for inventory control, prescription labeling, specimen identification, and inpatient identification. Picker (1993) reported that the Lackland Air Force Base Hospital used PDF417 bar codes placed on personnel identification cards for emergency room registration. PDF417 bar codes are a two-dimensional bar code symbology that can represent more information than traditional one-dimensional bar codes. Employee identification and extensive medical information is represented in the PDF417 bar code. This program enables quick and accurate identification and data retrieval for the approximate 58,000 emergency room patients using their hospital each year. Also, Bellows (1994) reported that the Mayo Clinic was using bar codes on patient wristbands for use in patient identification. This automatic data collection system is used to assure that blood products are administered properly and that this critical activity of patient care is assured of safety through accurate patient tracking and identification. Concerning the use of the computer as a tool in the emergency department from a broader view, Walrath (1983) describes a clinical information system that enables nurses to analyze trends in patient utilization and use those trends as a basis for scheduling. More generally, the field of medical informatics studies the use of information science and technology in a broad range of medical applications (Greenes & Shortliffe, 1990; Shortliffe & Perreault, 1990).

Miller and Jones (1995) reported the use of bar codes for a patient tracking system to facilitate hospital bed management. Patients are tracked from admission to a room to discharge from the hospital via bar codes. By knowing which rooms are occupied and when rooms become available, the hospital housekeeping staff is able to clean rooms and make them available for incoming patients. This system alleviated the substantial problem of long patient queues for placement in inpatient rooms. This work is the most closely related work found in the literature to a patient tracking and control system. However, there is not any publication of follow-up literature to this work.

Because of the highly competitive healthcare environment, emergency department management must endeavor to meet customer expectations and thus the patient's view of how the emergency department should operate (Hansagi et al., 1992). This inevitably leads to a cycle of improvement and change in the emergency department. The embrace of change by emergency department management not only improves the quality of care of patients but also allows for the survival of the hospitals and the emergency departments contained therein. Widra and Fottler (1988) predict that a lack of strategic change in the management of the emergency department will precipitate failure. They go on to state that, "the panorama of change sweeping the emergency sector of healthcare requires the mobilization of multiple input factors to yield a timely, appropriate, and efficacious response."

A form of automatic data collection technology that is gaining wider usage is radio frequency identification. Radio frequency identification systems have three main components: readers, antennae, and tags. The reader interrogates the tag by means of an energy burst in the form of a radio wave signal sent from the antenna. A low frequency passive transponder is embedded inside of the tag. The signal from the antenna charges the transponder in a matter of milliseconds. The transponder then returns a signal that carries information. This signal and its information is captured by the antenna and, thus, read by the reader (Zarate, 1993; IR-12E Reader, 1994). Information is then sent to the host computer through a standard computer connection or interface.

Due to their flexibility, radio frequency identification systems are preferred in many environments in which other automatic data collection technologies are not feasible. They are useful in dirty, dusty, or dark conditions, or conditions where data collection would be hazardous to humans (Pinkerton, 1994). One reason for this is that radio frequency identification systems do not require line-of-sight for the reading and collection of data. This makes the technology applicable for situations in which time or other constraints make it impossible for individuals to physically acquire data. This is true in the emergency department where clinicians must concern themselves with the care of patients and cannot spend time collecting auxiliary management information.

Due to the unobtrusiveness and accuracy of data collection with radio frequency identification technology, it was chosen for the collection of data in the experimental patient tracking and control system created in this research.

PATIENT TRACKING AND CONTROL

The transformation of the traditional emergency department "room board" to a computerized graphical display improves the effectiveness of the room board as an information source by enabling additional and more dynamic information to be displayed. This information should provide the emergency department staff with insight into the ongoing status of the emergency department and allow for more proactive management of the emergency department.

Although the room board has been utilized for quite a while in the emergency department environment, the thought of it as a graphical display is novel. Carswell and Wickens (1987) describe the term "object display" as any graphical technique that uses several dimensions of a single perceptual object to present multiple sources of information. Additionally, Wickens (1990) states that symbolic categorization tasks (i.e., tasks that enable the user to interpret a symbol into two or more levels of information) are utilized by the object display. Thus, the object display aids in the decision-making process by exploiting advantages such as pattern recognition, redundancy, and the user's memory and organizational structure, also known as the user's mental model.

These advantages infer that there should be a shorter learning curve for using an emergency department room board and greater efficiency in the everyday use of the room board. For example, an advantage is expected in the common task of the retrieval of patient location information. A patient tracking and control system would thus require less training for emergency department staff in the task of patient management. A reduction in training costs is especially important given the statement by Tivig and Meier (1991) that, "because of economic pressures on the healthcare system and clinical personnel shortages, especially in nursing, less time is available for in-service training."

Graphical displays provide a much more effective means of information display than the traditional room board through both the organization and the dynamic nature of the information presented. Designing room board displays as graphical displays exploits the user's mental information organization structure. This involves designing graphical representations of actual physical locations, a map of the emergency room for example, to be accurate and consistent in scale.

These organization structures allow for redundant information presentation which Sanders and McCormick (1987) describe as "an advantageous display strategy." Redundancy was also utilized in the control signals that the control system makes when reporting any unfavorable management conditions in the emergency department. The signals, redundant to the time in room board displays, will alert the emergency department staff that situations exist or are impending which need to be rectified.

CASE STUDY: AN EXPERIMENTAL PATIENT TRACKING AND CONTROL SYSTEM

In an effort to gauge the utility of automatic data collection tools for the tracking of patients, an experimental patient tracking and control system was designed in a laboratory setting for the purpose of testing its utility (Puerzer 1997). The experimental patient tracking and control system was developed in a laboratory in order to test its potential use in an actual emergency department. The experimental patient tracking and control system consists of three main components: the data collection system, graphical user interface, and a control system. A radio frequency identification system was selected to obtain data concerning the movement of patients through the model emergency department, since the data can be collected unobtrusively without interfering with the care process. This tracking information increases the awareness of the emergency department staff and, thereby, improves the control of patients in the emergency department.

The first task in the creation of the experimental patient tracking and control system was the specification of requirements. This process focused on what information is necessary for the tracking and control of patients in an actual emergency department and was developed by using an implementation model designed specifically for the creation of an information system integrated with an automatic data collection system.

An actual emergency department was used for the development of requirements definition for the experimental patient tracking and control system. The value of using an actual emergency department in the development of the experimental system was that the experimental system, although designed and tested in a laboratory, would be developed with an understanding of its real world requirements. For instance, the testing of the experimental patient tracking and control system allows for a determination of whether or not its components, specifically the radio frequency identification tools, can be implemented in the real world. The investigations into an actual emergency department help to bridge the gap between the laboratory and the real world in this research.

There are significant differences in the physical environment of an actual emergency department and the environment in the laboratory in which the experimental patient tracking and control system was designed and tested. This was recognized in the requirements definition of the experimental patient tracking and control system. When necessary, the tools used in determining the requirements of a patient tracking and control system were scaled down for the development of the experimental patient tracking and control system created for this research.

Information on all patients concerning their location and duration of time spent in the emergency department system is provided to the staff via a graphical computer display. This display is made up of multiple screens. One screen resembles the "room board" that is typically used in most emergency departments as a repository for location information. Another screen provides a physical layout representation of the emergency department and provides location information to emergency department staff about all patients. The remaining screens allow information to be entered and edited. The information provided by this graphical user interface would provide the staff with a complete system and status view of the entire emergency department.

In addition to displaying location and time information, the control system embedded in the experimental patient tracking and control's graphical user interface will provide graphical feedback to the emergency department staff concerning any possible, impending, and/or existent managerial problems in the emergency department. In summary, testing of the experimental patient tracking and control system can show if it can facilitate more effective management by enabling decisions to be made with full knowledge of all the events taking place in the emergency department.

The physical makeup of the experimental patient tracking and control system consisted of radio frequency identification tools (readers and tags) from the Indala Corporation (a division of Motorola), a PC utilizing a Windows-based operating system, Visual Basic programs, and an ACCESS database.

The created patient tracking and control system would be made up of the three readers attached to one personal computer. Two of the readers selected were Indala model IR-36E long-range readers. The other was an Indala model IR-12E short-range reader. These three readers each provide a decimal output at 9600 baud to an RS232 connector making them easy to use with a personal computer. They and their corresponding power supplies could be individually connected to the serial ports of a personal computer. The three readers each have an independent power supply. The IR-12E reader is wired directly to the power supply and the computer. The two IR-36E readers require electronic units, small boxes used to wire the reader, power supply, and personal computer together. The technical information provided by Indala stated that for the best results, the layout of the system should place the electronic units 10 feet from the IR-36E reader panels. It also stated that all readers and electronic units should be 10 feet from any computer monitors or equipment. Radio frequency identification equipment is very susceptible to interference from any electronic equipment as well as from metal objects within the read range. Efforts were made when laying out the equipment in the laboratory for any testing procedures to avoid interference that would adversely affect the tested read ranges. The effects of interference on the radio frequency identification equipment would have serious consequences for a patient tracking and control system utilized in an actual emergency department. Emergency departments are quite harsh environments with respect to electrical interference due to all of the electrical medical equipment. However, the potential for improvements on this weakness of radio frequency identification equipment motivates research on their use.

These read ranges depend on the size of the tag, the size of the reader, and whether the tag is an active or passive tag. Maximal read range is tested by orienting the face or flat side of the tag parallel to the face or flat side of the reader, and allowing minimal interfering conditions, e.g., electrical components, in the environment.

These system design considerations were taken into account when creating the layout for the experimental system. The IR-12E short-range reader serves as a registration reader, thus its proximity to the computer. The other two IR-36E long-range readers serve as room readers monitoring the movement of patients.

Additionally, three types of tags were utilized: IB-11E active tags, IT-21E passive tags, and IT-54 passive tags. The IB-11E tags are large tags, approximately the size of a hockey puck, with a very large read range. The IT-21E tags are approximately the size of a credit card, and have a medium read range. The IT-54 tags are small button sized tags with a small read range. A quantity of four IB-11E tags, five IT-21E tags, and six IT-54 tags were used. These three types of tags represented the spectrum of sizes and abilities of tags that Indala offered at the time of the acquisition of the radio frequency identification tools. The different types of tags were procured in order to test different types, sizes, and abilities of tags and to demonstrate their advantages and disadvantages.

The second task in the creation of the experimental patient tracking and control system was the creation of the graphical displays. As was previously stated, for the purposes of this research, the emphasis in the creation of graphical displays was simply to create a functional interface for the experimental patient tracking and control system. A personal computer was used. The graphical displays take signals from the data acquisition tools and display them in the form of patient location and time in the model emergency department. The graphical displays also incorporate signals from the patient control system to provide additional feedback on the duration each individual has been in the model emergency department.

The creation of an interface was necessary to convert the information received by the readers into information meaningful to the emergency department staff. The radio frequency identification readers provide information to the computer only when they identify a tag. The readers essentially serve as dumb terminals, constantly searching for tags and reacting when one comes within range.

The patient tracking and control computer interface was required to turn this basic identification information into a meaningful description to users of which tag/patient is identified and where that tag/patient is physically located. Additional information can be obtained from the interface regarding time, both of the identified events and of the time in the system for that patient, as well as the status of the patient.

Three main screens make up the user interface system. These screens are a data input screen, an emergency department map screen, and a patient status screen. Additionally, several other support screens were created to view patient data. These include a screen to display individual patient information, a screen to exit a patient from the system, and an online reports screen. All of these screens interact with each other, with buttons and menus available for transition from screen to screen.

The experimental user interface was designed to model an emergency department, which was set up in the Automatic Data Collection Laboratory at the University of Pittsburgh. The model system had three rooms: a registration room, a treatment room, and an x-ray room. A radio frequency reader was used to monitor the movement of patients in and out of each room. Each patient tracked in the model emergency department was assigned a radio frequency tag. As the patient passed through the model emergency department, he or she was tracked by the patient tracking and control system. This tracking was monitored through the user interface.

In order to determine the utility and the effectiveness of the experimental patient tracking and control system, the reliability and validity of the system were tested.

Through a series of tests, information was collected concerning the viability of the use of a patient tracking and control system, given the current state of radio frequency technology.

The reliability of the experimental patient tracking and control system was examined through tests of the capabilities of the radio frequency identification components. These tests included a determination of radio frequency identification reader read ranges and of the effects of radio frequency identification tag orientation and distance from the reader. The validity of the graphical displays of the patient tracking and control system was also tested. This was accomplished by testing the integrity of the graphical data displayed and by performing a physical simulation of using the system.

LESSONS LEARNED FROM
THE CASE STUDY

The results of the testing conducted on the experimental patient tracking and control system indicate that two major improvements must be made before implementation in an actual emergency department would be practical. First, the state of the art of radio frequency identification equipment would need to be advanced. The current read range was too small to realistically track human beings in the often chaotic environment of the hospital emergency department. Likewise, the sensitivity of the radio frequency equipment to electronic interference would be a major weakness in an emergency department filled with equipment such as heart monitors, portable x-ray equipment, and pagers. An implemented patient tracking and control system would require that tags be detected virtually 100% of the time to ensure the complete tracking of patients. As the reliability tests indicate, this would be a difficult task in an actual emergency department given the currently available equipment. However, the technical staff at Indala predicts that the state of the art in radio frequency identification equipment will rapidly advance in read range and general flexibility in the very near future.

The second change necessary for the patient tracking and control system is an increase in the complexity of the control logic. The model emergency department contained only three rooms. An actual emergency department will have additional rooms requiring tracking. These additional rooms will necessitate much more data input from radio frequency readers and, thus, the creation of more extensive control software. Likewise, the control system will have to accommodate the needs of an existing emergency department. Additional and customized control systems will require additional programming. However, this task is feasible. The complexity of the task would depend primarily on the actual emergency department.

The changes to the patient tracking and control system with regard to the data collection system would require a great deal of work and improvement in the radio frequency identification field. In fact, the improvements may require breakthroughs in the technology.

However, these deficiencies should not preclude the use of automatic data collections systems, including radio frequency identifications systems, from use in future knowledge management applications in healthcare. The need for massive data collection in healthcare virtually necessitates the use of such tools. With modest advances in technology, coupled with a concerted effort in the application of these tools in real-world settings, it is envisioned that automatic data collection tools will become an integral part of knowledge management in healthcare.

CONCLUSIONS

The most obvious future research stemming from this work is the implementation of a patient tracking and control system. Given improvements in the radio frequency identification technologies, the experimental patient tracking and control system could be expanded as necessary and implemented in an actual emergency department or other healthcare setting. Several major changes regarding the programming of the system, specifically concerning the graphics provided and the controls used, would require revision and adaptation specific to the environment in which the implemented patient tracking and control system will be used. These changes will be necessary for implementation in any specific healthcare environment, as each would feature different layouts, personnel, and patient populations.

Despite these inevitable customization requirements, a framework is in place for the implementation of an automatic data collection system such as that used in the experimental patient tracking and control system. Likewise, all of the information necessary for the tracking and control of patients has been identified. Thus, it would be up to the developers to collect the essential information specific to the environment in which implementation will occur. The implementation team would then prepare the patient tracking and control system specific to their own emergency department environment.

It is indisputable that the revolution in automated data collection has had and will continue to have a massive impact on knowledge management in healthcare. Unobtrusive real-time data collection can facilitate the monitoring of a variety of aspects of patient care resulting in greater accuracy in care analysis and treatment trends as well as in basic functions, such as billing. The implementation of such a system will require the knowledge of both healthcare systems and the technologies to be employed. Although the engineering involved in such an undertaking is daunting, the benefits in the knowledge management of the healthcare systems are considerable.

REFERENCES

Andrulis, D., Kellerman, A., Hintz, E., Hackman, B. & Weslowski, V. (1991, September). Emergency departments and crowding in United States teaching hospitals. *Annals Of Emergency Medicine*, 73-79.

Baker, D., Stevens, C. & Brook, R. (1991, August). Patients who leave a public hospital emergency department without being seen by a physician. *Journal Of The American Medical Association*, 1085-1090.

Bellows, B. (1994, January). Bar code operates at the Mayo Clinic. ID Systems, 31-34.

Bindman, A., Grumbach, K., Keane, D., Rauch, L. & Luce, J. (1991, August). Consequences of queuing for care at a public hospital emergency department. *Journal Of The American Medical Association*, 1091-1096.

Carswell, M. & Wickens, C. (1987, March). Information integration and the object display: An interaction of task demands and display superiority. *Ergonomics*, 511-527.

Gedde, T. & Gupta, Y. (1992, November). Patient-focused hospitals: Creating a competitive edge. *Industrial Engineering*, 62-66.

Greenes, R. & Shortliffe, E. (1990, February). Medical informatics: An emerging academic discipline and institutional priority. *Journal of The American Medicine Association*, 1114-1120.

Hagland, M. (1991, July). ED overcrowding spurs interest in quality and credentialing issues. *Hospitals*, 33-36.

Hansagi, H., Carlsson, B. & Brismar, B. (1992, Spring). The urgency of care need and patient satisfaction at a hospital emergency department. *Health Care Management Review*, 71-75.

IR-12E Reader. (1994). *Motorola Technical Report No. K01866-00* Rev. A. San Jose, CA, 1-3.

Kellerman, A. (1991, August). Too sick to wait. *Journal of The American Medical Association*, 1123-1124.

Kellerman, A. & Lynn, S. (1991, March). Critical decision making: Managing the emergency department in an overcrowded hospital. *Annals of Emergency Medicine*, 287-292.

McCabe, W. (1992, April). Total quality management in a hospital. *Quality Review Bulletin*, 134-140.

Miller, C. & Jones, D. (1995). Automated patient tracking solves bed management problem. Quest for Quality and Productivity in Health Services: 1995 Conference Proceedings. *Institute of Industrial Engineers*, 77-83.

Picker, D. (1993, May). Life-saving symbologies. *ID Systems*, 76-77.

Pinkerton, S. (1994, February). RF/ID puts a royal bedmaker's mind to rest. *ID Systems European Edition*, 18-20.

Puerzer, R. (1997). *The development of a patient tracking and control system for use in an emergency room.* Doctoral Dissertation, University of Pittsburgh.

Ranseen, T. (1991, July). ED use down 1%; urgent care use shows 2% rise. *Hospitals*, 14.

Sanders, M. & McCormick, E. (1987). *Human factors in engineering and design* (6th Ed.). New York: McGraw-Hill, 212-224.

Shortell, S. & Reinhardt, U. (1992). *Improving health policy and management: Nine critical research issues for the 1990's.* Ann Arbor, MI: Health Administration Press, 374.

Shortliffe, E. & Perreault, L. (eds.). (1990). *Medical informatics: Computer applications in health care.* New York: Addison-Wesley.

Tivig, G. & Meier, W. (1991, October). Patient monitor human interface design. *Hewlett-Packard Journal*, 29-37.

Walrath, J. (1983, July-August). Computer-assisted management in the emergency department. *Journal of Emergency Nursing*, 235-236.

Wickens, C. (1990). *Engineering psychology and human performance* (2nd Ed.). New York: HarperCollins, 112-122.

Widra, L. & Fottler M. (1988, Summer). Survival of the hospital emergency department: Strategic alternatives for the future. *Health Care Management Review*, 73-83.

Winters, J. (1990, October). State of the art technology: Improving the quality of patient care. *Scan-Tech 90 Proceedings,* 1-13.

Zarate, J. (1993). *Radio frequency identification.* Internal Report: University of Pittsburgh, 12.

Chapter VII

Data Mining and Knowledge Discovery in Healthcare Organizations:
A Decision-Tree Approach

Murat Caner Testik, Cukurova University, Turkey

George C. Runger, Arizona State University, USA

Bradford Kirkman-Liff, Arizona State University, USA

Edward A. Smith, University of Arizona and Translational
Genomics Research Institute, USA

ABSTRACT

Health care organizations are struggling to find new ways to cut healthcare utilization and costs while improving quality and outcomes. Predictive models that have been developed to predict global utilization for a healthcare organization cannot be used to predict the behavior of individuals. On the other hand, massive amounts of healthcare data are available in databases that can be used for exploring patterns and therefore knowledge discovery. Diversity and complexity of the healthcare data requires attention to the use of statistical methods. By nature, healthcare data are multivariate, making the analysis difficult as well as interesting. In this chapter, our intention is to classify individuals that are future high-utilizers of healthcare. In particular, we answer the question of whether a mathematical model can be generated utilizing a large claims database that will predict which individuals who are not using a service in a yet untested database will be high utilizers of that health service in the future. For this purpose, an integrated dataset from enrollment, medical claims, and pharmacy databases containing more than 150 million medical and pharmacy claim line items and for over four million patients is analyzed for knowledge discovery. A modern data-mining tool, namely decision trees, which may have a broad range of applications in healthcare organizations, was used in our analyses and a discussion of this valuable tool is provided. The results and managerial aspects are discussed. Several approaches are proposed for the use of this technique depending on the health plan.

INTRODUCTION

Many predictive models have been developed in healthcare in the past (Ash, 1999; Dunn, 1998; Dunn et al., 1995; Epstein & Cumella, 1988; Newhouse, 1986, 1995, 1998; van Vliet & Lamers, 1998; Weiner et al., 1995). However, for the most part, these models focused on how manipulation of plan design (deductibles, pays, etc.) will influence utilization behavior and to adjust for case-mix and risk for the purpose of predicting global costs and setting capitated reimbursement rates. Until recently, there has been little interest in applying prediction tools to individuals for the purpose of reducing costs and improving individual care. This lack of interest was mostly due to the absence of tools that can accurately predict future individual patient utilization, especially for patients who have had no current utilization. In general terms, current utilization of a particular kind of health service is the best predictor of future utilization of a particular kind of health service. Methods to predict future utilization of a particular service when there is no current utilization of the same service tend to produce results that are not meaningful for program managers.

Today, with the rapid increase in the generation and collection of data, researchers are able to explore patterns hidden in large databases. Massive amounts of healthcare data are also available in databases that can be used for knowledge discovery. Diversity and complexity of the healthcare data requires attention to the use of statistical methods. By nature, healthcare data are multivariate, making the analysis difficult as well as interesting.

The main objective of this research is to answer the question of whether a mathematical model can be generated utilizing a large claims database that will predict which individuals who are not using a service in a yet untested database will be high utilizers of that health service in the future. For this purpose we used a massive dataset containing more than 150 million medical and pharmacy claim line items and for over four million patients.

This research differs from previous related studies in a number of ways: (a) The focus is on identifying individuals for targeted interventions who currently have no use of the service under study; (b) An integrated dataset from commonly available data found in enrollment, medical claims, and pharmacy databases is used; (c) A model that is built on more advanced "episodes of care" cost groupings rather than merely raw claims data; and (d) A modern data mining technique, namely a decision tree, is used for knowledge discovery.

DATASET, DATA PREPROCESSING AND ANALYSES

Two blinded healthcare datasets — Census/Medical/Pharmacy (main) and Eligibility (supplementary)— were obtained from a private vendor, Symmetry Health Data Systems, Inc.

Note that the data protection legislation prohibits a health plan from providing patient-identifiable data to outside parties not directly involved in patient care. However, usage of data from patients by the health plan itself to monitor quality and to proactively intervene in statistically identified "high-risk" cases is allowed.

The main dataset includes more than 150 million claims (28.7 GB disk space) belonging to over four million insurance policyholders for the years of 1997, 1998, 1999, and 2000. The supplementary dataset (918 MB disk space) was first used to select the patients that are eligible for both the years of 1999 and 2000. The most recent two years of data was retained for analysis after cleaning those records that were believed to contain some sort of an error. The dataset consists of records for over 614K policyholders. For managing the data and analyses, the SAS v8.0 (statistical analysis software) was used (Scerbo, Dickstein & Wilson, 2001). Some of the demographic factors are provided in *Table 1* and *Table 2*.

Table 1: Demographics-Age Groups vs. Genders

Age Group	Male	Female	Total
[0-20]	72,524	70,471	142,995 (23.25%)
[20-30]	16,582	23,816	40,398 (6.57%)
[30-40]	34,574	45,177	79,751 (12.97%)
[40-50]	40,156	50,223	90,379 (14.70%)
[50-60]	30,681	36,171	66,852 (10.87%)
[60-...]	50,633	65,090	115,723 (18.82%)
Total	245,150 (39.87%)	290,948 (47.32%)	536,098 (87.19%)

Missing = 78,793

Table 2: Demographics-Regions

Region	Frequency
Southeast	0
Northwest	0
Midwest	113,474 (18.45%)
West	143,428 (23.33%)
Total	256,902 (41.78%)
Missing =	357,989 (58.22%)

Many different analyses of the data could be explored to begin to understand healthcare costs. However, one of the sponsors of this research was particularly interested in mental health costs. Current utilization of mental healthcare strongly predicts future use of mental healthcare: but can persons who have never used mental healthcare be identified before they have initial use? Consequently, our initial analysis was to isolate any predictors of future mental health costs in the absence of current use. Such predictors could be used for proactive intervention using counseling outreach, case management and other methods with subsequent improved clinical outcomes along with improved cost management.

The raw data set was typical of many transactional datasets, and far different from the final data set needed for data mining algorithms. Substantial preprocessing was required to transform the claim-focused data to a policyholders' domain (with each row corresponding to a policyholder). The data-preprocessing step is illustrated in *Figure 1*.

We describe this transformation to approximately 100 predictor variables in order to approach our analysis objective. The merged dataset contain several thousands of unique ICD-9 (International Classification of Diseases, ninth revision) and NDC (National Drug Code) codes. Each ICD-9 code was classified into one of 18 major diagnosis category (MDC). See *Table 3* for MDC categories and *Figure 2* for the frequencies of each MDC. Each MDC encompasses similar clinical problems.

For each policyholder, both MDC cost and count variables were created by totaling the corresponding costs and number of occurrences, respectively in each MDC category. Furthermore, for each policyholder each of the NDC codes were classified into one of 29 drug categories. Similarly, both drug cost and count variables were created by accumulating the associated costs and number of occurrences. See *Table 4* for drug categories.

Because this research is particularly concerned with the mental health category (MDC 5) and it is a known fact that patients who already have mental health problems are likely utilizers of the mental health treatments in the future, the focus is on policyholders who do not have any claims or records related to MDC 5, but might be potential utilizers in the future.

Figure 1: Overview of Data Management, Processing and Knowledge Discovery

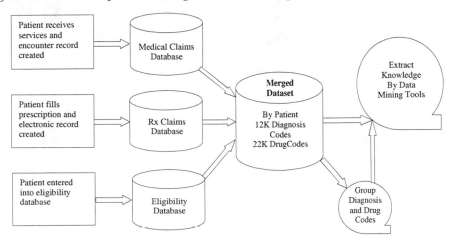

Table 3: Major Diagnosis Categories

ICD9	Description	MDC
001-139	Infectious and Parasitic Diseases	1
140-239	Neoplasms	2
240-279	Endocrine, Nutritional and Metabolic Diseases	3
280-289	Diseases of the Blood and Blood-Forming Organs	4
290-319	Mental Disorders	5
320-389	Inflammatory Diseases of the Central Nervous System	6
390-459	Circulatory System	7
460-519	Respiratory System	8
520-579	Digestive System	9
580-629	Genitourinary System	10
630-677	Pregnancy, Childbirth and Puerperium	11
680-709	Integument	12
710-739	Musculeoskeletal and Connective	13
740-759	Congenital Anomalies	14
760-779	Perinatal Period	15
780-799	Symptoms, Signs and Ill-Defined Conditions	16
800-999	Injury and Poisoning	17
-	Others	18

Figure 2: Major Diagnostic Categories' Frequencies

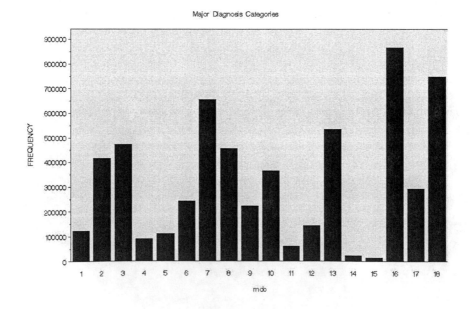

Table 4: Drug Categories

Drug Category	Description	Drug Category	Description
1	Antibiotics	16	Endocrine
2	Antivirals	17	Pulmonary
3	HIV Drug	18	Dermatological
4	Antineoplastic	19	ENT
5	Biologicals	20	Immunosupressive
7	Vaccines	21	Renal
8	Cardiovascular	22	Ophtalmologic
9	Neruologic	23	TB
10	Analgesics	24	Immunologic
11	Psychopharmaceuticals	25	GU
12	Anesthetics	26	Misc
13	Musculoskeletal	27	Illicit
14	Hemotalogical	28	Alternative
15	Gastrointestinal	29	Uncategorized

Table 5: Cut-Off Values and Frequencies of High-Utilizers and Low-Utilizers for Year 2000

Threshold Value	High Utilizers	Low Utilizers
$1,000	2,276 (0.40%)	569,289 (99.60%)
$2,500	798 (0.14%)	570,767 (99.86%)
$5,000	377 (0.07%)	571,188 (99.93%)

Some of the other variables used for the analyses are age, gender, region, time between emergency room visits, frequency of emergency room visits, total medical cost, provider type (clinician, facility, others), and service type (ancillary, medical/surgical, room/board, others).

DECISION TREES

A data-mining tool that may have a broad range of applications in healthcare organizations is a decision tree. Tree-based methods are structured on a conditional partitioning of the predictor variable space and then fitting a simple model such as a constant into each partition. Specific examples include, classification and regression trees known as CART (Breiman, Friedman, Olshen & Stone, 1984) and C4.5 (Quinlan, 1993).

Decision trees regress/classify observations by sorting them down the tree from the root node to some terminal node. Each node in the tree specifies a test of some predictor variable and each branch descending from that node corresponds to one of the possible values for this predictor variable. An observation is classified by starting at the root node of the tree, testing the predictor variable specified by this node, then moving down the

Figure 3: A Tree-Structure for Two Predictor Variables

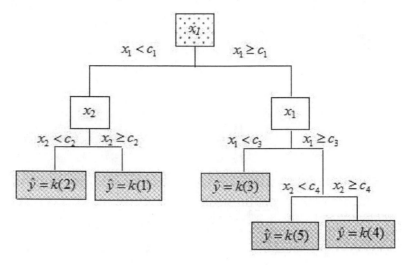

tree branch corresponding to the value of the variable. A tree structure is given in *Figure 3*. Here, the node with the dotted pattern is called the root node and the gray colored nodes are called terminal nodes. Lines represent the branches and inequalities are the tests of the predictor variables.

In this research, we consider the popular tree-based regression and classification method CART. We explain the CART algorithm with respect to classification trees because they accommodate categorical output variables rather than regression trees that are used for numerical output variables. Either method accommodates both categorical and numerical predictor variables.

It should also be noted that this technique could be used within a managed care organization using "unblinded" data to assess the future behavioral health needs of currently enrolled members. The usage of data for purposes of assessing the needs of members of a health plan is allowed under the Health Insurance Protection and Privacy Act (HIPPA).

Let y_i denote a categorical output variable taking values $k = 1, 2, ..., K$. Furthermore, let $x_i = (x_{i1}, x_{i2}, ..., x_{iq})$ represent predictor variables (either continuous or categorical). Here, the subscript i ($i = 1, ..., n$) is the index for the observations, n is the total number of observations, and q is the number of predictor variables. The CART algorithm is a recursive binary partitioning (splitting) of the predictor variable space. An example of recursive binary partitioning of the predictor space for two predictor variables is given in *Figure 4*. The x_1 space is initially split into two regions at the value $x_1 = c_1$ as shown in (a). At the next recursions one of the regions is partitioned further into other regions until a stopping rule is applied as seen in (b), (c), and (d).

The three key steps for constructing a classification tree are: (1) select the best partition of each node, (2) determine if a node is terminal, and (3) classify the terminal node to one of the output values.

The tree-based partition is found with a greedy algorithm. Starting with n observations, consider a splitting variable j and a split cutpoint c. Let R denote the regions created from a split such that:

Figure 4: Recursive Partitioning Algorithm of the Predictor Space

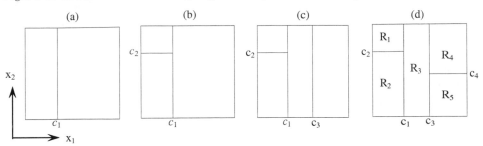

$$R_1(j, c) = \{x | x_j \le c\} \text{ and } R_2(j, c) = \{x | x_j > c\}$$

Note that the binary split of each node creates two regions: one containing those observations with the value of predictor variable less than a specified cutpoint c, and the other containing those with the predictor variable greater than c. The splitting variable j and the split cutpoint c are selected to minimize the average impurity of the output variable in the children nodes. A common measure of impurity at a node is the Gini index (Brieman et al., 1984).

$$\sum_{k=1}^{K} \hat{p}_{mk} (1 - \hat{p}_{mk})$$

where in a node m representing a region R_m with n_m observations

$$\hat{p}_{mk} = \frac{1}{n_m} \sum_{x_i \in R_m} I(y_i = k)$$

i.e., the proportion of class k observations in node m. Here, $I(.)$ is the indicator function taking the value 1, if $y_i = k$, and 0, otherwise. The split cutpoint c can be feasibly determined for each splitting variable and the optimal (j, c) pair may be found. By partitioning the data into the resulting two regions, this process is repeated on all of the regions.

A stopping rule is needed when growing a tree. A large tree might overfit the data, where as a small tree might not model the data well. A preferred strategy is to grow a large tree until a minimum node size is reached. Then this large tree maybe pruned to a desired subtree by collapsing any number of its non-terminal nodes. There are several popular pruning alternatives (Esposito, Malerba & Semeraro, 1997), but we used the standard cost-complexity method in CART. Finally, the observations at each terminal node m may be classified to class:

$$k(m) = \arg \max_{k} \hat{p}_{mk}$$

For observations with missing values, one approach is the construction of the surrogate variables. This approach considers a predictor variable for a split by only using the observations for which that predictor is not missing. After an optimal pair of the split variable and the split cutpoint is chosen, a list of surrogate predictor variables and cutpoints is formed. The first surrogate is the predictor variable that best mimics the split of the data achieved by the primary split. The second surrogate is the predictor variable and the corresponding cutpoint that does second best and so on.

For details of the decision trees and applications, interested readers is referred to Hastie, Tibshirani and Friedman (2001) and Wisnowski, Runger and Montgomery (1999, 2000).

RESULTS

SAS Enterprise Miner Version 4.0 was used to implement the CART algorithm to the policyholders dataset. Gini index was preferred as the splitting criteria. Three surrogate rules were saved in each node and missing observations were treated as an acceptable value. The first analysis included all 570K patients who did not have any costs for MDC 5 for 1999 but did in 2000. The dataset was randomly partitioned as 50% training and 50% validation. That is, 50% of the policyholders were used to construct the tree, and the other 50% were used to validate the findings.

In *Figure 5*, we show the SAS classification tree for the cut-off value $2,500. Note that the decimals of the percentages are rounded by the software. Starting from the root node, this tree may be interpreted easily. Consider the training data. Of the policyholders in the training dataset (285,783 policyholders) that had more than 4.5 emergency visits during 1999 (393 policyholders), 1% (about four policyholders) had mental health-related costs greater than or equal to $2,500 in the year 2000.

Figure 5: Classification Tree

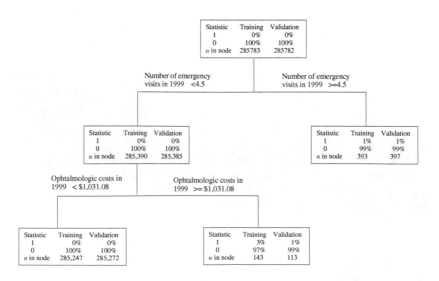

Policyholders who had less than 4.5 emergency room visits during 1999 (285,390 policyholders) consists of 0% (due to round-off, we did not get the actual number) of the mental health patients in 2000.

Of the policyholders who had less than 4.5 emergency room visits and had ophtalmologic costs greater than or equal to $1,031.08 during 1999, 3% had mental health costs greater than $2,500 in year 2000 (about five policyholders). The policyholders who had less than 4.5 emergency room visits and ophtalmologic costs less than $1,031.08 during 1999 (285,247 policyholders) but had mental health costs more than or equal to $2,500 in 2000 consists of 0% of policyholders who had less than 4.5 emergency room visits in 1999. The validation data can be interpreted similarly.

One of the key advantages of the tree-based methods is their interpretability. The variable, number of emergency room visits in 1999, is found to be the most significant variable for a classification of the future high and low utilizers. Although, the interpretation was easy, the tree just described does not classify the future high utilizers of the mental health services well. The main reason for this is the rareness of the modeled mental health patients compared to the total number of policyholders. Note that a classification algorithm that classifies all the policyholders as being future low utilizers will almost have a success rate of nearly 100%. Therefore, weights of the high utilizers relative to the low utilizers should be adjusted in order to force the CART algorithm to classify high utilizers better.

Different weight adjustments for the observations may be done. For our dataset, a proportion of 10% high utilizers and 90% low utilizers was useful. Therefore, a dataset containing all of the policyholders that had mental health costs greater than $2,500 in 2000 (798 policyholders) was mixed with a random sample of 7,182 policyholders from the remaining dataset.

We used several such created datasets and constructed classification trees. Approximately 30 trees were constructed in this manner. This form of stability analysis is important for data of this type. This analysis indicated that constructed classification trees were stable in selecting the same set of significant variables. One of the constructed classification trees is shown in *Figure 6*.

A similar objective could be approached with cross-validation (Breiman et al., 1984). Also, software that facilitates specifying prior probabilities or adjustment of costs (or loss) for different errors could also be used to put more importance on rare cases. We used a simplistic, but straightforward, alternative for our stability analysis.

The results of this classification are good as well as interesting. Note that we did not include any predictor variables that are directly related to MDC 5 and tried to predict future high utilizers that did not have any history of MDC 5 associated claims. One may also interpret this classification tree in terms of conditional probabilities. Of the 6,966 policyholders who had less than 0.5 (equivalently 0) emergency room visits in 1999, only 595 (approximately 9%) have MDC 5-related costs less than or equal to $2,500 in 2000. However, of these 6,966 policyholders who had less than 0.5 emergency room visits, there were 165 who had more than 116.5 hospital inpatient services in 1999 and 42 (approximately 25%) of these were to be high utilizers ($2,500 cut-off). Consequently, policyholders who had less than 0.5 emergency visits and more than 116.5 hospital inpatient services in 1999 had a probability of 0.25 for being high utilizers in 2000.

Figure 6: Classification Tree from the Weight-Adjusted Dataset

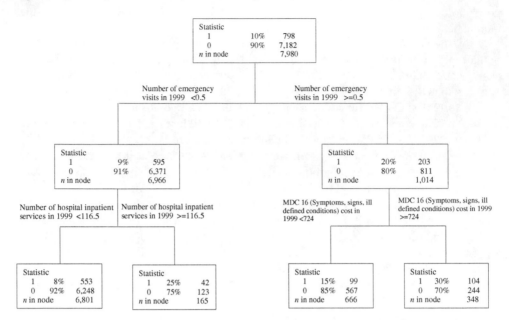

Furthermore, from the right branch of the tree, approximately 20% of policyholders who had more than 0.5 (equivalently one or more) emergency visits in 1999 were high utilizers in 2000. Furthermore, of the policyholders who had more than 0.5 emergency room visits and more than $724 of MDC 16-related costs in 1999, 104 (approximately 30%) were high utilizers. On the other hand, of the policyholders who had more than 0.5 emergency visits and less than $724 of MDC 16-related costs in 1999, 99 (approximately 15%) were high utilizers in 2000. It is seen that numerous questions could be explored from further analyses such as these.

The predictor variables selected by the CART algorithm may also be thought of as the significant variables for modeling the data. Moreover, these significant variables may be used in other statistical tools, such as logistic regression rather than using all predictor variables.

The use of this technique would vary by health plan, but several approaches can be proposed. First, physicians who provide primary care to identified patients who are at a high likelihood of needing behavioral health services would receive a notification explaining the methodology and encouraging them to be sensitive to the needs of these patients for referrals for behavioral health. Second, the identified patients could receive information packets on the availability of behavioral health services and encouraging them to call for an appointment if they felt depressed or anxious over recent health events. The number provided to them would go to a behavioral health provider or clinic, which would receive a list of the identified patients. Third, behavioral health providers using a list of the identified patients could make outreach calls.

CONCLUSIONS

An integrated healthcare dataset from enrollment, medical claims, and pharmacy databases containing more than 150 million medical and pharmacy claim line items and for over four million patients was processed for data mining. This chapter describes our approach to use a decision tree in such a complex domain. There are unique aspects to the interpretation of such trees when the number of cases of high importance is quite low. Furthermore, there are important issues related to stability and validity of the trees that we attempt to incorporate. The details of our experience along with some interesting success for predictions are described in detail. Decision trees present unique challenges in data analysis — very different from linear regression methods. The trees also provide unique models that are especially suited to this type of analysis.

These analyses demonstrate that CART data mining techniques can be used to extract knowledge from an integrated healthcare dataset concerning future mental health utilization in a population that has no current mental health utilization. Such a tool could be used to identify patients likely to have future mental heath usage based upon non-mental health usage, prior to their entry into the mental health system.

Managerial aspects of this technique would vary by health plan, but several approaches can be proposed. Such identification could be used to notify case managers and others for the need for early intervention, identified patients could receive information packets on the availability of behavioral health services and encouraging them to call for an appointment if they felt depressed or anxious over recent health events, and behavioral health providers using a list of the identified patients could make outreach calls. Such interventions can both reduce costs and improve the quality of life for those with serious physical and mental health conditions.

REFERENCES

Ash, A. (1999). Medicare risk adjustment: A status report. *1999 Medicare Managed Care Source Book*. New York: Faulkner & Gray.

Brieman, L., Friedman, J. H., Olshen, R. A. & Stone, C.J. (1984). *Classification and Regression Trees*. Belmont, CA: Wadsworth.

Dunn, D. (1998). Applications of health risk adjustments: What can be learned to date? *Inquiry*, 35, 132-147.

Dunn et al. (1995). *A Comparative Analysis of Methods of Health Risk Assessment: Final Report*. Cambridge, MA: Harvard School of Public Health.

Epstein, A. M. & Cumella, E. J. (1988). Capitation payment: Using predictors of medical utilization to adjust rates. *Health Care Financing Review*, 10, 51-69.

Esposito, F., Malerba, D. & Semeraro, G. (1997). A comparative analysis of methods for pruning decision trees. *IEEE Transactions on Pattern Analysis and Machine Intelligence*, 19, 476-491.

Hastie, T., Tibshirani, R. & Friedman, J. H. (2001). *The Elements of Statistical Learning: Data Mining, Inference, and Prediction*. New York: Springer Verlag.

Newhouse, J. P. (1986). Rate adjustors for medicare under capitation. *Health Care Financing Review Annual Supplement*, 8, 45-56.

Newhouse, J. P. (1996). Reimbursing health plans and health providers: Efficiency in production versus selection. *Journal of Economic Literature*, 34, 1236-1263.

Newhouse, J. P. (1998). Risk adjustment: Where are we now? *Inquiry*, 35, 122-131.

Quinlan, J. R. (1993). *C4.5: Programs for Machine Learning*. San Mateo, CA: Morgan Kaufmann.

Scerbo, M., Dickstein, C. & Wilson, A. (2001). *Health Care Data and the SAS System*. Cary, NC: SAS Institute.

Van Vliet, R. C. J. A. & Lamers, L. M. (1998). The high costs of death: Should health plans get higher payments when members die? *Medical Care*, 36, 1451-1460.

Weiner, J. P., Parente, S. T., Garnick, D. W., Fowles, J., Lawthers, A. G. & Palmer, R. H. (1995). Variation in office-based quality. A claims-based profile of care provided to Medicare patients with diabetes. *Journal of American Medical Association*, 273, 1503-1508.

Wisnowski, J. W., Runger, G. C. & Montgomery, D. C. (1999, 2000). Analyzing data from designed experiments: A regression tree approach. *Quality Engineering*, 12, 185-197.

Chapter VIII

Engineering Dependable Health Information Systems

Khin Than Win, University of Wollongong, Australia

Peter Croll, Queensland University of Technology, Australia

ABSTRACT

Effective and appropriate implementation of health information systems assists with an organization's knowledge management. To enhance a user's trustworthiness and full adoption, a health information system needs to be dependable. This chapter reviews the different development methodologies available for engineering dependable solutions and their application by citing two case studies as an example. Health information systems cover a diverse set of applications. The focus in this chapter is on the development of electronic health record systems, the importance of dependability, and the relationship between dependability and data quality of the health record systems.

INTRODUCTION

Knowledge management assists people to be more capable contributors to an organization's strategic plans (Wilson & Snyder, 1999). The success of an organization depends on the quality of that knowledge. To support Knowledge management successfully, health information systems must provide both information and guidance to the organizations. Health information systems are complex and diverse. They involve computer-stored databases containing patient information to support medical order entry, results reporting, decision support systems, clinical reminders, the pharmacy system, management information system, epidemiological surveillance system, communications and networking systems and other healthcare applications (Anderson & Aydin, 1994; Wiederhold & Perreault, 1990). It is widely recognized within the health industries that effective and appropriate usage of health information systems would greatly assist in creation of successful knowledge-based organizations.

Health information systems either contain or make direct reference to sensitive health data for individual patients. It is of utmost importance that such data is both secure and free from error. Inaccurate or insecure information can be detrimental to the individual and subsequently to the company or organization responsible. Any computer system where failure could have an impact on a person's health or be life threatening should be regarded as a safety-related system (IEC 61508, 2000). Privacy is now regarded as a pertinent area of growing concern, as more health information is available electronically online. Hence, it is essential to develop health information systems that can be trusted and are dependable. Such systems do not evolve over time but must be developed with sufficient rigor using appropriate engineering methods. To assist the reader in understanding what is required, this chapter will outline the essential criteria for developing dependable systems and detail some recent experiences from relevant health information case studies. The development of successful knowledge management health information systems will depend on how well these techniques are applied.

HEALTH INFORMATION SYSTEMS

Health information systems cover a wide-ranging and diverse set of applications. These include: electronic health record systems, hospital information systems, nursing information systems, laboratory information systems, pharmacy systems, radiology systems, patient monitoring systems, office systems, bibliographic retrieval systems, clinical decision support systems, clinical research systems, medical education systems and health assessment systems (Wiederhold & Perreault, 1990). It is difficult and could be misleading to generalise across the full spectrum. Hence, this chapter will focus on one of the key areas of development, the Electronic Health Record.

PURPOSES OF ELECTRONIC HEALTH RECORD

Schloeffel and Jeselon have categorised the purpose of Electronic Health Records as either primary or secondary (Schloeffel & Jeselon, 2002).

Primary Purpose

Its primary purpose is to provide a documented record of care, by means of communication among clinicians, contributing to the patient's care for the benefit of patient and clinicians. It will support the present and future care by the same or other clinicians.

Secondary Purpose

Its secondary purpose is for medical-legal purposes, quality management, education, research, public and population health, policy development, health service management, billing, finance and reimbursement.

Primary and Secondary Users of Health Data

The users can also be categorised as primary or secondary. Physicians, nurses, nursing assistants, therapist and allied health professionals are primary users of health data. Researchers, educators, third-party payers, business administrators, legal representatives, auditors, employers, public health officials, quality assurors and utilization review staff are the secondary users (Win et al., 2002). Yet users, particularly primary users, may access the record for either purpose as applicable.

IMPORTANCE OF REQUIREMENTS ENGINEERING IN DEVELOPING DEPENDABLE HEALTH INFORMATION SYSTEMS

User requirements need to be fulfilled for the system to be successfully implemented. The system may be perfect technologically, but if the system could not meet the user requirements, healthcare dollars spent will be wasted due to inefficiencies or low adoption rates. Hence, it is vital to undertake appropriate requirement elicitation for the various stakeholders. *Who are these stakeholders?* Stakeholders are people who will be affected by the system and who have a direct or indirect influence on the system requirements. For example, stakeholders for the electronic medical record systems include the subject of the record, the record keeper, overseeing regulatory bodies, third-party contributors who may provide expert reports or other materials of relevance and others who may wish to use the record for research (Wheatley, 2000). As there are many stakeholders involved, their goals may conflict and vary. The health information systems developed need to prioritise goals according to the strategic plans of the organization for maximum success, plus they need to assist the actual patient care process for a given work situation. Ideally, such a system should be easy to use and should require little or no training (Drazen et al., 1995).

Failure to identify the end user's requirements and the production of implementations that do not meet the needs of the user would lead to failure of the system. For example, an expert system developed in the UK, Computerised Coloscopy, was designed by the technical staff, with insufficient involvement of the actual users and hence failed to meet the requirements (Heeks et al., 1999). A reluctance to change on the part of the healthcare professionals who are the intended users of the system (Moczygemba & Hewitt, 2001) also lead to the failure of the system.

CHOOSING THE APPROPRIATE METHODOLOGIES IN DEVELOPING HEALTH INFORMATION SYSTEMS

Different software processes are available to assist in the development of new software systems. The software development process can be based on the traditional model, such as the Waterfall model, which is procedural oriented. This process can also be based on the iterative software development model, such as the Rational Unified Process, which is object oriented or agile development methodologies, such as extreme programming, paired programming and Scrum, which are people and changed process oriented. This section reviews the more popular development methods and following their application in two health systems used as case studies some recommendation as to the their applicability in engineering dependable solutions is discussed.

Waterfall Model

The waterfall model is the software development process that cascades from one phase to another (Sommerville, 2001). The requirement definition involves the system's services, constraints and goals, which are defined in detail and serve as a system specification after consultation with system users. As the development process is essentially sequential in nature, in practice it is progressively more difficult to accommodate changes after the process is underway.

Iterative Software Development Model

With the iterative software development model the system develops through incremental release. The advantage is that it can provide the stakeholders with progressively more operating functions and more capable versions of a system at regular intervals (Scacchi, 2001). Successful iterative development can provide management

Figure 1: Waterfall Model (Sommerville, 2001)

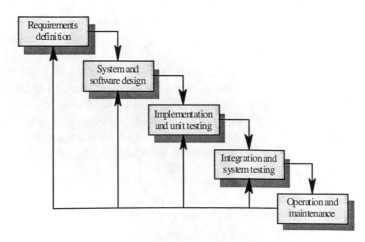

Figure 2: Rational Unified Process (Kruchten, 2000)

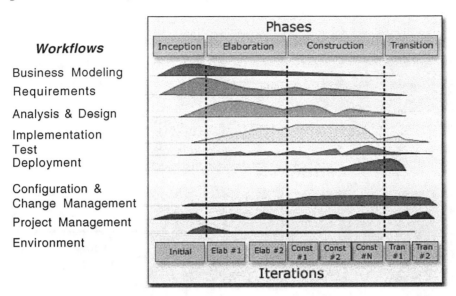

with a means of making tactical changes, allows the development process to improve along the way, provides better control of complex projects, improves software quality and customer satisfaction (Kruchten, 2000). The Rational unified process is an example of a well-known iterative software development method that is highly visually and permits control changes.

Spiral Model

The spiral model includes elements of a specification-driven, prototype-driven process and the classic software life cycle. Inner cycles of the spiral model include early system analysis and prototyping. Outer cycles include a classic software life cycle.

Agile Development Technology

In agile development, the highest priority is given to satisfying the customer through early and continuous delivery of valuable software. These development methods embrace changing requirements rather than the tradition of opposing them, even late in the development. The idea is that agile processes harness change for the customer's competitive advantage (http://www.agileAlliance.org). Agile software development stresses quality in design, recommends short iterations with feature planning and dynamic prioritisation. Turbulent, high-change environments work well with the agile development methodology (Highsmith & Cockburn, 2001).

Cockburn and Highsmith have stated, "Agile development excels in explanatory problem domains, extreme, complex, high-change projects and operates in a people-centered, collaborative, organised culture" (Cockburn, 2001).

Figure 3: Spiral Model (Boehm, 2001)

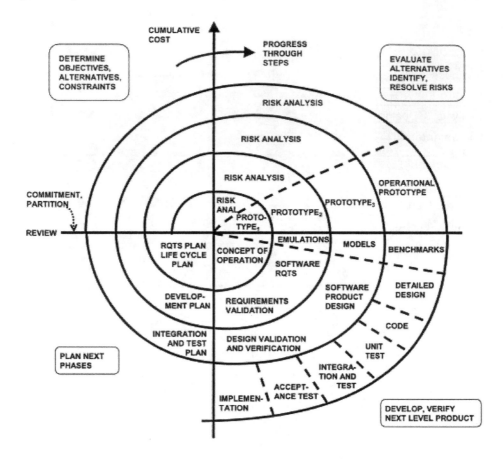

Boehm (2002) has compared the agile methods and plan-driven methods. Traditional methods, iterative models, and spiral models can be considered as the plan-driven methods.

Each method has its advantages and will ultimately depend on the project characteristics and the skills of the particular development team. Stakeholders need to decide which development methods suit them most in implementing a given health record system.

CASE STUDIES

Two case studies will now be discussed in turn in order to illustrate the respective advantages of these different development methodologies in facilitating the engineering of a dependable health information system.

Table 1: Comparison of Agile Methods and Plan-Driven Methods (Boehm, 2002)

Home-ground area	Agile methods	Plan-driven methods
Developers	Agile, knowledgeable, collocated, and collaborative	Plan-oriented; adequate skills; access to external knowledge
Customers	Dedicated, knowledgeable, collocated, collaborative, representative, and empowered	Access to knowledgeable, collaborative, representative, and empowered customers
Requirements	Largely emergent; rapid change	Knowable early; largely stable
Architecture	Designed for current requirements	Designed for current and foreseeable requirements
Refactoring	Inexpensive	Expensive
Size	Smaller teams and products	Larger teams and products
Primary objective	Rapid value	High assurance

Case Study 1

One of the healthcare centres in Australia needs to conduct research for primary care purposes from the health data available to them. It resides in different legacy databases and needs to be integrated for the healthcare research. If the data is not properly linked, the data quality and hence the health research outcome is seriously compromised.

At the start of the development of the linkage process, the development team had chosen a fairly traditional sequential approach: that of engineering the user requirements first before any development. The stakeholders did not have a clear idea of the requirements until the development was underway. As the project progressed, the stakeholders progressively realised that due to poor documentation the data currency, such as different units, were used in different databases for the age such as months and years, chronology of events and different data standards (Alcock et al., 2001). Hence the requirements of the system kept changing during the development. Furthermore data cleaning and standardisation needed to be done before linking and matching could take place. The development team and the stakeholders had to agree to abandon the contract-driven approach and towards the end of the project, find ways to work together more closely to gain a satisfactory outcome.

Case Study 2

One of the Divisions of General Practice in Australia has developed a health information system that can facilitate different healthcare providers to access patient's data stored in a central server without compromising the privacy, ownership and confidentiality of the patient. After consulting with the stakeholders, the software was developed, when it was demonstrated to the stakeholders at the end of the development, the development team found out that the software developed did not meet all the requirements and needed to develop a new program to meet them (Bomba et al., 2002).

- It can be seen that changing requirements in health record systems   implementation are common.
- Multiple stakeholders are involved in both projects.

- Both are health information systems projects focusing on the different aspects according to the needs of the stakeholders.
- Projects are focusing on not all of the dependability attributes.
- Communication and collaboration with stakeholders are needed for successful development of the project.
- Changing requirements are unavoidable in the development of complex systems and if the stakeholders know the different software development methodologies available, they can choose the project team appropriately to suit the requirements to develop dependable health information systems.

There may be changing requirements along the system development life cycle, so the waterfall model approach will not be suitable. Depending on the situation, the RUP or Agile development methodology can be chosen.

It is very difficult to have a clear vision of large projects from the beginning. It is difficult to follow the waterfall model for the development of the health information systems, as systems developed are complex systems. Requirements may not be fully realised until the user sees part of the proposed solution. Thus it is important for collaboration between all stakeholders and the technical team throughout the process. If the customer and developers work together throughout the process, complex systems with changed requirements can be overcome and the project will succeed.

As is the case with any endeavour involving people, there are conflicting goals. These differing views need to be resolved if the project is to be successful. It is essential to communicate effectively between the project groups, and it is a critical management task to put together a group that works effectively (Sommerville, 2001).

It appears that documenting the requirements assists the development team and stakeholder not only in terms of communication, understanding of the problems, and maintenance after the system is developed, but also to analyse the changes of project direction.

In system development, it is important that the development team and stakeholders collaborate to have the project succeed. Choosing the appropriate methodologies in developing health information systems also depends on how much commitment stakeholders can contribute to the project. As health information systems are complex systems, the technical team also needs to have a clear vision of all the requirements of the system.

It is unsuitable to suggest the fixed development process for a particular health information system. Less experienced development teams would be looking for a prescriptive simple solution. Depending on the complexity of the system and experience of using the particular development process, the development team needs to choose the suitable process. The software process needs to be according to the type of software, the familiarity of team members with the software process, and the appropriateness of the requirements for the software. Quality issues depend on the team's experience in using the particular method chosen. The standards do not prescribe the methods, for example the IEC 61508 functional safety of electrical/electronic/programmable safety electronic safety-related system (IEC 61508, 2000) does not recommend any particular software development method for safety-related systems, yet it lists all the approved methods available. Likewise, the development of dependable health information systems also needs to apply the range of applicable methods. Each application, each development team and the environment will be different.

Electronic health record systems consist of invaluable data, which are important for primary care, diagnosis, treatment, research, administrative, and financial purposes. Dependable electronic health record systems would improve the quality and safety of healthcare. It is important to implement dependable electronic health record systems. As in the case studies described above and as in the authors' experience, implementing an electronic health record system is a complex task to explore and fulfill stakeholders' requirements. The development team and stakeholders need to understand the importance of dependability of electronic health record systems so that the system developed would assist in improving the quality and safety of the healthcare provided.

KEY CONSIDERATION FOR DEPENDABLE HEALTH INFORMATION SYSTEM

It has been established that since electronic health record systems include patients' health information, it is important that such systems are both trusted and dependable (Win et al., 2002). The consequence of errors or incomplete information can have minor to significant impact on an individual's life, ranging from embarrassment to loss of life.

Dependability

Dependability can be categorised into availability, reliability, security and safety from software engineering perspectives (Sommerville, 2001). In context of the Electronic Health Record Systems, dependability can be explained as follows:

Availability

This refers to the total number of hours a system is operational, e.g., non-availability could result in delays in accessing critical health data.

Reliability

This refers to how often a system fails. An unreliable system may at best exhibit poor availability or in some circumstances supply incorrect health data.

Security

This refers to how difficult it is for an unauthorised user to gain access to a system and its data. For the electronic health record system, a secure system will have adequate access control, authentication and encryption measures in place to ensure adequate privacy and to prevent tampering.

Safety

This refers to the risk that an electronic health record system can cause harm to an individual.

Data Quality And Dependability

Electronic Health Record Systems consist of system resources and the organizational rule. System resources include primary and secondary users of health data, hardware such as computers, a network, and software such as application programs.

Designing or redesigning the Electronic Health Record Systems would need to address information processing and the management structure (Lippeveld & Sauerborn, 2000).

Data Quality

Arts et al. defined data quality as, "the totality of features and characteristics of a data set, that bear on its ability to satisfy the needs that result from the intended use of the data" (Arts et al., 2002).

Wherever possible, data quality should not be compromised because low quality health data will have a great impact on the decision-making process and a tremendous effect on patient management. Data quality is important because appropriate information available will assist in the decision-making process. Processing, analysing and interpreting the information would lead to new knowledge and interpretation of this knowledge would lead to decision-making (Sauerborn, 2000).

Wang and Strong (1996) identified data quality as data that are fit to be used by data consumers. Electronic Health Record System consists of aggregated data for diagnosis, treatment, research, finance or planning (Rector et al., 1991) and it is important to maintain the data quality. The American Health Information Management Association data quality management model has identified characteristics of data quality, which includes accessibility, accuracy, consistency, comprehensiveness, currency, definition, granularity, relevancy, precision and timeliness (AHIMA, 1998).

Arts et al. have identified accuracy and completeness as the most cited data quality attributes. Based on their literature review, there are data errors at the different steps in the data collection process. Data errors from incomplete data entry for medical databases is 4%; inaccurate extraction 1.7%; incomplete extraction 1.4%; inaccurate data transfer 0.9%; 2% inaccuracy for automatically collected data; 6% incompleteness in automatically collected data for central registry databases (Arts et al., 2002).

Table 2 presents characteristics involved in data quality, how it could be related to the dependability and the appropriate measures needed to ensure the data quality.

The quality of data cannot be taken in isolation, but is related to the software and hardware resources involved. This requires whole-system dependability to support the decision-making process and ensure that risks to patients are minimised. Implementing dependable health record systems comes at the cost of additional effort in design process plus validation overheads. With a safe system, reliable information would be available to authorised users in a timely manner and that will support the knowledge management successfully.

Data quality is important because appropriate information available will assist in the decision-making process. Processing, analysing and interpreting the information would lead to new knowledge and interpretation of this knowledge would lead to decision-making (Sauerborn, 2000).

Table 2: Relationship of Health Data Quality and Dependability

Appropriate	Inappropriate	Dependability	Measures
Accuracy of healthcare data	Inaccurate information by mistake	Reliability	Validation check
	Inaccurate information by software	Security, Reliability	Quality control
	Inaccurate information by intention	Security	Proper security measures
Accessibility of health information	Data not accessible due to destruction of data	Availability, Security, Safety	Security measures
	Data not accessible due to accidental destruction	Reliability	Authentication check, safety procedures
	Data not accessible due to intentional manipulation	Security, Reliability	
	Data inaccessible due to malfunction in hardware or software	Availability, reliability	
	Data inaccessible due to location of information unknown	Availability	
Consistency of health data	Different value to same logical data Different units Inconsistent semantics	Reliability	Implementing data standards Interoperability checks
Comprehensive health data	Missing data	Availability, reliability	Ensure data integrity
	Incomplete data due to incomplete transfer	Reliability	
	System not functioning properly	Availability, reliability, safety	
Data currency	Inaccurate data value	Reliability	Appropriate data field

Inaccurate or incomplete information can have an impact on research and disease surveillance (Cushman, 1997).

Inaccurate Information by Software

In the UK, because of the millennium bug error, incorrect Down Syndrome test results were sent to 154 pregnant women. Because of that, four Down Syndrome babies were born to mothers to whom their tests put them in the low risk group. Two terminations were carried out as a result of mistaken test report (Wainwright, 2001).

Inaccurate Information by Mistake

A woman in Dusseldorf, Germany, was erroneously informed that her test results showed she had incurable syphilis and had passed that on to the daughter and the son. As a result, she strangled her 15-year-old daughter and attempted to kill her son and herself (Neumann, 1995).

Table 3: Examples of Cause-and-Effect (Win et al., 2002)

Cause	Effect
- Inaccurate information by software - Data not accessible due to destruction of data - Data not accessible due to malfunction in hardware or software - Incomplete data due to incomplete transfer - System not functioning properly - Mismatched records - Missing results	- Wrong diagnosis - Wrong medication - Wrong dosage administration - Unnecessary repetition of laboratory tests - Misdiagnosis - Poor public health information - Unnecessary spending of health care dollars - Late diagnosis - Late timely treatment

Impaired data quality can result from a fault in the system. Therefore, data entry, data capture, data storage, integration of data, communication, data retrieval and data security all play an important role in the data quality for the health information system. As stated previously, impaired data quality can have a direct impact on a patient's health. *Table 3* outlines some of the cause–and-effect of impaired data.

RELATIONSHIP FRAMEWORK FOR DATA QUALITY AND DEPENDABILITY

It can be proposed that dependability and data quality are important for the decision-making process. The following figure is the framework of how dependability and data quality are related for the decision-making process in the electronic health record systems.

As shown in *Figure 4*, inappropriate data (*Table 2*) can occur in any steps involved in information processing: data entry, data collection, data processing and data transmission.

A data verification and data validation check during the data entry should be included to improve the reliability of the data. For example, adding algorithms that check against the patient's age and weight can prevent erroneous entry of patients' data. If the person's age and weight entered is in the unacceptable range, the system will prompt the alert message so that the care provider will know and decide immediately whether it is the wrong data entry or whether patient is in the abnormal weight range. In The Medical Director Software, which is widely used in General Practices in the Illawarra Region of New South Wales, the system will prompt the normal weight range, if the weight entered is in the abnormal range so the healthcare personnel can validate the entry.

As electronic health record systems need to integrate different processes both among different healthcare institution and within the same organization, interoperability, integrity and comparability of the data should be considered essential to the integration. Data standards play an important role in integration of different health record systems. Message format standards organizations have developed standards for integration of electronic health record systems. Data linkage and integration projects have been implemented in different healthcare institutions around the world.

Figure 4: Data and Decision-Making

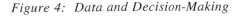

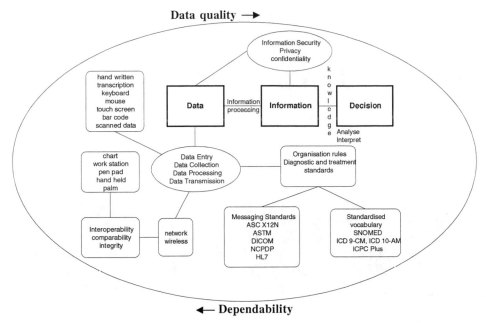

The National Electronic Task Force of Australia has identified two approaches in integration of electronic health records. These are: a federated system and a standard health record architecture approach. Data from different standards are integrated in real time and displayed to the patient and healthcare providers in the federated system approach. In a standard architecture approach, data is aggregated in the information storage level. New Children's Hospital in Westmead Sydney, NSW, has a whole institution electronic health record federated system available at bed site (A Health Information Network for Australia, 2000).

Privacy and Confidentiality

As electronic health record systems become more computerised and integrated among different healthcare providers, data can be accessible from different places by different users and invasion of privacy is at a higher risk. To maintain the privacy and confidentiality of the system, the system needs to be secured. Security is one of the attributes of dependability. Issues of confidentiality and abuse of data cause many healthcare providers to oppose the coordination of medical databases despite the potential benefits (Gaithersburg, 2000).

Data users have the duty to maintain the confidentiality of the data and systems developed need to deter access by unauthorized users. Users should abide by the law of healthcare privacy legislation and legislation should be implemented according to the changing technology. Advances in technology increase user accessibility and privacy protections involve use of technology.   Healthcare providers' reluctance to share

Figure 5: VennDiagram — User, Technology, Legislation (Win et al., 2002)

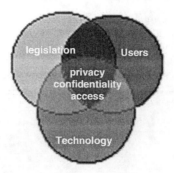

information in local area networks can be overcome by providing adequate technology to support security measures and privacy legislation to protect health data (Amatayakul, 1998). Protection of patient records can be achieved by implementing security policies to control access appropriating authorization before releasing the health data and providing additional security measures to more sensitive data (American Academy of Pediatrics, 1999).

Safety

For safer, higher quality care, it is needed to redesign systems of care, including the use of IT to support clinical and administrative purposes (Institute of Medicine, 2001). After the release of the report "To Err is Human: Building a Safer Health System" (Kohn et al., 2000), the importance of safety has been emphasised in healthcare. Reports of medical misadventures, such as 98,000 Americans dying each year as a result of preventable medical errors (Kohn et al., 2000), show why this focus is long overdue. The Institute of Medicine estimates the number of lives lost to preventable medication errors alone represents more than 7,000 deaths annually, i.e., more than the number of injuries in work place (Institute of Medicine, 2000). The National Survey from New Zealand has

Figure 6: Directive Graph of Medical Errors

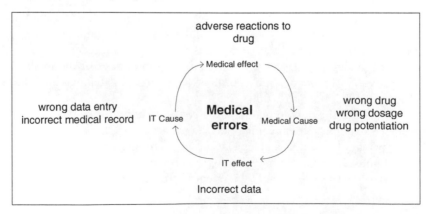

documented 4.5% of all admissions were associated with highly preventable adverse events (Davis et al., 2001). Adverse medical events can be mapped into medical cause, IT effect, IT cause and non-IT cause.

As described above, errors can occur in any stage because both causes and effects are interrelated, as illustrated in the directive graph. What is needed is a more definitive method to track back the cause from the known effects. The adverse events of medical errors can be more comprehensively traced back using the fault tree analysis.

Fault Tree Analysis

Fault tree analysis is one of the different approaches of the risk analysis methods and is the most widely used method in system reliability analysis. It is a deductive top-down method of analysing system design and performance. It involves specifying a top event to analyse, followed by identifying all of the associated elements in the system that could cause the top event to occur (www.fault-tree.com). The following are examples of fault tree analysis for adverse drug reactions, hypersensitivity to drug and wrong dose of medication. As seen in the example fault trees, the top event, adverse event wrong dose, hypersensitivity can be traced back to the bottom nodes. In other control systems, failure or hazardous events are machine failures, either from software or hardware causes.

Medical errors can be from communication errors, human errors, or system errors. It is important to mitigate errors as much as possible to have dependable health information systems.

Figure 7: Fault tree — Hypersensitivity to Drug

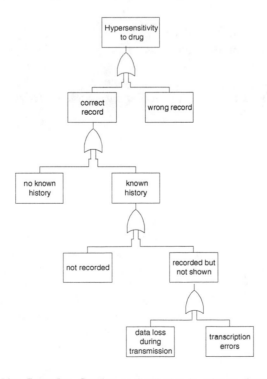

Figure 8: Fault Tree — Wrong Dose Medication

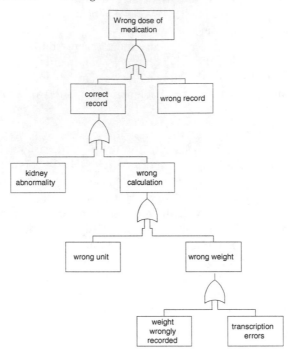

Health information system resource management is as equally important as data quality. Choosing the appropriate technology to implement a dependable health information system is important for the success of the organization. Knowledge of available software process development methodology by healthcare management, healthcare providers, and users would achieve the goal of creating a knowledge-based healthcare organization.

CONCLUSIONS[1]

Data, information processing, and decision-making are all essential for the success of an organization. Data in health information systems are invaluable assets of the organization. Successful information processing and data management contribute to better research, disease surveillance, prevention of disease, promotion of health, better treatment, depending on the type of health information system.

Dependable health information systems would assist the knowledge management of the organization. Knowledge of software development methodologies available would assist the healthcare providers in better decision-making to choose the appropriate health information systems development which would also lead to improvement of promotion of health, prevention of disease, and better healthcare.

REFERENCES

A Health Information Network for Australia. (2000). Report to Health Ministers by the National Electronic Health Record Taskforce, Commonwealth of Australia. Retrieved October 2000 from: http://www.health.gov.au/healthonline/ehr_rep.pdf.

AHIMA Data Quality Task Force. (1998, June). *Data Quality Management Model, Journal of AHIMA.* Retrieved May 2001 from: http://www.ahima.org/journal/pb/98.06.html.

Alcock, C., Burgess, L., Cooper, J., & Win, K.T. (2001). The rise of e-health in Australia: Electronic health records and privacy legislation. In *Proceedings of the Fourth International Conference on Electronic Commerce Research (ICECR-4),* Dallas, Texas, USA, November 8-11, vol. 2, pp. 466-474.

Amatayakul, M. (1998, October). The state of the computer based patient record, *Journal of American Health Information Management Association.* Retrieved February 2001 from: http://www.ahima.org/journal/features/feature9810.1.html.

American Academy of Pediatrics: Pediatric Practice Action Group and Task Force on Medical Informatics. (1999). *Privacy protection of health information: Patient rights and pediatrician responsibilities,* 104, 973-977.

Anderson, J. G. & Aydin C. E. (1994). Theoretical perspectives and methodologies for the evaluation of health care information system. In J. G. Anderson, C. E. Aydin & S. J. Jay (Eds.), *Evaluating Health Care Information Systems: Methods and Applications* (pp. 5-29). Sage Publications.

Arts, D. G. T., Keizer, N. F. D. & Scheffer, G. J. (2002). Defining and improving data quality in medical registries: A literature review, case study, and generic framework. *Journal of American Medical Informatics Association,* 9, 600-661.

Boehm, B. (2001, May). *The spiral model as a tool for Evolutionary Acquisition, Cross Talk.* Retrieved from: http://www.stsc.hill.af.mil/crosstalk/2001/05/boehm.html.

Boehm, B. (2002, January). Get ready for agile methods, with care. *IEEE Computer,* 64-69.

Bomba, D., Fulcher, J. & Dalley, A. (2002). Lessons Learnt from the UoW-IDGP Smart_ID Project, *Proceedings of HIC2002. The 10th Annual Health Informatics conference,* Melbourne Convention Centre, August 4-6, 2002, Melbourne, Australia, ISBN: 0 958537097.

Cockburn, A. (2001, November). Agile software development. *The people factor. Computer,* 131-133.

Cushman, R. (1997). Serious technology assessment for health care information technology. *Journal of the American Medical Informatics Association,* 4(4), 259-265.

Davis et al. (2001, December). Adverse events in New Zealand Public hospitals: Principal findings from a national survey (occasional paper). The Ministry of Health, Wellington, New Zealand.

Drazen, E. L., Mezger, J. B., Ritter, J. L. & Schneider, M. K. (1995). Patient Care Information Systems: Successful design and implementation. In K. J. Hannah & M. J. Ball (Eds.), *Computers in Health Care.* New York: Springer-Verlag.

Gaithersburg, I. V. (2000, March). Electronic medical records and patient privacy. *The Health Care Manager,* 63-69.

Heeks, R., Mundy, D. & Salazar, A. (1999). *Why Health Care Information Systems Succeed or Fail.* Information Systems for Public Sector Management Working

Paper Series, Working paper No.9, Institute for Development Policy and Management, ISBN: 19025 1825 X.

Highsmith, J. & Cockburn, A. (2001, September). Agile Software Development: The Business Innovation. *Computer*, 120-122.

IEC 61508. (2000). Functional safety of electrical/electronic/programmable electronic safety related systems. Retrieved December 2000 from: http://www.iec.ch/61508/

Institute of Medicine. (2000). *Doing what counts for patient safety: Federal Actions to reduce medical error and their impact*. Report of Quality Interagency Coordination Task Force to the President. Retrieved from: http://www.quic.gov/report/mederr2.htm.

Institute of Medicine, Committee on Quality of Health Care in America. (2001). *Crossing the quality chasm: A New Health System for the 21st Century*. Washington, D.C.: National Academy Press.

Kohn, L. T., Corrigan, J. M. & Donaldson, M. S. (2000). *To Err is Human: Building a Safer Health System*. Washington, D.C.: National Academy Press.

Kruchten, P. (2000). *The Rational Unified Process* (second edition). Addison-Wesley.

Lippeveld, T. & Sauerborn, R. (2000). A framework for designing health information systems. In T. Lippeveld, R. Sauerborn & C. Bodart (Eds.), *Design and Implementation of Health Information Systems* (pp. 15-32). Geneva: World Health Organisation.

Moczygemba, J. & Hewitt, B. (2001). Managing clinical data in an electronic environment. *The Health Care Manager*, 19(4), 33-38.

Neumann, P. G. (1995). *Computer Related Risks*. Addison Wesley, ACM Press.

Rector, A. L., Nolan, W. A. & Kay, S. (1991). Foundations for an Electronic Medical Record. *Methods of Information in Medicine*, 30, 179-86.

Sauerborn, R. (2000). Using Information to make decisions. In T. Lippeveld, R. Sauerborn & C. Bodart C. (Eds.), *Design and Implementation of Health Information Systems* (pp. 33-48). Geneva: World Health Organisation.

Scacchi, W. (2001). Process models in software engineering. In Marciniak (Ed.), *Encyclopaedia of Software Engineering* (second edition). John Wiley.

Schloeffel, P. & Jeselon, P. (2002). ISO/TC 215 Ad Hoc Group Report, Standards Requirements for the Electronic Health Record and Discharge. Referral Plans: Final Report. Retrieved April 22, 2003 from the World Wide Web: http://www.gpcg.org/publications/docs/ISO_HER_FinalReport.pdf.

Sommerville, I. (2001). *Software Engineering* (sixth edition). Addison-Wesley.

Wainwright, M. (2001). *NHS faces huge damages bill after millennium bug error. Guardian*. Retrieved September 17, 2001 from: http://www.guardian.co.uk/Archive/Article/0,4273,4257065,00.html.

Wang, R. Y. & Strong, D. M. (1996). Beyond accuracy: What data quality means to data consumers. *Journal of Management Information Systems*, 12(4), 5.

Wheatley, I. (2000). The Attitude of Referring Doctors to Hospital Electronic Medical Records. *Proceedings of the First Australian Information Security Management Workshop,* Australia. Retrieved September 2002 from: http://www.cm.deakin.edu.au/mwarren/secman/pdf/12.pdf.

Wiederhold, G. & Perreault (1990). Hospital information systems. In E. H. Shortliffe, L. E. Perreault, G. Wiederhold & L. M. Fagan (Eds.), *Medical Informatics: Computer Applications in Health Care* (pp. 219-243). Addison-Wesley.

Wilson, L. T. & Snyder, C. A. (1999, March/April). Knowledge Management and IT: How are they related? *IT Professional*, IEEE, 73-74.

Win, K. T, Croll, P. & Cooper, J. (2002). Setting a safety standards for electronic medical records. *Proceedings of HIC 2002, The 10th Annual Health Informatics Conference, Melbourne Convention Centre*, August 4-6, 2002, Melbourne, Australia.

Win, K. T., Croll, P., Cooper, J. & Alcock, C. (2002). Issues of privacy, confidentiality and access in electronic health record. *Journal of Law and Information Science*, 12(1), 24-25.

ENDNOTE

[1]   Further Reading: (a) *Software Engineering* (6th edition). The book covers comprehensive revision of software engineering techniques that can be applied to practical software project development (Sommerville, 2001). Addison Wesley, ISBN 0 201 39815 X. (b) *The Rational Unified Process: An introduction* (2nd edition). This book explains clearly about the iterative software development model and analysis of software lifecycles. (Kruchten, 2000). Addison-Wesley. (c) *Agile Software Development.* It presents the principles of agile methodologies and explains the methodologies and which methodologies fit for different projects. (Cockburn). Addison- Wesley.

Chapter IX

e-Health with Knowledge Management:
The Areas of Tomorrow[1]

Sushil K. Sharma, Ball State University, USA

Nilmini Wickramasinghe, Cleveland State University, USA

ABSTRACT

The main purpose of this chapter is to bring out and discuss the central facts pertaining to the importance of incorporating knowledge management in the area of e-health. This is accomplished by focusing on the application of knowledge management in e-health and its effects.

INTRODUCTION

The evolution of the "Information Age" in medicine is mirrored in the exponential growth of medical web pages, increasing number of online data sources, and growing services and publications available on the World Wide Web. The Internet started with a few computers linked by the predecessor in 1969 and has grown to more than six million web sites today, of which at least 2% have health-related content. More than 150 million people currently communicate over the Internet with medical information being amongst the most retrieved information on the web. Health information providers on the web mostly consist of private companies offering medical information, individual patients and health professionals, patient self-support groups, non-governmental organizations, universities, research institutes and governmental agencies. Thus, the importance of e-health has grown tremendously these days and providing e-health coupled with the concept of knowledge management will only serve to enhance the efficiency of e-health initiatives.

e-HEALTH

E-health is a very broad term that encompasses many different activities related to the use of the Internet for healthcare. The rate at which health professionals are using the Internet as a source of consumer information about health and medicine is rapidly increasing. It has been reported by healthcare professionals that large numbers of patients arrive at their offices either with questions related to online medical information or a large variety of health products on the Internet. Some of this content may prove extremely helpful to the health and recovery of a patient. Prior to 1999, e-health was barely in use. Now it seems to be a general "buzzword," used to characterize not only "Internet medicine," but also virtually everything related to computers and medicine (E-Health in the Medical Field, 2003).

Intel, for example, has referred to e-health as "a concerted effort undertaken by leaders in healthcare and hi-tech industries to fully harness the benefits available through convergence of the Internet and healthcare." As the Internet has created new opportunities and challenges to the traditional healthcare information technology industry, the use of this new term to address these issues seems appropriate. The latest challenges for the healthcare information technology industry with respect to e-health fall primarily into the following categories:

1.   Institution-to-institution data transmission possibility (B2B = "business to business");
2.   Consumers' capability to interact with their systems online (B2C = "business to consumer"); and
3.   Peer-to-peer consumer communication possibility (C2C = "consumer to consumer").

E-health can be described as an emerging field at the intersection of medical informatics, public health and business, referring to health services and information delivered or enhanced through the Internet and related technologies (Eysenbach, 2001). In a broader sense, the term characterizes not only a technical development, but also a state-of-mind, a way of thinking, an attitude, and a commitment for networked, global thinking to improve healthcare locally, regionally, and worldwide by using information and communication technology (ibid).

The E's in e-Health

The preceding definition of e-health is broad enough to apply to the dynamic environment of the Internet and at the same time acknowledge that e-health encompasses more than just "Internet and Medicine" (Eysenbach, 2001). It is useful to think of the "e" in e-health not just standing for "electronic," but also a number of other "e's," which together perhaps best characterize what e-health is all about.   Specifically, we now present some of the "e"s that serve to represent the "e" in the e-health that have been identified by Gunther Eysenbach, editor, Journal of Medical Internet Research in his editorial comments on what is e-health, as follows:

Efficiency – E-health aims to increase efficiency in healthcare, thereby decreasing costs, in particular transactions costs. This can be realized by avoiding redundant or unnecessary diagnostic or therapeutic interventions, through enhanced communication possibilities between healthcare establishments, and through patient involvement.

Enhancing Quality of care – Increasing efficiency improves quality along with reducing costs. In addition, e-health provides a vehicle for trying to decrease the myriad of medical errors which in turn naturally impact the quality of healthcare treatments in a positive fashion.

Evidence Based – E-health interventions should be evidence-based thus they should be proven by rigorous scientific evaluation and thus no assumptions need be made in this area with respect to treatments.

Empowerment of Consumers and Patients – E-health facilitates patient-centered medicine, and supports wiser patient choice. This is accomplished by making the knowledge bases of medicine and personal electronic records accessible to consumers over the Internet.

Education of not only physicians but also consumers – Today's healthcare sector is complex and physicians must contend with continually updating of their medical knowledge base to keep abreast with new treatment protocols etc e-health offers an effective avenue for this. Education however is not just limited to physicians but all medical and healthcare professional as well as healthcare consumers.

Extending the scope of healthcare in both a geographical sense as well as in a conceptual sense – Via e-health, it is possible for patients to access key knowledge and reach experts who maybe located in different countries for primary or even second opinions. In addition, the area of telemedicine in particular helps to provide needed and a broad range of healthcare services to remote and typically inaccessible areas.

Ethics – E-health involves new forms of patient-physician interaction and poses new challenges and threats to ethical issues such as online professional practice, informed consent and privacy issues. It is important that many of the ethical dilemmas presented by e-health initiatives are to some extent no different to the ethical dilemmas generally created by e-commerce technologies with which all organizations must contend.

Equity – To make healthcare more equitable is one of the promises of e-health, but at the same time there is a considerable threat that e-health may deepen the gap between the "rich" and "poor" and increase the digital divide (Journal of Medical Internet Research, 2001).

THE ROLE OF CONSUMERS

Today, a large number of patients and consumers already use the Internet to retrieve health-related information, to interact with health providers and even to order pharmaceutical products. Physicians mainly use the web to access science databases like PUBMED or MEDLINE, but they lag behind other professions in their use of online information. On the other hand, consumers have taken the lead in adopting the Internet media for the retrieval and exchange of health information. Informed and Internet-savvy patients will play a crucial role in being a major driving force for clinicians to "go online" and for evidence-based medicine. Patients will undoubtedly increase the pressure on physicians to use timely evidence by accessing online information. They also will encourage them to adapt themselves to information technology in order to deliver high quality health services. For the first time in the history of medicine, consumers have equal access to the knowledge bases of medicine — and they are heavily using this access. It has been noted that "the number of Medline searches performed by directly accessing the database at the National Library of Medicine increased from 7 million in 1996 to 120 million in 1997, when free public access was opened; the new searches are attributed primarily to non-physicians" (Sieving PC Factors Driving the Increase in Medical Information on the Web, 1999). Thus, the Internet will act as a catalyst for evidence-based medicine in two ways: First, it enables health professionals to access timely evidence. Second, it enables consumers to draw information from the very same knowledge base, leading to increased pressure on health professionals to actually use the evidence (PricewaterhouseCoopers Healthcare Practice, 2003).

By 2005, 88.5 million adults will use the Internet to find health information, shop for health products and communicate with affiliated payers and providers through online channels, according to Cyber Dialogue (Online Health Information Seekers Growing, 2003). Today, the e-health consumer demands include the need for specific health services, such as obtaining information when faced with a newly established diagnosis.

Some key challenges must be met to develop optimal partnerships between consumers and other groups of decision-makers. Some of these include the need for:

- Meaningful collaboration with patients,
- Preparation for upcoming technological developments,
- Efficient strategies to monitor patterns of Internet use among consumers,
- Balance between connectivity and privacy factors,
- Better understanding of the balance between real and virtual interactions, and
- Equitable access to technology and information across the globe.

e-HEALTH ISSUES

Three important issues must be carefully considered in the field of e-health (The Higher the Connection Speed, 2001). These issues tend to be similar to all aspects of e-commerce and typically comprise the areas of procurement, connectivity, and benefits. We discuss each in turn briefly.

e-Procurement

Health systems must begin to consider how their organizations are going to adapt and leverage Internet-based tools to manage their medical supplies.

Procurement in healthcare products must move toward an online business platform for data interchange. Producers and consumers also must work together toward standardization, including a universal product numbering system. As shown in *Figure 1*, in the US, e-procurement of medical supplies is estimated to grow to 15% of medical supply spending in the US by 2003, according to Deutsche Banc Alex Brown (PricewaterhouseCoopers Healthcare Practice, 2003).

e-Connectivity

Healthcare is local, and so is connectivity. Finding that they can not boil the ocean, connectivity companies must pragmatically assess what the industry can reasonably move to on a step-by-step basis. Technology is a tool, but it will not pay for itself unless organizations deploy it in practice and track how their clinicians and administrative workers are using it. To do so, managers must design processes and metrics for productivity. Otherwise, it's like expecting someone to drive a car when his previous experience is limited to a 10-speed bicycle. However, healthcare organizations will find that getting this work stream web-enabled offers the most opportunity now, and that other functions like disease management and demand management can also be Internet-enabled.

Health plans and hospitals are beginning to migrate to the web for claims-related transactions as the first step of a broader Internet strategy. This can be clearly depicted by *Figure 2*. Because many organizations continue to use Electronic Data Interchange (EDI) for claims submissions, transactions surrounding claims — eligibility, referrals, etc., they will be the first to be adopted for e-health connectivity. Those health plans that are adopting Internet connectivity for these functions view them as the foundation upon which to build other Internet-enabled partnerships with patients and providers.

Figure 1: e-Procurement Market Sales

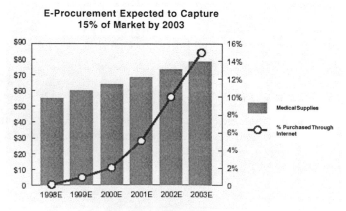

Source: Odyssey Research, 2003

Figure 2: Increase in the Percent of Electronically Filed Claims

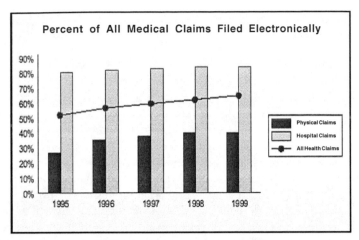

Source: Odyssey Research, 2003

The critical need for automation has risen as the number of healthcare transactions is outpacing the growth of health spending. The number of claims submitted increased by about 7% during the past five years, according to the Health Data Directory. In contrast, healthcare spending has increased at between 5% and 6% during the past five years. Many of the functions associated with claims submissions and payment are repetitive tasks that are more efficiently done by computers. The most expensive processes are not the claims submissions themselves, but the tasks surrounding the claims process, such as eligibility checks and referrals. Coupling that with increasing labor shortages, the onus is on organizations to re-engineer (PricewaterhouseCoopers Healthcare Practice, 2003).

Health plans must understand physicians' needs when designing Internet-based solutions. First-mover advantage is not as important as a system that works. Many e-business companies have benefited from a first-mover advantage, which means they get the most capital, the best partners and brand recognition. However, healthcare is a "show-me" business and successful models will replicate market by market.

e-Benefits

The health industry has discovered the benefits of online business. Like the conundrum of the chicken-and-the-egg, many employers and health plans are awaiting the development and implementation of e-benefits and e-insurance products. Health plans don't want to deliver web-based products if employees are not ready to use them. Employers can not deliver e-benefits products until health plans develop them. However, starting with online benefits enrollment, e-health is evolving in incremental stages. A by-product of this evolution is the combination of employee responsibility and authorization. Paternalistic urges aside, employers will gradually grant more control for health benefits to employees themselves. One of the primary drivers of e-benefits is the possibility of self-service tools through which employees can customize their own insurance plans and have ready access to them, just as they do with their other online accounts. Employees may become more fiscally responsible about their benefits once their insurance information is made more easily available to them. Finally, they may want complete exposure over all the issues of their benefits.

The process of moving toward an online system cannot be an all-at-once process. Employers will gradually shift responsibility to their employees and proceed further depending on how the new system is being adopted and implemented. The national research conducted by PricewaterhouseCoopers (PricewaterhouseCoopers Healthcare Practice, 2003) indicates that few employers are willing to adopt self-directed, otherwise known as defined contribution, health plans today. However, as they adopt more web-enabled functions, they will move more responsibility for choices to employees. As that balance of responsibility shifts, some employers will need to determine how ready their workforce is to accept increasing levels of responsibility.

Physicians are among the first ones to be directly and adversely affected when a significant portion of the healthcare insurance market moves to self-directed, Internet health benefits accounts. Some defined contribution health plans have medical savings accounts as a centerpiece. In these, employees pay out of a medical savings account for routine expenses up to $1,500 or $2,000. Physicians must be prepared to deal with patients who are paying cash for their visits and who may shop around for the best value. *Figure 3* shows the statistics of the probability of customers using the Internet when they have access to a PC (Odyssey Research, 2003).

The insurers should come up with new e-quote products to assist consumers using the Internet for healthcare benefits. They also must follow the growing and changing needs of people and develop products that assist consumers going through the online process.

Standardization can be chosen as the ascendant theme of Healthcare in the near future. Proper steps are to be taken to penetrate this e-business niche so that employees and employers can make apples-to-apples comparisons. Offering more options without proper insight into the standard benefits may just add more confusion.

Figure 3: Internet Usage Among Customers

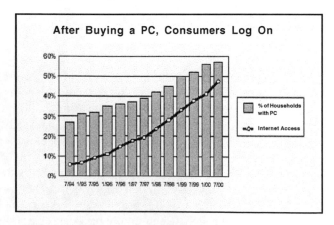

Source: Odyssey Research, 2003

e-HEALTH: A CASE EXAMPLE[2]

Let us take the e-health department at a large healthcare organization in the Midwest of North America (ABC Healthcare Organization) as an example to see how the Internet can be used for healthcare and the benefits that can be derived. The ABC Healthcare Organization is one of the world's largest and busiest health centers. It was founded in the early 1920s as a not-for-profit group practice, integrating clinical and hospital care with research and physician education. The ABC Healthcare Organization has more than 1,000 salaried physicians on staff, representing approximately 120 specialties and subspecialities. Last year, they provided for almost 2 million outpatient visits and almost 50,000 hospital admissions. Patients came to ABC Healthcare Organization from across America and from more than 80 nations.

The demand for web-based health will increase rapidly as the Internet is branching out its roots into common households. From 1999 to 2001, there was a 67% increase in the number of people who had requested health information via ABC Healthcare Organization's web site. In 2001, they received an average of 1,500 web mail inquiries per month, including an average of 270 requests for appointments. People requested various types of information online, including second opinions, general health information, and appointment requests.

Many e-mails and phone calls were received by the clinic staff requesting quality second opinions from the famous physicians at ABC Healthcare Organization. Looking at the high volume of requests for second opinions, the organization decided to enter into the e-market.

E-health is one of the important divisions in the Information Technology Department of ABC Healthcare Organization. It has the primary responsibility of making sure that secure and trustworthy information is presented online. It also has to ensure that online patients are getting the same amount and quality of information that regular patients receive.

e-Health Second Opinion

When patients are faced with a serious medical problem, obtaining a second opinion has long been an accepted medical practice. With the rise of consumerism since the late 70s, both patients and healthcare providers adopted the practice of second opinions to get maximum satisfaction from the treatment. Consider this accepted practice juxtaposed against the technology advances with computers, coupled with the phenomenal growth of the Internet. In 2000, 52 million American adults, or 55% of those with Internet access, sought health information online, many of these people seeking specific information about their own or a family member's condition (Efficient Knowledge Making, 2003). As the use of these online medical resources continues to grow exponentially, healthcare organizations have a unique opportunity to leverage consumer interest in the Internet to advance e-market services. Specifically, the demand for medical second opinions, coupled with the acceptance of the Internet, created an opportunity to develop and offer a web-based second opinion service that meets the public's demand for convenient access to credible, quality, patient-directed healthcare while also increasing the efficiency of the physicians who provide these services. In February 2002, ABC Healthcare Organization, launched its e-health Second Opinion Program, an Internet-based service for patients with a life-threatening or life-altering diagnosis who wish to obtain a second opinion from physicians at ABC Healthcare Organization.

The Development

Development of the operational plan for the Internet-based second opinion program was facilitated by the experience of ABC Healthcare Organization with an 80-year history for providing specialty consultations and second opinions. For approximately 65 years, the only portal to the doctor was through the front door of the hospital and clinic and these patients came primarily from the Midwest and its contiguous states.

A fundamental shift occurred in the mid-1990s. Patients and potential patients began using technology to gain greater access to healthcare information and healthcare providers, bypassing traditional geographic barriers to service. Additionally, many patients in other countries expressed a desire to have ABC Healthcare Organization physicians render a second opinion when they were faced with a new diagnosis or medical problem. Typically, these requests and the data were sent by fax and overnight courier service. Although connectivity at home is increasing and getting faster — 18% of e-health users have broadband connections (The Higher the Connection Speed, 2001) — the ability to respond to this demand for health information was challenged by the many different methods used for responding to remote patient's inquiries that also integrated existing operational processes and information systems.

E-health second opinion represents in its basic form the transformation of a traditional medical service into an e-health service. The program was designed to handle only second opinions and to require the data upon which the primary diagnosis was based. Each clinical department and the physicians identified the diagnoses in their practices for which second opinions were requested. Since rendering a second opinion is considered by the regulations of most state medical boards as the practice of medicine, an early decision in the development of the second opinion program was to license those physicians who were to participate in the program throughout the States. Since ABC Healthcare Organization is a multi-specialty group practice in which the physicians are credentialed through a single office, this office facilitated the licensing of the ABC Healthcare Organization physicians participating in the e-health program in each state in which the program was being offered.

Integration of Online Second Opinions with the Existing System

ABC Healthcare Organization has a vigorous information system for fast and convenient access to patient information. This makes it necessary that the integration of the e-health second opinion program into current operational systems should be efficient and seamless. To achieve this, any patient's visit through the Internet is handled in the same way as a physical visit at ABC Healthcare Organization.

Integration of e-health second opinion should not cause any kind of efficiency and response time problems to the current IT system. To ensure this, the same methods of online registration, appointment, e-mail, results reporting, statistical reporting and financial reporting systems are integrated with the online second opinion request forms and requester contact information gathering process. Hence the overall infrastructure is not disturbed. *Figure 4* provides a schematic of the logical architecture for the e-health second opinion program.

During the process of requesting a second opinion online, the patient can stop the process at any stage and resume at a later time. The information is saved so that the patient need not start from the beginning when returning within the specified time interval. This feature also gives the patient the ability to talk to experienced nurse practitioners on the team. This has proven to be very useful to the patients and allows them to submit complete and informative second opinion requests. The patients are given the full list of the nurses and their e-mail and telephone contacts to contact at any point during the e-consult process if they have any questions. A registered nurse contacts the patient directly by telephone one to two days following completion of the consultation to ensure the patient understands the content of the second opinion information and that all questions have been answered. Should the patient have further questions, the clinical staff facilitates the discussion with the physician who completed the second opinion. Once all of the steps of the process are completed, the medical records are filed with the Health Data Services department for further action.

Online Healthcare Provision to Patients

With the entrance of the health industry into the World Wide Web, the ability of patients to communicate with physicians or healthcare providers changes radically. In a time of great need, such as when patients have been diagnosed with a life-threatening or life-altering diagnosis, quality information from a trusted source is paramount. Second opinions offer the reassurance and peace of mind that a prescribed course of treatment is the best for each individual. Most importantly, second opinions provide a safeguard against unnecessary or inappropriate treatment.

Various factors both externally and internally were considered before launching second opinion requests in e-space. Integration of the second opinion process into existing operational and information technology systems at ABC Healthcare Organiza-

Figure 4: Logical Design of the Online Second Opinion

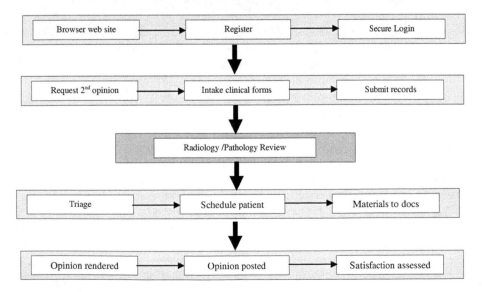

tion minimized the operational impact of a new clinical offering. In fact, adding the web expression to already existing services permitted consolidation of many different processes into a unified method by which a second opinion could be rendered remotely for selected diagnoses. By incorporating e-appointments into the physician's routine medical practice, by complying with disparate state licensing regulations, and by communicating the program's features and benefits to providers and patients, ABC Healthcare Organization has launched a second opinion program that satisfies internal constituents whiles responding to external market demands for quality service and convenience. When the consultation is real and the visit is virtual, greater access and value is created for all concerned. Future developments will continue the integration of technology into existing healthcare processes, in addition to the creation of new processes that will more effectively address the clinical needs of patients.

DRAWBACKS OF USING e-HEALTH AND POSSIBLE SOLUTIONS

At the core of the e-health debate is the tension between access and quality assurance. Access to healthcare becomes less hierarchical and nonlinear with e-health as it destroys the single-point, gatekeeper model of access, allowing multiple entry points. Thus on the surface it seems that these technologies should decrease costs and improve access. But, in reality heath information online poses serious issues for quality assurance systems. Systems based on licensure or malpractice law are premised on a single point of entry identifiably located in physical space. These systems will be ineffective to police a delivery system that is no longer based on physicality or the preeminence of the traditional patient-physician relationship.

Lack of physicality can be considered as a major problem in the e-health world. Physically meeting a patient will give the physician a better chance to interact and find out more about the problem. For example, consider the online second opinion: For each diagnosis, sets of questions are predefined and the patient has to fill in the answers. But sometimes some further questions may arise depending on a given answer. Physically, the physician changes his questions depending on the response of the patient, but this is not possible when the patient is being asked questions online. Even if it is made interactive, it cannot be as efficient as asking the patient in person.

As e-health provides more choice and communication (aided by the promise of extracting administrative costs from the healthcare delivery system), access should be dramatically improved. Yet, e-health's lack of physicality, its depersonalization, anonymity, and even coldness challenge usual conceptions of competence and compassion. Further, multipoint entry into the delivery system makes continuity difficult to achieve, while health advice sites based on e-commerce paradigms involve considerable conflicts of interest. Finally, e-health marketing practices and privacy concerns frequently seem to involve the commodification of patients and patient data.

Despite the challenges discussed above, e-health has great potential for good. Highly efficient national medical markets, around-the-clock service and the seamless integration of products and services no longer should be the stuff of dreams. The ability to heavily personalize computer-mediated relationships may rehabilitate patient-physician relationships eroded by years of managed care, while the web's ability to deliver rich information directly to consumers could reverse centuries of damaging informational asymmetry between patient and physician.

To achieve the promise of e-health, ethical and legal structures must be refurbished to further demand the provision of quality medical information, untainted by patient-sorting costs or provider self-interest. Regulatory systems must be changed so that they are no longer premised on ties with some physical place. Legal and ethical constructs must be informed by e-health codes of conduct and computer mediated data quality solutions.

The US Department of Health and Human Services has sought valiantly to reconcile cost extraction and patient rights in its privacy regulations. This is a positive sign for e-health. In the e-health environment, as information, diagnosis, treatment, and care are delivered through inconversant channels, serious challenges posed by e-health should not be underestimated. However, there is still time to re-engineer legal and ethical codes to marry increased access to quality assurance and avoid the abyss of a computer-mediated sequel to the worst and most dehumanizing aspects of managed care.

INCORPORATING KNOWLEDGE MANAGEMENT IN E-HEALTH

Incorporating the concepts, looks, and strategies of Knowledge Management (KM) can only reveal the full value of e-health. In order to understand this, we now introduce KM before discussing how KM helps e-health. Specifically, we provide the context for why knowledge management is now necessary and briefly discuss the value of knowledge management as well as seven basic considerations for embracing knowledge management in any organizational setting.

Quality of Medical Information

Sometimes the information displayed on the Internet will not be of good quality. This is a major setback, as both the consumers and healthcare providers will not be ready to use and rely on such a system. Studies assessing the quality of health-related web sites, newsgroups or evaluating interactive venues using the method of posing as a fictitious patient have demonstrated that important aspects of quality — like reliability, accessibility, and completeness of information and advice on the Internet — are extremely variable. Though this problem also exists in media which are not web-oriented, like magazines, newspapers, and television, some extra problems — such as the originators of messages and their credibility — are difficult to assess by readers and are more troublesome when it comes to the use of the Internet. Solutions for these concerns — such as the widespread use of evaluative meta-information — have been proposed (Alberthal, 1995) and will, once adopted, help to make the web a more useful tool for patient education. Furthermore, the Internet will open new ways for professional medical education (Knowledge Management, 2003). Knowledge management will provide a great way to achieve good quality, as all the actions will become organized using it.

The e-Knowledge Market as an Enabler of e-Health

The e-knowledge market concept can be a powerful, next generation platform for enabling e-Healthcare.

Knowledge management offers ideas and approaches that can be valuable to disability researchers and service providers. A consumer or patient — centered orientation, a belief that "healthcare is an information business," and a focus on obtaining maximum value from information resources are all important concepts with broad applicability.

In an era of user involvement, consumer empowerment, and the wide dissemination of information on health and health services, it is important that we identify who the consumers of online health information are, what their information needs are, and understand why and how they seek information online. Following this method will enable information to be provided in ways that will have benefits from the worldwide to the individual level. It will also inform current debates over the quantity and quality of information that is provided and issues of privacy and security. Using knowledge management in this process will obviously improve the way in which the data is shown to customers online and thus increases customer satisfaction, which is one of the primary concerns of e-health sites.

Health Knowledge Management

So far, most (if not all) of the technology-based applications to promote knowledge management in health have been a mere transition from paper-based to electronic-based means to process and distribute information in text form. Most of the efforts to date have been developed for and by healthcare providers. The belief remains that in the future the bandwidth of knowledge management will increase and this will allow consumers to communicate more effectively. With these developments one will be to go beyond text to more "natural" or primal ways of representing and exchanging knowledge.

To make knowledge management grow to its full extent and be more useful, projects and applications that will explore innovative ways to synthesize, distill, package, integrate and deliver different types of information (e.g., clinical data, anecdotes, rules of thumb, or intuitive statements) in more engaging and more efficient ways need to be developed.

CONCLUSIONS

From the above discussion we highlight that knowledge management can be a tremendous factor in developing the infrastructure and outcome of e-health. Using the Internet as one of the media to promote health conditions can be of great use if proper security and other issues are taken care of.

The second opinion e-health program at ABC Hospital discussed earlier, also points out the ease with which healthcare is reachable to people using the Internet. Adding web applications to an existing healthcare organization's activities will increase awareness among patients and also spread the news faster and in a more convenient way. Given the rate at Internet use is increasing, it is definitely useful to provide health information online. However, e-health also brings with it many challenges. Knowledge management, when incorporated into e-health applications, can serve to make e-health better and make the process even faster with its efficient organization of critical information and relevant knowledge, thereby providing solutions to many of the current challenges facing e-health initiatives.

The Internet will not be the same in the next millennium. Important developments are likely to improve not only the speed but also the quality of information and retrieval possibilities. The web could evolve into a global medical knowledge base, where diverse medical Internet applications and resources are interconnected and integrated beyond manual "linking." Moreover, the Internet will revolutionize science itself by opening new ways of scholarly communication and electronic publishing. The Internet and related new communication technologies will enable health professionals to reach larger populations with interactive applications, which in turn will open enormous opportunities and challenges. The need for research is clear. "Cyber medicine" research should go beyond the mere development and provision of technical solutions. It should also address social and human factors and evaluate the impact of the Internet on society, healthcare, and public health. As researchers, one has the responsibility not to follow blindly the general Internet hype, but to help physicians and consumers to maximize the use of the Internet by carefully evaluating our interventions and revealing determinants that influence the effectiveness and efficiency of Internet communications in healthcare. Many of these evaluation methods are yet to be developed.

REFERENCES

Alberthal, L. (1995). *Remarks to the Financial Executives Institute.* Dallas, Texas, October 23, 1995.

Efficient Knowledge Making. (2003). Retrieved from the World Wide Web at: http://www.jmir.org/2000/3/index.htm.

E-Health and the Practicing Physician. (2003). Retrieved from the World Wide Web at: www.medscape.com.

E-Health in the Medical Field. (2003). Retrieved from the World Wide Web at: http://www.americantelemed.org/ehealth/ehealthH.htm.

Eysenbach, G. (2001). *Journal of Medical Internet Research*, 3(2), e20.

Eysenbach, G. & Diepgen, T. L. (1998). Towards quality management of medical information on the Internet: Evaluation, labeling, and filtering of information. *BMJ*, 317, 1496-1500.

Knowledge Management - Emerging Perspectives. (2003). Retrieved from the World Wide Web at: www.outsights.com.

Odyssey Research. (2003). Retrieved from the World Wide Web at: www.odysseyresearch.org.

Online Health Information Seekers Growing Twice as Fast as Online Population: Cyber Dialogue. (2000). Retrieved May 23, 2000 from the World Wide Web.

PricewaterhouseCoopers Healthcare Practice. (2003). Retrieved from the World Wide Web at: www.pwchealth.com.

Sieving PC Factors Driving the Increase in Medical Information on the Web — One American Perspective. (1999). *Journal of Med Internet Research.* Retrieved from the World Wide Web at: www.jmir.org/1999/1/e3.

Terry, N. P. (2000). Structural and legal implications of e-Health. *Journal of Health Law*, 33, 605-613.

The Higher the Connection Speed, the Higher the Value: Broadband Use as an Indication of Value amongst e-Health Users. (2001). *Cyber Dialogue Cybercitizen Health Trend Report 2001*, 49.

Tiwana, A. (2002). *The Knowledge Management Tool Kit — Practical Techniques for Building a Knowledge Management System.*

ENDNOTES

[1]   The authors are most appreciative to the work of Harsha P. Reddy in collecting much of the data for this chapter.

[2]   The data was collected from on-site visits, discussions with key actors and evaluation of numerous internal documents.

Chapter X

Evidence-Based Medicine:
A New Approach in the Practice of Medicine

Nilmini Wickramasinghe, Cleveland State University, USA

Sushil K. Sharma, Ball State University, USA

Harsha P. Reddy, Cleveland State University, USA

ABSTRACT

The ongoing tension between certainty over uncertainty is the main force that is driving the evidence-based medicine movement. The central philosophy of this practice lies in the idea that one can never take for granted one's own practice, but by using a structured, problem-based approach, practitioners can logically manoeuvre their way through the obstacle course of clinical decision-making. Attending postgraduate educational events and reading various science journals are no longer sufficient to keep healthcare practitioners aware of all the new developments in practice. To gain this knowledge they need to accept that there are questions they have to ask about their practice. Having posed a number of questions, answers should be found to the most important, practitioners should appraise the quality of the resulting evidence and, if appropriate, practitioners should implement change in response to that new knowledge.

INTRODUCTION

Evidence-based medicine (EBM) can be thought of as the conscientious, explicit and judicious use of current best evidence in making decisions about the care of the individual patient. It means integrating individual clinical expertise with the best available external clinical evidence from systematic research (Sackett, 2003).

Medical practitioners see an overwhelming number of patients. Several questions concerning diagnosis, prognosis, treatment and general care may arise during each session. Hence, it is quite possible for a medical practitioner to make many thousands of clinical decisions a year. As per Covell (Covell & Manning, 1995), when asked, general practitioners say that they generate on average two questions per three patients. Forty percent of the questions were factual (e.g., What dose?), 43% were concerned with medical opinion and 17% were nonmedical. On average, the clinician is left with four unanswered questions per surgery or clinic. A colleague typically meets only 30% of physicians' information needs during the patient visit. Further, the reasons for not using printed resources includes lack of knowledge of appropriate resources, office textbook collections are often too old, as well as a lack of time to search for needed information. In addition, there is no proof that the information obtained is 100% up-to-date. Evidence-based practice can be of great help in this scenario of the background of information needed and clinical overload and the general feeling of helplessness. EBM aims to provide the best possible evidence at the point of clinical (or management) contact.

As per the study by Lundberg (1992), in 1900 there were about 10,000 scientific journals; in 1990 there were more than 100,000 scientific journals. Ninety percent of all major scientific advances are in only 150 of those 100,000 publications; 80% of the citations noted by Science Citation Index are to less than 1,000 journals. Not all of this information is valid or useful for patient care. There is a need to be able to identify relevant information and to be able to critically evaluate the scientific methodology and conclusions of the information.

Evidence-based medicine then focuses on converting the abstract exercise of reading and appraising the literature into the pragmatic process of using the literature to benefit individual patients while simultaneously expanding the clinician's knowledge base (Bordley, 1997).

The primary objective of this chapter is to discuss this new approach of practicing medicine. The need for evidence-based medicine becomes even more pronounced in an environment focusing on lowering healthcare costs. However, it is our thesis that in order to realize the full power and potential of EBM we must integrate the strategies, processes, tools, techniques and technologies of knowledge management. Given that the focus of this entire book is on creating knowledge based healthcare organizations, the goal of this chapter is to familiarize readers with the new and growing area of EBM. From this chapter we believe it will then be possible to appreciate the key role of both information and more importantly knowledge to EBM and thus why it is indeed imperative to incorporate a KM focus in EBM.

STEPS IN EVIDENCE-BASED MEDICINE

The practice of evidence-based medicine can be divided into the following components:

1.   Ascertaining a problem or area of uncertainty.
2.   Converting information into a focused, clinically important question that is likely to be answered.
3.   Efficiently tracking down and appraising the best evidence.

4.   Estimating the clinical importance of the evidence and the clinical applicability of any recommendations or conclusions.
5.   Unifying the evidence with clinical expertise, patient preferences and applying the results in clinical practice.
6.   Summarizing and caching records for future reference.

Ascertaining a Problem or Area of Uncertainty

This is the first step within EBM and must be done with utmost care, especially since all the other steps almost completely rely on this step. A bad identification will lead to form an irrelevant question and an incorrect clinical appraisal that leads directly to a wrong conclusion. This wrong conclusion can be very dangerous and even be harmful to the patient.

A considerable amount of time then should be spent to find the area which needs a literature search. The area of uncertainty should be properly focused and narrowed down before proceeding to the process of formulating the question.

Converting Information into a Focused, Clinically Important Question

The amount of work that the practitioners have to complete is sometimes overwhelming and they forget to ask what they are doing. The questioning attitude is what makes good professionals. Medical practitioners must think through carefully if they in fact are doing the right things and if so are they being done in the right way and at the right time. Further, they should be very accurate when forming a question because in extreme cases a question can be so badly formed that its answer is either unrelated or even meaningless.

Consider the following clinical scenario:

John is a new patient who visits a clinic for a routine physical exam. His medical records from his previous physician are available. John is in good health, although he has had hypertension for many years. There is a family history of stroke. He is 67 years old and he goes on long walks almost every day.

John's hypertension has been successfully controlled by Beta-blockers and he expressed satisfaction with this therapy and he has a feeling that he is getting better. However, John's daughter, who sees another physician, has recently been diagnosed with hypertension and was given Captopril. John wants to know if he can use Captopril. So the problem is whether or not Captopril would be a better medication for John.

A relevant question has to be formed for the above problem. Answers may be found more efficiently by structuring the question. It is, therefore, important to try to break the question down into several parts. This process is also known as "anatomy." The question should be framed in such a way that it facilitates the answer.

The question can be broken into:
- Patient or problem
- Intervention

- Comparison intervention
- Outcomes

Patient or Problem

The first part is to identify the problem or the patient. Healthcare problems may not always seem to be about patients. Sometimes the question may be regarding administrative work, other times the "problem or patient" may be the out of hours of the nurses. It is critical in EBM that the question being described is the patient or problem that is seen. The question must not be too specific at this stage as some important evidence might go unnoticed. There is also a balance to be struck between getting evidence about exactly the group of patients and getting all the evidence about all groups of patients.

Intervention

Intervention may in fact be a postponement of an action such as an operation. Most interventions are more straightforward such as types of dressings, drug therapies or counseling. Alternatively, there can be the provision of differing environmental factors. This portion of the question is important as it confirms the future action to be taken regarding the treatment.

Specificity must be as accurate as possible at this stage as there might be a need to back track if any evidence is not found. The way in which the treatment is offered to patients varies from both within and between primary and secondary care.

Comparison Intervention

Sometimes there is a comparison of intervention. For example, a search can be made for papers comparing the use of head lice lotion in children compared with placebo. Most of the treatments come to practice after performing such comparison tests. Comparative studies offer a great deal of information and help when searching for the evidence.

Outcomes

Outcome measures are particularly important when considering the question. It is worth spending some time working out exactly what it is you want. In some life-threatening or life-altering diseases, most of the times it happens that by concentrating on the mortality, important aspects of morbidity might be neglected. For example, the use of toxic chemotherapies for cancer may affect both aspects (Evidence-based Medicine, 2003).

In the case of John, in the example above, the question structure is detailed in *Table 1*. Using this anatomy, the focused question for John would be:

"In elderly patients, are ACE inhibitors more effective than beta blockers in controlling high blood pressure and minimizing adverse effects?"

Efficiently Tracking Down and Appraising the Best Evidence

One of the questions is formulated. The next step in EBM is tracking down the evidence. This again requires attention to several key steps as described here.

Table 1: Structure of the Question

Patient / problem	High rate of blood pressure, elderly
Intervention	Beta blockers
Comparison intervention	ACE inhibitors
Outcomes	Reduce blood pressure, minimize adverse effects

Finding the Evidence

It is important that the most relevant and best available resources are to be searched and utilized for the different types of questions. Best information reserves can be gathered by following a systematic approach. The following five questions can be used as a guide for this process (*Evidence-based Medicine*, 2003).

- *Type of question being asked:* It is useful and also necessary to decide the category in which the question fits into. "Clinical findings," "Therapy," "Prevention," "Prognosis," "Harm or risk" and "Quality of life" are some of the varieties of questions.

- *Choice of information that would provide evidence to answer this type of question:* Careful consideration must be given to the issues of qualitative and quantitative evidence. Sometimes qualitative factors that are impossible or difficult to quantify are involved for some types of questions, including some therapy questions. Though cultural perceptions, values, customs or other types of soft complexity make generalization between groups or population difficult, evidence is needed for decision-making.

- *Type of study that would provide such information:* For each particular type of question, various studies and investigations, which supply the information that can be used as strongest evidence to weakest evidence, must be accumulated. Qualitative research may provide information for complex health policy decisions.

- *Varieties of resources that would give access to the results of the above studies:* Resources can be classified into two fundamental types "primary" and "secondary." Primary sources are the ones in which the original studies are published, while the secondary sources are the ones which refer to or give bibliographical access in the form of references to material in primary sources. Among the primary sources, textbooks along with journals and publications occupy the most important position. With the growth of the Internet, the Web as a source of information is becoming a vital resource. Online information with the aid of powerful search engines such as MSN, Google, Altavista, Yahoo, OMNI, etc., provides links to various sites that have relevant primary and secondary sources of information in an organized way, while computer bibliographic databases like PubMed, MedLine, CINAHL, and EMBASE, etc., are the most important types of secondary resources. These online data sources have links to thousands of electronic journals and research papers from all around the world.

- *How can the best use of the available resources be obtained?* A search can be of two types:
  - High Sensitivity/Low Specificity Search — This search gives importance to comprehensiveness — finding everything of any relevance at all.
  - Low Sensitivity/High Specificity Search — This search gives importance to selectivity — finding only the most highly relevant material.

Clearly there exists a trade-off between the above two categories.

Appraising the Evidence

The main goal of a critical appraisal is to identify the quality of the article. There are three key issues to think about when appraising any paper:
- The validity of the results of the study.
- The actual results.
- The relevance of the results.

Estimating the Clinical Importance of the Evidence

In this step, records are verified to see if the evidence obtained is relevant to the patient's problem and also to verify if the evidence or information obtained is of any clinical importance. Any evidence that is not clinically recognizable must be set aside. It can be considered as supplementary information, but must not be taken as the primary source of information to extract evidence.

The following section will describe how to make a decision regarding the usage of the acquired data.

Deciding Whether or Not to Act on Evidence

The process of evidence-based medicine is one that requires change to be monitored (*Evidence-based Medicine*, 2003). The evidence that supports the validity or truthfulness of the information is found primarily in the study methodology. Here, investigators address the issue of bias, both conscious and unconscious. The investigators or the patients must not overly influence the study results. To ensure this, study methodologies such as randomization, blinding and accounting are applied for all patients. To facilitate the rigor of the methodology, the audit cycle as depicted in *Figure 1* is often utilized.

Evaluating the medical literature is a complex undertaking. Once it is determined that the study methodology is valid, the results and their applicability to the patient must be examined. Clinicians may have additional concerns such as whether the study represented people similar to his or her patients, whether the study suggested a clear and useful plan of action, and whether the study covered those aspects of the problem that are most important to the patient.

Distinct sources and techniques can be used to achieve and access the clinical importance. Randomized controlled trails are one of the widely used methods. The following are important considerations:
- For the prevention of bias, the groups must be randomized.
- The comparison groups must be similar as different groups might have different characteristics that may lead to bias.

Figure 1: The Audit Cycle

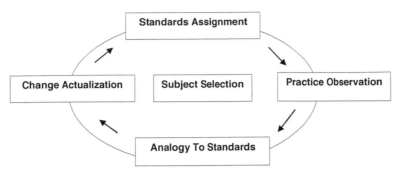

- Patients must be unaware of whether their treatment is experimental or placebo. This is to be considered important as it affects the mental confidence of the patient and may even lead to an altogether different result.
- The length of study must reflect the type of study. It is necessary to have an idea of the natural progress of the disease for determining the appropriate length for a study.
- A good clinical trail requires a complete follow up of both groups. If less than 80% of the patients adequately followed up, then the results may be invalid.
- Appropriate outcome measures must be used in the research of the treatment. It must also be seen that the outcome measures are as accurate as possible.

Unifying the Evidence with Clinical Expertise, Patient Preferences and Applying it to Practice

The final step in the EBM process is to return to the patient and discuss the evidence and suggestions for further treatment.

Suppose, for example, the analysis shows that the evidence is evaluated and accepted and that it meets the criteria for validity. To complete the analysis a review of the results must be performed. Care must also be taken to determine if they are applicable to the particular patient.

Let us return to the example given earlier for the patient John. The following treatment can be suggested. Suppose the results of this study indicate that ACE inhibitors are not more effective than beta-blockers in treatment of hypertension and that they lead to an increased risk of stroke. For John (based on his situation, the physician's clinical judgment, and the evidence) it does not seem appropriate to change to ACE inhibitors. Since there is a family history of stroke, his daughter is not a good candidate for ACE inhibitors, either. A copy of the study can be sent to her to share with her physician so that her physician will have a chance to go through the study to determine if the treatment being offered to John's daughter needs any improvements.

Summarizing and Caching Records for Future Reference

This is the last step in the evidence-based practice. It is not a mandatory step but is highly recommended. As there is a high probability for that physician to get cases very similar to the one he conducted research on, it is always better for him to store and organize all his research. His own work can become the most important resource of information for his future research.

MISAPPREHENSIONS ABOUT EVIDENCE-BASED MEDICINE

Misapprehensions arise naturally regarding any issue. They must be discussed and clarified. In addition, it is important that any of the unintended negative effects must also be taken care of and rectified immediately. While practicing or considering the practice of evidence-based medicine, the nature of the new paradigm is sometimes misinterpreted.

Recognizing the limitations of intuition, experience, and understanding of pathophysiology in permitting strong inferences may be misinterpreted as rejecting these routes to knowledge. Specific misinterpretations of evidence-based medicine, and their corrections, are provided in *Table 2*.

Table 1: Evidence-Based Medicine and Their Corrections

Misinterpretation	Correction
Evidence-based medicine ignores clinical experience and clinical intuition.	This is not true. Untested signs and symptoms should not be rejected out of hand. They may prove extremely useful, and ultimately be proved valid through rigorous testing. Diagnostic tests may differ in their accuracy depending on the skill of the practitioner.
Understanding of basic investigation and pathophysiology plays no part in evidence-based medicine.	The dearth of adequate evidence demands that clinical problem solving must rely on an understanding of underlying pathophysiology.
Evidence-based medicine ignores standard aspects of clinical training such as the physical examination.	A careful history and physical examination provides much, and often the best, evidence for diagnosis and directs treatment decisions. Evidence-based practice considers the physical conditions of the patient while evaluating the evidence and also before applying treatment to the patient.

Source: Campbell, 1987

BARRIERS TO PRACTICING EVIDENCE-BASED MEDICINE

There are some difficult challenges to be faced regarding the practice of EBM. These include but are not limited to: (1) the appropriate literature may not be readily available; (2) economic constraints and counterproductive incentives may compete with the dictates of evidence as determinants of clinical decisions; and (3) sometimes the evidence obtained may be capacious, and there might not be a sufficient amount of time for careful revision relevant to a pressing clinical problem.

Some solutions to these problems are already available. Optimal integration of computer technology into clinical practice facilitates finding and accessing evidence. Reference to literature overviews meeting scientific principles (Oxman and Guyatt, 1998) and collections of methodologically sound and highly relevant articles (Haynes, 1991) can markedly increase efficiency. Evidence-based summaries are becoming increasingly available. Using online health information for obtaining evidence is already in practice. Furthermore, it is gaining importance. Increasingly, scientific overviews will be systematically integrated with information regarding toxicity and side effects, cost, and the consequences of alternative courses of action to develop clinical policy guidelines. The prospects for these developments are both bright and exciting. It is with respect to capturing key knowledge, in particular tacit knowledge, and storing this knowledge so that it can be easily and efficiently accessed and hence used and reused that we believe the strategies, processes, tools, techniques and technologies of knowledge management have the greatest value in facilitating EBM, addressing its key barriers and enabling it to reach its full potential.

CONCERNS REGARDING ADOPTION OF EVIDENCE-BASED MEDICINE

Although EBM has heightened awareness of the most effective management strategies, much of the evidence is not acted on in everyday clinical practice. In particular, five main themes have been identified that affect the implementation process (Freeman and Sweeney, 2001). These include:

Personal and Professional Experiences of the General Practitioners

Doctors' personal and professional experiences influence how clinical evidence is implemented. Despite being a relatively homogeneous group, the general practitioner's enthusiasm for the evidence and the way in which they implemented it varied. Thus, there is no proof that whatever approach is assumed as the best depending on the evidence is actually the best or not.

The Patient-Doctor Relationship

Implementation is influenced by the relationships that doctors developed with their patients. Perceived patient characteristics could have a positive or negative effect on implementation. It also depends on the confidence of the patient in the physician and also in the treatment.

A Perceived Tension between Primary and Secondary Care

Implementation is also influenced by the relationships of doctors with secondary care doctors. Specialists approached evidence-based practice differently, treating "diseases rather than patients." Based on the same evidence, a general practitioner may think one approach as the best one, while a cardiologist might think the same approach as the least approachable.

General Practitioners Feeling about their Patients and Evidence

Clinical evidence is not just an intellectually celibate commodity that is lifted out of medical journals and transferred to a patient. It has an emotional impact on practitioners and patients. Sometimes the knowledge that the evidence existed, waiting to be applied, was seen as a burden in itself. It may make the patient more anxious. Some practitioners may forgo applying the evidence due to the patient's unwillingness to a new kind of treatment.

The Logistical Problems

Some tricky logistical problems make the doctors less enthusiastic about implementing clinical evidence. Many physicians find it risky and a hassle both for doctors and patients to start a new treatment. Some patients might feel the same. Many of the problems can be resolved by the incorporation of knowledge management. For some problems, using the knowledge management concepts can reduce the intensity of its effect.

CONCLUSIONS

Based on an awareness of the limitations of traditional determinants of clinical decisions, a new paradigm for medical practice has arisen. Evidence-based medicine deals directly with the uncertainties of clinical medicine and has the potential for transforming the education and practice of the next generation of physicians. These physicians will continue to face an exploding volume of literature, rapid introduction of new technologies, deepening concern about burgeoning medical costs, and increasing attention to the quality and outcomes of medical care. The likelihood that evidence-based medicine can help ameliorate these problems should encourage its dissemination.

EBM is still in its infancy. Further, it requires new skills of physicians and other medical practitioners. While strategies for inculcating the principles of evidence-based medicine remain to be refined, initial experience has revealed a number of effective approaches. An evidence-based approach is robust, informative and feasible. It also promotes the quality and consistency of healthcare delivery, and it ensures that the services are cost effective. This chapter has served to highlight the key issues pertaining to EBM. By doing so, it highlights the integral role for KM within any EBM initiative to facilitate the generation, capture, storing, use and reuse of critical medical knowledge. We close by calling for further research into this key area of healthcare in today's 21st Century.

REFERENCES

Bordley, D. R. (1997, May). Evidence-Based Medicine: a Powerful Educational Tool for Clerkship Education. *American Journal of Medicine*, 102(5), 427-432.

Campbell, E. J. (1987, April). The diagnosing mind. *PubMed, Lancet*, 1(8537), 849-851.

Covell, D., Uman, G. & Manning, P. R (1995, October). Information Needs in Office Practice: Are They Being Met? *Annals of Internal Medicine*, 103(4), 596-599.

Dawes, M., Davies, P., Gray, A., Jonathan, M., Seers, K. & Snowball, R. (2003). Evidence-based practice — A primer for healthcare professionals. *Evidence-based medicine electronic tutorial*. Retrieved from the World Wide Web: http://www.hsl.unc.edu/lm/ebm/welcome.htm.

Evidence-based Medicine Working Group. (2003). Retrieved from the World Wide Web: www.med.ualberta.ca/ebm/ebmintro.htm.

Freeman, A. C. & Sweeney, K. (n.d.). *Why General Practitioners Do Not Implement Evidence: Guidelines for Reading Literature Reviews.*

Haynes, R. B. (ed.). (1991, January/February). ACP J Club: A18. *Annals of Internal Medicine,* 114, S1.

Introduction to Evidence-Based Medicine. (2003). Retrieved from the World Wide Web: www.hsl.edu/lm/ebm/welcome.htm.

Lundberg, G. D. (1992, April). Perspective from the editor of JAMA. *The JAMA Bulletin of the Medical Library Association*, 80(2), 110.

Oxman, A. D. & Guyatt, G. H. (1988, April). Qualitative Study. *CMAJ*, 15, 138(8), 697-703.

Sackett, D. (2003). Evidence-based medicine — What is it and what it isn't. *The Origins and Aspirations of ACP Journal Club.* Retrieved from the World Wide Web: www.minervation.com/cebm/ebmisisnt.html.

Chapter XI

Moving to an Online Framework for Knowledge-Driven Healthcare

Bruce Shadbolt, Canberra Clinical School, Australia

Rui Wang, National Health Sciences Centre, Australia

Paul S. Craft, Canberra Hospital, Australia

ABSTRACT

The acquisition of knowledge in healthcare is mostly piecemeal and irregular. Consequently, we believe that the integration of science and patient care into a seamless framework is the key to establishing widespread knowledge-based healthcare organizations. Over the last five years, we have developed a dynamic methodology that completes the full information cycle using a generic online framework that merges science with clinical practice over the continuum of care. Called Protocol Hypothesis Testing (PHT), the framework is an extremely flexible web-enabled system that provides authors (expert groups) with the ability to instantly modify the structure of the system to meet the changing needs of clinical practice and incremental knowledge generation. The fully relational, centralised approach caters to the diversity of local needs whilst providing a global focus. The PHT System:
- *helps drive collaboration between clinicians, researchers, patients, and healthcare organizations to continually improve and use the latest and best evidence;*
- *interfaces between clinical practice and bio-technology research;*

- *conducts randomised clinical trial research;*
- *centrally runs local clinical investigations and health service research;*
- *provides clinicians and patients with user-generated, decision-support algorithms and evidence-based summaries that are applicable to specific patients and their treatment choices;*
- *manages individual patient's information, automatically distributing information to where it is needed, and providing patients with probable paths their treatment may follow; and*
- *provides a process to explore improvements in cost-effectiveness.*

In sum, the PHT system creates a centralised, seamless framework between research and clinical practice that is responsive to instant change based on hypothesis testing (science), data mining (exploration & thresholds) and expert opinion (authors) — all in the context of the needs of different diseases, clinical specialties and healthcare organisations.

INTRODUCTION

Knowledge is a critical resource in the provision of healthcare (Ayres and Clinton, 1997), guiding improvements to clinical decision-making, patient care, health outcomes, workforce quality, and organizational behaviour and structure. In this chapter, we have focused on knowledge acquisition associated with clinical decision-making, patient care and health outcomes. Improvement in these aspects of healthcare is based on our ability to generate and incorporate new knowledge into clinical practice, while maintaining existing sound clinical processes. In reality, the generation of knowledge is mostly piecemeal and irregular, and healthcare organizations are slow at incorporating this new knowledge (Phillips, 1998). Consequently, we believe that the integration of science and patient care into a single framework is the key to establishing widespread healthcare improvement. Current approaches tend not to support this integration, and are inadequate to cope with the rapid rate of change in health technology and advances in medical science (Rosser, 1999; McDonald, 2000; Malterud, 2001).

Over the last five years, we have been developing an online approach to integrate scientific investigation with decision-support methods and quality improvement processes (Shadbolt & Craft, 1998). This integration also incorporates the structure and processes of local healthcare organizations (*Figure 1*), while relying on a global, centralized IT design that operates on the Internet. Called Protocol Hypothesis Testing (PHT), it is a generic online framework that creates a seamless approach between research and clinical practice, completing the full information cycle to enhance our capacity to create, share and use knowledge.

At an organizational level, the model revolves round the literature, with the PHT approach supporting locally relevant research and the incorporation of new knowledge into clinical practice, creating a balance between external and internal information (Davies, 2001). This knowledge can be used in decision-making, and in organizational policy and planning. On the other hand, the global structure of the PHT framework allows organizations to belong to larger groups not bound by their institutional "walls," enabling a natural process for sharing expertise and standardizing care.

Figure 1: A Knowledge-Based Healthcare Model Incorporating the Protocol Hypothesis Testing (PHT) Framework at an Organizational Level

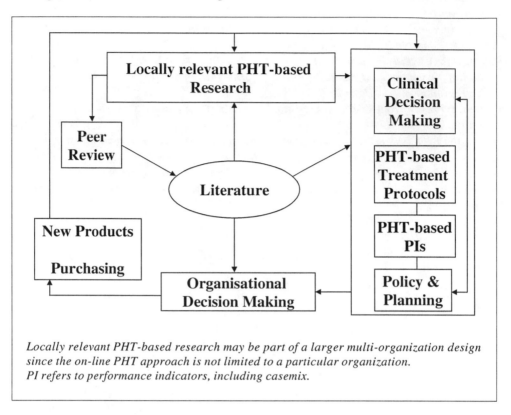

Locally relevant PHT-based research may be part of a larger multi-organization design since the on-line PHT approach is not limited to a particular organization.
PI refers to performance indicators, including casemix.

In the remainder of this chapter we further explore the need for a framework like the PHT, and examine the development of the PHT approach as a case study.

KNOWLEDGE MANAGEMENT

Over the last two decades, there has been a major shift in the world economy from an industrial economy to a knowledge economy (Sveiby, 1997). Managing knowledge has become a major concern for many organizations, and is increasingly being seen as a source of sustainable competitive advantage (Moody and Shanks, 2002). The main objectives are to make more effective use of "know-how" and expertise.

Like other industries, healthcare organizations compete to exist. Advantage comes from cost-effective quality services. On the other hand, in addition to financial reward, the drivers of the clinical workforce are mostly saving or improving human life. As a result, a divergence exists between management and clinical practice, especially in the public sector. Managers have attempted to better align this difference through a focus on developing processes to better improve patient outcomes and quality of care in the hope of gaining more interest from clinicians (Shortell et al., 1998; Savitz & Kaluzny, 2000; Lee et al., 2002). However, these processes of knowledge acquisition are mostly inwardly focused — a situation that runs counter to the formal structures clinicians typically use to acquire knowledge, and creates a practical problem in the capacity for a single organization to properly evaluate clinical care.

Currently, clinicians' experience is variable across the knowledge continuum. Clinicians' exposure to the conduct of experimentation is very selective, with those trained with a research focus and positioned within academic healthcare organizations typically being the ones involved in research (Ross et al., 2001). Clinical areas vary in the extent to which treatment protocols or guidelines are used (Ward et al., 1998). Thus, our knowledge of "best practice" varies considerably between individuals and organizations. Recent efforts to improve this situation include the emergence of *evidence-based medicine* (Sackett et al., 1996) and *quality improvement* (Berwick, 1998).

Evidence-Based Medicine

Evidence-Based Medicine (EBM) is the "use of current best evidence in making decisions about the care of individual patients" (Sackett et al., 1996). The practice of EBM entails a process of lifelong, self-directed learning in which caring for patients creates the need for clinically important information. The process requires an individual or group to (Craig et al., 2001):

- Convert these information needs into answerable questions
- Track down efficiently the best evidence with which to answer them
- Critically appraise that evidence for its validity and usefulness
- Apply the results to patient care in light of preferences and clinical data

Evidence databases exist that add value to the literature by providing more efficient access to appropriate evidence. The notion of using the vast literature resource to provide clinicians with a relatively standard source of information to assist clinical decision-making has merit. It may assist in the quicker uptake of "proven" new treatments (Moody and Shanks, 2002). The majority of clinicians, however, do not use a formal EBM approach. Regardless of advancing technology, we believe the main barrier to the widespread adoption of EBM is a fundamental flaw in the concept.

Evidence bases come from research studies that tend *not* to be designed for clinical decision making. The information within the literature is best suited to supporting decision making about experimentation, often driven by research sponsors (Djulbegovic et al., 2000; Evans & Pocock, 2001). Similarly, the knowledge within the literature is often not readily generalised to everyday clinical practice (Britton et al., 1999). Also, the "written down knowledge" is not likely to identify enough of the information needed to obtain a reasonable replication of the outcomes within clinical practice.

Consequently, the best use of EBM is for clinical decisions about "well-defined" treatments. However, such treatment options are small compared to the variety of clinical decisions. It is estimated that about 70% of treatments do *not* have sufficient evidence to support their use over alternatives (Chalmers, 1993). This poor coverage of evidence is despite a massive growth in the medical literature (McDonald et al., 2002).

We believe a solution to the above issues will not solely come from technology or from conducting more systematic reviews or meta-analyses to synthesise the literature. The answer may lie in creating broadly accessible evidence that is built on the foundations of scientific inquiry (hypothesis-driven, controlled trials) but engineered to meet everyday clinical need and decision making. Research studies would be inclusive of clinicians and patients, with the broader coverage of study designs increasing the extent of valid finding generalisation. By facilitating the participation of more clinicians and service-focused facilities, broad clinical research access will also improve knowledge, both tacit and explicit within the healthcare industry.

From this perspective, EBM would become less of an opportunistic approach to support clinical decision making, and become more a formal part of a purpose–built, knowledge generation infrastructure that supports both the scientific generation of clinical practice evidence and the application of that evidence to individual patients.

Clinical Quality Improvement

There are many variations of improvement processes for healthcare. However, most have their roots in traditional quality assurance methods (Shamoo, 1994) (e.g., continuous quality improvement — CQI; clinical practice improvement — CPI; quality and patient safety; total quality management; knowledge management; decision support).

Clinical quality assurance, typically through audit, has been part of the health system for many years. The movement to quality improvement (especially CQI and CPI) has emerged about the same time as EBM — almost existing as competing approaches. Certainly, the groups using each approach have a different set of philosophies about what is valid and reliable evidence, even though their overall goals are similar — improving clinical decision making and patients' outcomes. Typically, clinical quality improvement processes involve identifying "what is trying to be accomplished" (aim), identifying and defining measures of success, and determining potential change strategies for producing improvement. Then the team follows a PDSA cycle (Langley et al., 1994). These concepts, principles and methods have been found to work effectively in manufacturing industries. In translating these to healthcare, the claim has been that at the core of quality improvement is serial experimentation using a scientific method (Berwick, 1998). We believe that this claim has both helped and hindered the adoption of quality improvement.

Over the last 10 years there have been a number of studies examining organizational clinical improvement approaches and uptakes. In addition to some evidence of improvement success, the reiterated conclusion is that:
- implementation of continuous clinical quality improvement requires strong ongoing organizational support (Solberg et al., 1998; Savitz and Kaluzny, 2000), including promotion and reminder systems and quality IT support (Lee et al., 2002)
- clinical quality improvement activity within an organization does not necessarily constitute a substantial change towards a continuous quality improvement culture (Boerstler et al., 1996), and that an organizational wide approach is needed to be successful (Shortell et al., 1998)
- the number of healthcare organizations with the necessary dimensions needed to facilitate clinical improvement programs is small (Huq and Martin, 2000)
- physicians are skeptical of the findings from these clinical data (Brailer, 1997)
- there is a lack of collaboration between organizations (Brailer, 1997)
- a significant factor influencing implementation of improvement approaches is the use of scientific skills in decision making and the adoption of quality information systems capable of producing precise and valid information (Lee et al., 2002)

Generally, clinicians want to feel they are making decisions with good scientific support. However, the "scientific" method used in quality improvement has too many differences to the methods required for clinical peer review journals (reference standard). As a result, clinicians do not feel part of a "proper" research study when asked to participate in quality improvement projects. This is reinforced by the lack of people with clinical trial experience involved or promoting these activities. Furthermore, despite a project specific methodology, the tools of CQI reinforce adherence rather than choice. Our experience and others suggests that many clinicians do not feel comfortable with this (James, 2002).

The move away from a centralised quality model to small groups conducting their own improvement activities within an organization has helped improve the application of the approach (Lakin et al., 1999), but has also created an irregular coverage within organizations (Shortell et al., 1998). Given that the quality improvement process requires substantial resources and personal effort, broad adoption is difficult using the current methods.

DEVELOPMENT OF THE PHT APPROACH

In this section, we examine the development of the Protocol Hypothesis Testing (PHT) framework as a case study. The increasing focus on healthcare improvement has led to a progressive increase in activities such as clinical trials, quality improvement projects, decision support systems and EBM. However, little has been done to develop frameworks to integrate these approaches for efficient and effective use in healthcare organizations (Rosser, 1999; McDonald, 2000; Malterud, 2001). They are mostly segregated, developing their own methods and IT systems, and yet the overall goals are similar — improving decision making and patients' outcomes.

In the previous section, we discussed EBM and quality improvement processes. We believe that the integration of their strengths may lead to a more effective and efficient framework that has broader acceptance among clinicians. The PHT methodology is designed to combine the conduct of clinical practice, clinical trials, EBM and continuous quality improvement into a single system, creating a seamless framework between research and everyday clinical practice.

The complexity and demands placed on a single, all-inclusive framework made it impossible to achieve the PHT approach without the use of online technology. Also, to achieve a sustainable system, we needed a dynamic business structure, instantly modifiable by the user, while maintaining the integrity of study and management designs. Consequently, we divided the PHT system into two subsystems: a Parameter Setting Module (Authors) and a Clinical User Module with patient access.

Typically, knowledge-based systems are driven by knowledge engineers, with users accessing the data and knowledge bases through a decision support engine (Gregor, 1996). Our approach allowed us to modify this component structure to include a knowledge generation engine with an author (user) interface (*Figure 2*). We replaced the knowledge engineer with an author assigned the task of continually and critically appraising the evidence and reaching consensus among other users about our explicit and tacit knowledge, what new knowledge needs to be generated and how best to generate this new knowledge using the PHT structure. An author is a representative of

Figure 2: Components of the PHT Knowledge-Based Approach

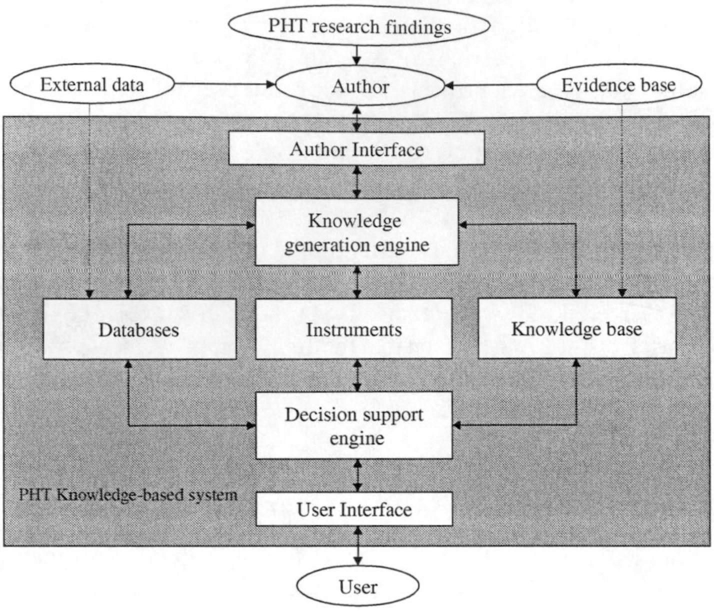

Author is defined as a representative of a larger group of clinical users (e.g., expert group). The web-enabled centralised PHT system is designed to accommodate multiple authors within and between organizations

a larger group of cooperative clinical users and other stakeholders. These users may choose to establish a committee or cooperative group as the author (or Expert Group), especially if the number of clinical users is large or multidisciplinary expertise is required.

The cooperative user design provides a group structure that fits within a larger, centralised, fully relational system. We believe that bringing together the different needs of smaller groups through a centralised structure will help overcome the variable implementation being encountered by quality improvement processes (Shortell et al., 1998; Hug et al., 2000; Lee et al., 2002) and the delivery of EBM (Moody & Shanks, 2002).

The PHT framework has three cyclic phases aimed at achieving incremental knowledge gain based on scientific methods and some aspects of data mining (see *Figure 3*). During the *Author design phase,* authors are given the responsibility of managing the knowledge generation and learning processes of the system. As part of this, authors are able to include external sources through reviewing and synthesising the literature, other data and clinical knowledge. Thus, a balance can be achieved between the use of internal and external information in the advancement of the system's knowledge base.

In the second phase (*Clinician and patient interface*), the system brings together the study designs, knowledge base and decision rules. By intelligently operationalising

Figure 3: The Continuous Improvement Process Cycle for a Cooperative Clinical Group and Author Using the PHT Knowledge-Based System

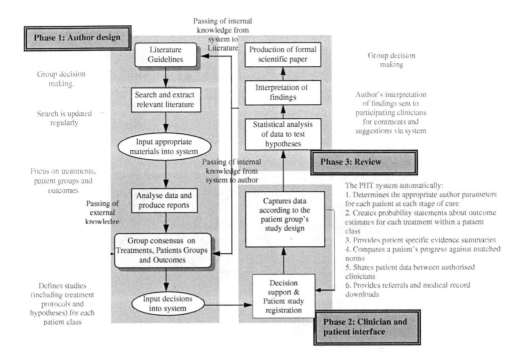

authors' parameters, the PHT system is capable of simultaneously dealing with the diversity of user requirements for different patient populations, clinical specialty, care settings, and states of patients' health and social condition. Basically, every patient seen by a clinician can contribute to new knowledge generation.

The third phase of the PHT framework is the *hypothesis review phase*. At this point, the *a priori* trial designed data can be instantly used when appropriate to test the hypotheses associated with classes of patients. This process is supported in part by data mining. During this review phase, authors interpret the findings and produce electronic journal-style information. The initial findings of the authors are distributed via the system to contributing clinicians for their input. The framework is focused on rapid knowledge generation through *a priori* research designs rather than the more time-consuming task of interrogating semi-structured databases. Authors then return to the first phase to continue the process. This cycle allows participating clinicians to feel part of an active process with clinically relevant aims that help them in their real-time decision making, filling a gap currently existing between research and our understanding of clinical practice.

Parameter Setting Module and the Role of Authors

PHT provides authors with the ability to create their own research studies, treatment management protocols, decision rules and evidence base using the parameter setting process (knowledge generation engine) for defined samples of patients. The underlying structure of the knowledge generation engine involves a specialised, fully relational, hierarchical step-down design to meet the needs of healthcare. At the top is the healthcare organizational coverage and clinical specialty of the authorship representation. The patient cohort, disease or health condition, and care setting follow. At the centre of the hierarchy is the formation of the patient groups. This process includes defining clinically relevant, evidence-based characteristics, decision rules and treatment histories. Under a patient group are the treatment/care protocols, randomization/ blinding options, study assessment parameters and hypotheses.

This step-down design allows authors to maximise the blending of scientific methodology with the delivery of routine healthcare and decision support for individual patient care. Nearly all types of research studies can be implemented by an author (supporting the CONSORT checklist) (Moher et al., 2001) within a "virtually" created healthcare process over time and the care continuum (*Figure 4*).

In terms of data standards, definitions and measurement, an author can define measurement instruments into the system, creating a centralised instrument repository for reuse (the instrument setting module). The measurement instruments attached to the treatment protocols are associated with a specific patient group. Thus, measures can be

Figure 4: The Parameter Setting Module is Multi-Dimensional Linking Patient Groups (PG) to Treatment Protocols (TP) to Study Assessments for a Specific Geographic Area, Disease and Cohort (Authorship)

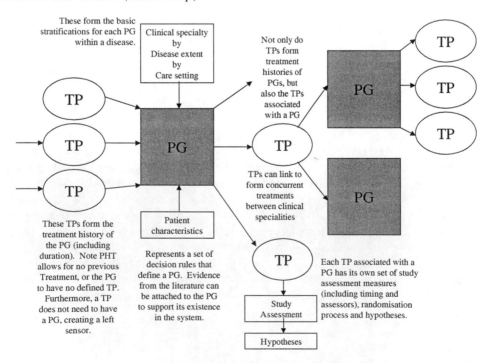

intelligently used to determine treatment effectiveness for specific groups of patients, reducing the inappropriate use of generic measures.

The PHT system is designed to deal with nearly any type of organizational coverage, including international, nested designs, or geographic overlaps between authors of different diseases. This flexibility is paramount to manage the diversity of needs associated with each author group. As the knowledge base builds, there will be incentives for authors to join into larger collaborations. Larger clinician membership broadens generalisation of the findings and increases patient recruitment speed. The by-product is broader standardisation of knowledge, definitions and measurement

Clinical User Module

The Clinical Module relies on a sophisticated, continually learning decision support engine (*Figure 2*). It automatically determines the appropriate author param-eters for each patient at each stage of care. The user interface is extremely friendly, requiring only a small number of pages to perform its main functions. Considerable effort was given to the human engineering and performance aspects to increase the technology uptake.

We designed the PHT system to facilitate relatively effortless classification of *all* patients into clinically relevant, evidence-based groups that are mutually exclusive. After classification, the actual study cohort a patient enters is defined by the treatment protocol that the patient chooses to receive (see *Figures 5a* and *5b* as an example). This treatment protocol may be a formal clinical trial, with or without randomization, routine treatment or modified treatment.

Figures 5: An Example of a Page from the Clinical Users Module - Treatment Protocol Selection for a Specific Patient Group of Advanced Colon Cancer
a) EBM Approach to Providing Relevant Evidence on Standard Treatments and RCTS

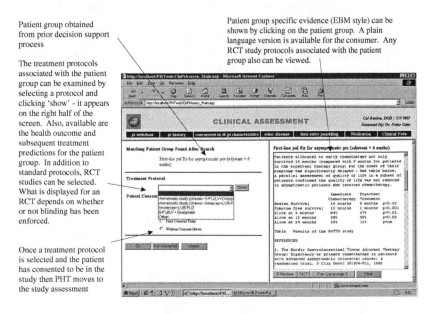

Figures 5: An Example of a Page from the Clinical Users Module - Treatment Protocol Selection for a Specific Patient Group of Advanced Colon Cancer
b) System Generated Health Outcome and Treatment Predictions, Specific to the Patient

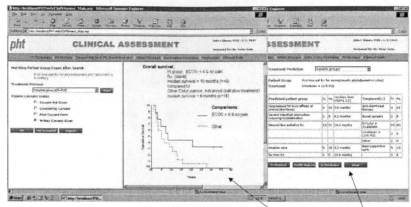

For each treatment protocol (apart from the RCTs), the health outcome predictions and treatment predictions using previous patients' experiences are dynamically generated. Access to these predictions is controlled according to the potential for bias.

The key to classification is the authorship-defined, parsimonious, and evidence-based set of rules for each clinical situation for rule improvement over time. Thus, each question in the classification module is based intelligently on prior answers for that patient type. As shown in *Figure 4*, the rules can be set to capture the complex network of interactions and transactions in clinical practice.

Once a patient becomes a member of a treatment group, outcome measures, including time points, flags/warnings and measurement methods specific to that treatment are available. As data are collected, an automated incremental approach is available for standard treatments to calculate and display probability estimates of health outcomes and subsequent treatment (see *Figure 5b* as an example). In addition to the scientific features, the system manages an individual's information, including real-time patient monitoring against matched norms, characterising a patient's history over the continuum of care, care plans and recommended referrals, reports for medical records, patient-specific flags and warnings to improve safety, and a communication process between health professionals.

Ethics and Consent

The PHT system has built-in clinician and patient consent support, with embedded consent procedures. The system is designed so that every clinician and patient can provide consent before entering a study, regardless of the treatment protocol chosen. This process is more detailed and specific in relation to treatment choice than that seen in many studies (Menikoff, 2003), and reflects a growing belief that every patient should receive detailed and appropriate information before consenting to therapy.

In relation to ethics committees, there are often critical delays in starting clinical research projects because of the approval process. Furthermore, ethics committees may have difficulty due to work loads in ensuring timely review of the progress and outcomes of ongoing studies. The generic framework of the PHT system with a built-in scientific structure may help improve these processes, providing indirect support to ethics committees. However, questions will need to be addressed about definitions and standards of PHT-generated studies, and how best to deal with ethics committee approval for multi-centre author group coverage.

CONCLUSIONS

The PHT system demonstrates that it is possible to integrate existing knowledge-based approaches into a single generic methodology. The potential benefits are:
- better organised knowledge creation, sharing and use;
- a seamless relationship between research and patient care;
- increased capacity to globalise healthcare knowledge;
- knowledge becomes more unified and less competitive;
- better balance between the use of internal and external information;
- better use of expertise and sharing of expertise;
- reduced costs of running clinical trials, EBM and quality improvement activities;
- efficient and effective use of IT.

The design of the PHT structure is based on an innovative, very flexible, generic, online, user-based relational framework that has important control processes in place to maintain the integrity of the system. This design is crucial to create a globalized approach capable of accommodating the needs of different local healthcare organizations, diseases and clinical specialties.

In turn, we envisage that the availability of this futuristic approach will result not only in dramatic and unique improvements in the creation, use and sharing of knowledge, but also dramatically reduce the cost and effort required to implement these activities. Patients will have more choices, clinicians will have valuable decision support and authors will have the tools to experiment and deliver patient-specific, clinical guidelines, creating a sustainable process for continual practice and outcome improvement in healthcare.

REFERENCES

Ayres, D. H. M. & Clinton, S. (1997). *The User Connection: Making the Clinical Information Systems Vision Work.* NSW Health, Health Informatics Conference, (HIC '97), Sydney.

Berwick, D. (1998). Developing and testing changes in delivery of care. *Annals of Internal Medicine*, 128(8), 651-656.

Boerstler, P. H. et al. (1996). Implementation of total quality management: Conventional wisdom versus reality. *Hospital and Health Services Administration*, 41, 143-52.

Brailer, D. (1997). Report on the Wharton Study Group on clinical performance improvement. *Journal Clinical Outcome Measurement*, 4(5), 37-43.

Britton, A., McKee, M., Black, N., McPherson, K., Sanderson, C. & Bain, C. (1999). Threats to applicability of randomised trials: Exclusions and selective participation. *Journal of Health Services Research Policy*, 4(2), 112-121.

Chalmers, I. (1993). The Cochrane collaboration: Preparing, maintaining and disseminating systematic reviews of the effects of healthcare. In K. S. Warren and F. Mosteller (Eds.), *Doing More Good Than Harm: The Evaluation of Health Care Interventions*. New York: Annals of the New York Academy of Sciences.

Craig, C. C., Irwig, L. M. & Stockler, M. (2001). Evidence-based medicine: Useful tools for decision making. *eMJA*, 174, 248-259.

Davies, H. T. (2001). Public release of performance data and quality improvement: Internal responses to external data by US health care providers. *Quality Health Care*, 10(2), 104-110.

Djulbegovic, B. et al. (2000). The uncertainty principle and industry-sponsored research. *Lancet*, 356(9230), 635-638.

Evans, S. & Pocock, S. (2001). Societal responsibilities of clinical trial sponsors. Lack of commercial pay off is not a legitimate reason for stopping a trial. *British Medical Journal*, 322(7286), 569-570.

Gregor, S. (1996) Expert systems. In E. Hovenga, E. Kidd & B. Cesnik (Eds.), *Health Informatics: An Overview* (pp. 149-160). South Melbourne: Pearson Professional (Australia).

Huq, Z. & Martin, T. N. (2000). Workforce cultural factors in TQM/CQI implementation in hospitals. *Health Care Management Review*, 25(3), 80-93.

James, B. (2002). *Interview with Brent James: How good is your healthcare?* Retrieved from The World Wide Web at: http://www.pbs.org/criticalcondition/program/brentJames.html.

Lakin, K. C., Bast, J., Hewitt, A. S., O'Nell, S. N. & Sajevic, P. (1999). A demonstration to test performance-based outcome measures as the foundation of a quality assurance/quality enhancement system. In J. F. Gardner & S. Nudler (Eds.), *Quality Performance in Human Services: Leadership, Values, and Vision* (pp. 285-312). Baltimore, MD: Paul Brookes Publishing.

Langley, G. J., Nolan, K. M. & Nolan, T. W. (1994, June). The foundation of improvement. *Quality Progress*, 81-86.

Lee, S., Choi, K. S., Kang, H. Y., Cho, W. & Chae, Y. M. (2002). Assessing the factors influencing continuous quality improvement implementation: Experience in Korean hospitals. *International Journal of Quality Health Care*, 14(5), 383-391.

Malterud, K. (2001). The art and science of clinical knowledge: Evidence beyond measures and numbers. *Lancet*, 358(9279), 397-400.

McDonald, I. G. (2000). Quality assurance and technology assessment: Pieces of a larger puzzle. *Journal of Quality Clinical Practices*, 20(2-3), 87-94.

McDonald, S., Westby, M., Clarke, M. & Lefebvre, C. (2002). Cochrane Centres' Working Group on 50 years of randomized trials: Number and size of randomized trials reported in general health care journals from 1948 to 1997. *International Journal of Epidemiology*, 31(1), 125-127.

Menikoff, J. (2003). The hidden alternative: Getting investigational treatments off-study. *Lancet*, 361(9351), 63-67.

Moher, D., Schulz, K. F. & Altman, D. G. (2001). The consort statement: Revised recommendations for improving the quality of reports of parallel-group andomised trials. *Lancet*, 357(9263), 1191-1194.

Moody, D. & Shanks, G. (2002). Using on-line medical knowledge to support evidence based practice: A case study of a successful knowledge management project. In

R. Grutler (Ed.), *Knowledge Media in Healthcare: Opportunities and Challenges* (pp. 187-204). Hershey, PA: Idea Group Inc.

Phillips, P. A. (1998). Disseminating and applying the best evidence. *Medical Journal of Australia*, 168(6), 260-261.

Ross, S., Grant, A., Counsell, C., Gillespie, W., Russell, I. & Prescott, R. (2001, December). Barriers to participation in randomised controlled trials: A systematic review. *Journal of Clinical Epidemiology*, 52(12), 1143-1156.

Rosser, W. W. (1999). Application of evidence from randomised controlled trials to general practice. *Lancet*, 353(9153), 661-664.

Sackett, D. L., Rosenberg, W. C., Gray, J., Haynes, R. B. & Richrdson, W. S. (1996, January). Evidence based medicine: what it is and what it isn't. *British Medical Journal*, 312, 71-72.

Savitz, L. A. & Kaluzny, A. D. (2000). Assessing the implementation of clinical process innovations: A cross-case comparison. *Journal of Healthcare Management*, 45(6), 366-80.

Shadbolt, B. & Craft, P. S. (1998). Merging science and clinical practice to evaluate cancer treatment protocols. In J. Sansoni and L. Tilley (Eds.), *Proceedings of Implementing the Health Outcomes Approach* (August 7-8). Canberra, NSW: Wollongong University.

Shamoo, A. E. (1994). Quality assurance. *Quality Assurance*, 1(1), 4-9.

Shortell, S. M., Bennett, C. L. & Byck, G. R. (1998). Assessing the impact of continuous quality improvement on clinical practice: What it will take to accelerate progress. *Milbank Quarterly,* 76(4), 593-624.

Solberg, L. I., Brekke, M. L., Kottke, T. E. & Steel, R. P. (1998). Continuous quality improvement in primary care: What's happening? *Medical Care*, 36(5), 625-35.

Sveiby, K. E. (1997). *The New Organisational Wealth: Managing and Measuring Knowledge-Based Assets*. San Francisco, CA: Berret-Koehler.

Ward, J., Boyages, J. & Gupta, L. (1998). Local impact of the NHMRC early breast cancer guidelines: Where to from here? *Med Journal of Australia,* 169, 292-293.

ENDNOTE

[1] The development of the Protocol Hypothesis Testing (PHT) System is supported by the Australian Capital Territory (ACT) Department of Health, The Canberra Hospital, the ACT Government, and the National Health Sciences Centre.

Chapter XII

Using the Malcolm Baldrige National Quality Award Criteria to Enable KM and Create a Systemic Organizational Perspective

Susan West Engelkemeyer, Babson College, USA

Sharon Muret-Wagstaff, Children's Hospital Boston, USA

ABSTRACT

Health care leaders face an intensifying array of changes and challenges that heighten the need for systematic approaches to knowledge management at the organizational level. Healthcare costs are rising, biomedical science and technological advances are burgeoning, and recent reports indicate that medical errors are widespread. In its report on strategies for achieving improvement in the quality of healthcare delivered to Americans, the Institute of Medicine recommends building organizational supports for change such as the redesign of care based on best practices, use of information technologies to capture and use clinical information, and incorporation of performance and outcome measurements for improvement and accountability (Institute of Medicine, 2001). The Baldrige National Quality Program and its Healthcare Criteria for Performance Excellence *(Baldrige National Quality Program, 2003) offer both the framework and the tools to guide organizations in building these critical supports. This chapter describes the Malcolm Baldrige National Quality Award and its framework, criteria, and scoring system. It provides insight into the pitfalls that stand between an organization and successful KM, as well as examples of ways in which healthcare groups and institutions are becoming learning organizations — successfully employing cycles of learning and effective knowledge management systems in order to enhance performance and better meet the needs of their patients and other customers. The Baldrige Healthcare Criteria for Performance Excellence offer a useful framework for developing a knowledge management system at the organizational level in an increasingly complex environment. Use of the Baldrige Criteria will enhance the knowledge assets of your organization and enable your organization to deliver more value to patients and other customers. These criteria will also improve organizational efficiency and effectiveness through the management of individual, team, and organizational knowledge.*

INTRODUCTION

Healthcare leaders face an intensifying array of changes and challenges that heighten the need for systematic approaches to knowledge management at the organizational level. Healthcare costs are rising, biomedical science and technological advances are burgeoning, yet recent reports indicate that medical errors are widespread (Institute of Medicine, 2000) and that US patients receive only about half of the care suggested by guidelines for common conditions and preventive care (McGlynn et al., 2003).

In its report on strategies for achieving improvement in the quality of healthcare delivered to Americans, the Institute of Medicine recommends building organizational supports for change such as the redesign of care based on best practices, use of information technologies to capture and use clinical information, and incorporation of performance and outcome measurements for improvement and accountability (Institute of Medicine, 2001). The Baldrige National Quality Program and its *Healthcare Criteria for Performance Excellence* (Baldrige National Quality Program, 2003) offer both the framework and the tools to guide organizations in building these critical supports. This chapter describes the Malcolm Baldrige National Quality Award and its framework, criteria, and scoring system. It provides insight into the pitfalls that stand between an organization and successful KM, as well as examples of ways in which healthcare groups and institutions are becoming learning organizations—successfully employing cycles of learning and effective knowledge management systems in order to enhance performance and better meet the needs of patients and other customers.

ABOUT THE MALCOLM BALDRIGE NATIONAL QUALITY AWARD

The Malcolm Baldrige National Quality Award was established by Congress in 1987 to raise awareness and recognize US companies that have developed successful quality management systems. Up to three awards in five categories may be given each year in manufacturing, service, small business, education, and healthcare. Organizations in healthcare and education have been eligible for the award since 1999. Since its inception,

51 organizations — 23 manufacturing firms, 13 small businesses, 11 service organizations, three educational institutions, and one healthcare organization — have been named as award recipients. The first healthcare award recipient, SSM Healthcare, was announced in 2002.

The Baldrige Award and its Criteria provide a systemic view of the organization. This view is a prerequisite to achieving organizational performance excellence. The organizational system is comprised of seven categories, including: category 1.0 leadership; category 2.0 strategic planning; category 3.0 patient, other customer, and market focus; category 5.0 staff focus; and category 6.0 process management. Measurement, analysis, and knowledge management — category 4.0 — provides a fact-based system for improving performance, and is the foundation for the performance management system. Category 7.0 — results — demonstrates the overall performance of the system (*Figure 1*).[1]

The Healthcare Criteria are designed to help organizations use an integrated approach to organizational performance management that results in:
- Delivery of ever-improving value to patients and other customers, contributing to improved healthcare quality;
- Improvement of overall organizational effectiveness and capabilities as a healthcare provider;
- Organizational and personal learning.[2]

Organizations that apply for the award undergo a rigorous examination process in three stages. In Stage One, seven to 10 examiners conduct independent reviews of the application. In Stage Two, a team of approximately seven examiners conducts consensus scoring and identification of strengths and opportunities for improvement in all seven categories. In Stage Three, a team of approximately seven examiners carries out a week-long site visit to verify processes and results and to clarify aspects of the organization's

Figure 1: Baldrige Criteria Framework (A System Perspective)

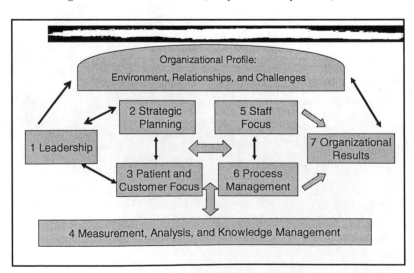

system for performance excellence. Those organizations that progress to a site visit have passed through a demanding screening process in which a narrowing field of applicants goes forward at each stage. For example, in 2002, 49 organizations applied for the award, 26 went to Stage Two (consensus), and 11 moved on in the process to a site visit. From this pool of 11 applicants, three 2002 Award recipients were named in November, 2002.

Although Baldrige is designated an "award," perhaps the greatest benefit to an organization that prepares an application is the self-assessment and learning that occurs throughout the application and feedback process. The Baldrige Criteria ask organizations to articulate "how" they address particular criteria elements. For example, Item 4.2: Information and Knowledge Management asks applicants to address *how* data and information are made accessible to staff, patients, and other customers, as appropriate. And it asks how organizational knowledge is managed to accomplish the collection and transfer of staff knowledge and the identification and sharing of best practices (Baldrige National Quality Program, p. 25). These types of questions force applicants to consider *if* they even have a process in place to address these aspects of the criteria and *what* constitutes the process to deliver on these elements. Imbedded in the criteria is also the concept of organizational improvement through cycles of learning. Applicants must address how they create and manage systems for evaluation, learning, and improvement. This learning approach relies on the analysis, synthesis, communication, and action through the management of individual, group, and organizational knowledge.

CHALLENGES AND PITFALLS

Healthcare organizations have encountered several challenges and pitfalls in designing effective knowledge management systems. It is generally conceded that capturing and disseminating innovations in healthcare is often slow (Berwick, 2003), and that most healthcare organizations have not yet matured to optimal levels of organizational development that move beyond detection and correction of errors to using performance measures to redesign and continually improve their work (Institute of Medicine, 2001; Davies and Nutley, 2000).

Many healthcare organizations are beginning to use the Baldrige Healthcare Criteria for Performance Excellence for self-assessment in order to develop effective organizational learning systems that go beyond individual approaches, and a growing number have applied for the Award each year since 1999. The following list of pitfalls that organizations in all sectors often encounter when beginning their quality journeys is derived from the authors' 12 years of collective experience with the Baldrige process and from the scoring criteria:

1. *Collection of much uncoordinated "stuff."* Low scoring applicants have a chaotic and uncoordinated approach to individual, group, and organizational learning. There is no systematic approach to coordination, synthesis, and communication of information.
2. *Lack of comparative/benchmark data.* An insular approach to information about markets, customers, and processes characterizes low scoring applications. Formal benchmarking initiatives and comparisons to other organizations are limited, both inside and outside of the organization's industry.

3. *Lack of alignment.*   The stovepipes are smoking in these organizations —
    communication and information sharing among work groups, departments, and
    divisions is limited. The "internal customer" concept is not evident in practice.
4. *Numerous activities but few processes.* Low scoring applicants have difficulty
    describing systematic processes within their organizations. Anecdotal stories are
    common responses to questions about how the organization accomplishes key
    functions (e.g., customer complaint management).
5. *Lack of customer definition and focus.* These organizations sometimes lose sight
    of the customer. They are not clearly customer focused in all they do. For example,
    the communication of current customer needs and expectations is not pervasive
    throughout the organization. In fact, some low scoring applications have difficulty
    articulating their customer segments and assessing the needs and expectations of
    different customer groups.
6. *Inconsistent management by fact.* Low scoring applicants manage by intuition and
    by "putting out fires," rather than by the carefully planned use of relevant data and
    information. Systematic review of key data by senior managers is limited.
7. *Delegation of improvement activities.* In these organizations, improvement
    activities — cycles of learning — are not the responsibility of all in the organization,
    particularly top management. Typically, something akin to an Office of Quality is
    expected to manage improvement processes.
8. *Failure to engage key stakeholders.* Organizations may overlook the input from
    the knowledge and experiences of frontline, customer-facing employees for pur-
    poses such as strategic planning and rapid cycle change. In other instances,
    nurses, physicians, and other clinical personnel are not engaged collaboratively
    with administrative leaders to target opportunities and to develop effective
    measures and improvement innovations aligned with the organization's mission.

These pitfalls indicate a lack of coordination of individual, group, and organizational knowledge through the systematic collection, analysis, and communication of
relevant data and information throughout the organization. Limited sharing and integration of key information inhibits an organization's ability to learn from others inside and
outside the organization, improve processes and systems in order to enhance efficiency
and effectiveness, and develop as an organization in order to provide more value to its
patients, other customers, and stakeholders.

SUCCESS STORIES

The potential to exploit knowledge management and information and communication technology to improve healthcare organizational performance is great (Stefanelli,
2002). Innovators in developing computer-interpretable clinical guidelines, which address the core function of healthcare organizations, are coming together to develop
international standards (Peleg et al., 2003). Quality leaders at Dartmouth-Hitchcock
Medical Center report use in various centers of a one-page health status report to
determine: if care and services are meeting the needs of patients with spinal problems;
real-time process monitoring of cycle time, quality, productivity, and customer satisfac-

tion by an emergency department; and a data system to monitor "wired" patients remotely (Nelson et al., 2003).

Others have incorporated knowledge management in microsystems within an overall organizational view using the Baldrige framework and criteria. At Baylor Healthcare System, for example, an internal, Baldrige-based survey of 98 top executives was used to determine information system needs to achieve critical success factors for all business units (Prybutok and Spink, 1997). The Veterans Health Administration (VHA) uses an internal Baldrige-based quality award open to all Veterans Integrated Service Networks within the VHA system to identify areas of achievement and areas for improvement within the VHA system (Shirks et al., 2002; Weeks et al., 2000). A recent analysis of data from 220 US hospitals provided empirical evidence that focusing on the content addressed in the Baldrige criteria leads hospitals to improvement on specific dimensions of performance (Goldstein and Schweikhart, 2002).

PROFILE OF SSM HEALTHCARE[3]

In 2002, SSM Healthcare (SSMHC) became the first healthcare recipient of the Baldrige National Quality Award since these organizations became eligible in 1999. SSM Healthcare is a not-for-profit Catholic health system with approximately $1.7 billion in revenue and 21 acute care hospitals and three nursing homes in Missouri, Illinois, Wisconsin, and Oklahoma. The system has approximately 22,200 employees and 5,000 affiliated physicians. Services provided include emergency, medical/surgery, oncology, mental health, obstetric, cardiology, orthopedic, pediatric, and rehabilitative care. Services are delivered via inpatient, outpatient, emergency, and ambulatory surgery settings within acute care hospitals.

What distinguishes this provider from many of its peers and competitors in the healthcare industry? The authors have identified seven aspects of SSMHC that provide insight into how it delivers value to its patients and other customers. These include: (1) alignment and cascading of plans with overall goals for the system; (2) extensive market analysis; (3) multiple methods for understanding patient needs, expectations, and satisfaction; (4) widespread dissemination and access to performance data; (5) focus on diversity; (6) a team approach to improved outcomes; and (7) a mission that extends beyond patients.

Alignment and Cascading of Plans with Overall Goals for the System

SSMHC's Strategic, Financial and Human Resource Planning Process (SFPP) begins with the Board of Director's review of vision and mission statements and Corporate Planning's survey of the key participants from the previous year. The process extends over a 12-month cycle and involves all of the organization's networks, entities, and departments. Three-year (long-term) and annual (short-term) planning horizons are used. System management sets and communicates system-wide goals to each entity and provides standardized forms and definitions to ensure a consistent format and alignment of plans with the system's overall goals. Department goals are further cascaded to the employees, with individual "Passports" reflecting individual goals that support the department goals.

Extensive Market Analysis

Every three years, during the SFPP, environmental scanning is used to identify and plan for potential customers, customers of competitors, and future markets. The scan includes market research, analysis of market share by product line, population trends, and an inventory of competitors, which includes their market share trends and competitive positions. In addition, data from annual medical staff surveys, patient satisfaction surveys, physician contacts, literature searches, telephone surveys, and focus groups of competitors' customers are used.

Multiple Methods for Understanding Patient Needs, Expectations, and Satisfaction

SSMHC has established formal and informal listening and learning tools for former and current patients and their families. Surveys are customized for each of the key segments. Tools include satisfaction surveys, market research, comment cards, a complaint management system, patient follow-up calls, and an Internet response system. In addition, SSMHC assesses potential patients and future markets through a variety of tools.

Widespread Dissemination and Access to Performance Data

SSMHC uses an automated system to make clinical, financial, operational, customer, and market performance information available to all of its sites. For example, SSMHC makes data available to physician partners from any location via multiple devices, including personal computers, personal digital assistants (PDAs), pagers, and fax machines.

Focus on Diversity

SSMHC has maintained a continuous focus on increasing the number of minorities in professional and managerial positions. Minorities in professional and managerial positions increased from almost 8% in 1997 to 9.2% in 2001, considerably better than the healthcare industry benchmark of 2%.

A Team Approach to Improved Outcomes

As part of SSMHC's "Clinical Collaborative" process, physicians work with other care-givers, administrators, and staff to make rapid improvements in clinical outcomes. Selection of clinical collaboratives occurs in alignment with system goals, such as improving patient outcomes, satisfaction, and safety. The results for SSMHC's clinical collaboratives for patients with congestive heart failure and ischemic heart disease demonstrate levels that approach or exceed national benchmarks. In addition, CARE PATHWAYS®, protocols, and standing orders are used to outline a standardized plan of care for SSMHC's patients. These tools are designed with patient input and are intended to create partnerships with physicians to improve patient care.

A Mission that Extends Beyond Patients

The SSMHC system-wide "Healthy Communities" initiative was launched in 1995 to leverage the system's resources with those of the communities it serves. SSMHC requires each of its entities to actively engage in one or more community projects such as free dental clinics and campaigns to reduce smoking and drinking among teens. It encourages and supports employees at all levels of the organization to participate in teams involved in identifying opportunities for community outreach. In addition, SSMHC provides a significant amount of charity care to improve the health of the communities it serves. Since 1999, SSMHC has exceeded its charity care goal of contributing a minimum of 25% of its operating margin from the prior year.

What are key results that demonstrate the effectiveness of SSMHC's approach? SSMHC has undertaken six quality collaboratives, involving 85 teams in 2002, up from 14 teams in 1999. Consequently, clinical care indicators and outcomes for patients with congestive heart failure and ischemic heart disease now approach or exceed national benchmarks. SSMHC's share of the market in the St. Louis area increased over each of the past three years to 18%, while three of its five competitors have lost market share. Connected physicians have increased steadily from 3,200 in 1999 to 7,288 in 2002. SSM has maintained "AA" credit rating by both Standard and Poor's and Fitch for four consecutive years, where less than one percent of US hospitals attain this level. Currently, SSMHC is providing in excess of 29% of the previous year's operating margin to provide care to communities that are economically, physically, and socially disadvantaged (compared to a goal of 25%).

These seven aspects highlight how SSMHC incorporates data from environmental scanning, patient and stakeholder surveys, and performance results to assess and improve organizational performance. And SSMHC's team approach allows all caregivers to learn from each other in order to improve clinical outcomes and the patient's experience. This knowledge-based system not only enhances SSMHC's performance results, it also enables the organization to reach beyond its walls and provide care to disadvantaged communities.

BALDRIGE ORGANIZATIONAL SELF-ASSESSMENT

Using Baldrige National Quality Program criteria and other tools to build an effective knowledge management system for a healthcare organization is challenging, but it need not be daunting.

The following mini-assessment is based on the 2003 MBNQA criteria. This assessment draws from elements that relate particularly to knowledge management and provides an organization with an understanding of where their strength areas and areas for improvement with respect to knowledge management exist. It also provides a starting point for discussions about creative ways to apply knowledge management concepts to achieve organizational improvement.

Baldrige Knowledge Management Mini-Assessment

The following questionnaire is based on the Malcolm Baldrige National Quality Award 2003 Criteria for Performance Excellence. Definitions of a few terms are included for clarification:

- *Senior Leaders* are those in the organization that have primary responsibility for organizational direction, strategies, management, and performance.
- *Benchmarking* refers to processes and results that represent best practices and performance for similar activities, inside or outside the organization's industry.
- *Stakeholders* might include patients, other customers, employees, suppliers, partners, and the community.

Below is a list of various statements about your organization. "Your organization" may be an entire healthcare system, a specific facility, or a department. Although there may be variability across facilities or departments, apply the statement to your organization in general as best you can. Read each statement carefully and decide the extent to which it applies to your organization.

Use the following scale:

3 = Applies to a great extent or completely applies to my organization
2 = Applies to a moderate extent in my organization
1 = Does not apply or applies to a small extent in my organization

In my organization...

_____ 1. Senior leaders review organizational performance and capabilities to assess organizational health, competitive performance, and progress relative to goals.

_____ 2. Senior leaders use organizational performance review findings and employee feedback to improve their leadership effectiveness.

_____ 3. Performance is compared to past performance, competitors, and key benchmarks.

_____ 4. Performance relative to plans is regularly tracked.

_____ 5. Key product/service features and their relative importance/value to customers influences current and future marketing, product planning, and other business developments.

_____ 6. Mechanisms are in place to facilitate the ability of customers to conduct business, seek assistance and information, and make complaints.

_____ 7. Customer satisfaction relative to competitors and/or benchmarks is obtained and used for planning and decision making.

_____ 8. Data collected are deployed to all users to support the effective management and evaluation of key processes.

_____ 9. Data collected are consistently evaluated and used for the improvement of key processes and services.

_____ 10. Appropriate sources of comparative data and information (including benchmarking and competitive comparisons) are used for improving organizational performance.

_____ 11. Results of organizational-level analysis are linked to work group and/or functional-level operations to enable effective support for decision making.

_____ 12. Data analysis supports organizational performance review and organizational planning by senior leaders of the organization.

_____ 13. Data analysis supports daily operations throughout the organization.

_____ 14. Performance data are regularly assessed against action plans and goals and translated into priorities for improvement.

_____ 15. The approach to education and training balances short- and longer-term organizational and employee needs, including development, learning, and career progression.

_____ 16. Formal and informal methods are used to determine the key factors that affect employee well being, satisfaction, and motivation.

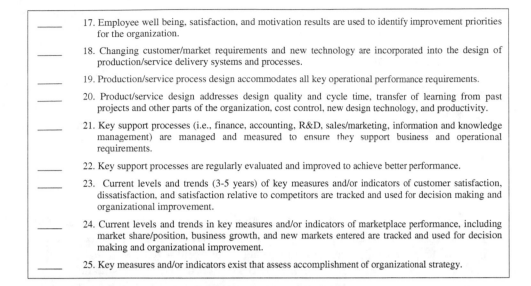

_____ 17. Employee well being, satisfaction, and motivation results are used to identify improvement priorities for the organization.

_____ 18. Changing customer/market requirements and new technology are incorporated into the design of production/service delivery systems and processes.

_____ 19. Production/service process design accommodates all key operational performance requirements.

_____ 20. Product/service design addresses design quality and cycle time, transfer of learning from past projects and other parts of the organization, cost control, new design technology, and productivity.

_____ 21. Key support processes (i.e., finance, accounting, R&D, sales/marketing, information and knowledge management) are managed and measured to ensure they support business and operational requirements.

_____ 22. Key support processes are regularly evaluated and improved to achieve better performance.

_____ 23. Current levels and trends (3-5 years) of key measures and/or indicators of customer satisfaction, dissatisfaction, and satisfaction relative to competitors are tracked and used for decision making and organizational improvement.

_____ 24. Current levels and trends in key measures and/or indicators of marketplace performance, including market share/position, business growth, and new markets entered are tracked and used for decision making and organizational improvement.

_____ 25. Key measures and/or indicators exist that assess accomplishment of organizational strategy.

Now, group your items into your three response categories — 1, 2, and 3. Items under Category 3 — Applies to a great extent or completely applies to my organization — are areas of strength for your organization. You should plan to celebrate and sustain your strengths, but carefully consider applying additional resources to that area at this time. Items under Category 2 — Applies to a moderate extent to my organization — indicate some level of maturity with that particular aspect of knowledge management and limited resources may enhance performance in these areas.

Review the items under Category 1 — Does not apply or applies to a small extent to my organization. These are the areas where you will want to examine most closely and determine priorities for improvement among these. For example, if you marked items #3, 7, 10, and 18 in Category 1 that would indicate your organization does not look outside itself to understand performance comparisons, benchmark information, and changing customer and market needs and requirements. This might generate a benchmarking initiative, the collection of comparative data, and environmental scanning. This data and information could then be incorporated into short and longer-term planning in your organization.

If you had a large proportion of items in Category 1 — Does not apply or applies to a small extent to my organization — you may want to consider taking the E-Baldrige Self-Assessment and Action Planning document which is available at http://www.quality.nist.gov/eBaldrige/Step_One.htm (accessed February 13, 2004). This provides an opportunity to complete a brief online questionnaire and answer questions about your organization. The questions are based on the Baldrige Criteria's Organizational Profile. The profile is a snapshot of your organization, the key influences on how you operate, and the key challenges your organization faces.

Your answers to the E-Baldrige questions indicate how "easy" it is to answer particular questions. For example, **"Easy to answer"** indicates questions that would be easy for your organization to provide an answer with widespread agreement and consensus. **"Could answer"** indicates questions for which data are not readily available, but your organization could produce data to provide a consensus response to address this question. **"Difficult to answer"** indicates questions that would be difficult or impossible to answer and/or to reach agreement and consensus on at this time. Below are two examples of questions in the E-Baldrige:

- What is your overall approach to organizational learning and sharing your knowledge assets within the organization?
- What are the principal factors that determine your success relative to your competitors and other organizations delivering similar healthcare services?

Answers to these questions provide information about areas for which conflicting, little, or no information is available. Areas in which limited information is available can be used for action planning in your organization to provide more clarity and direction. After completion of E-Baldrige, you'll receive a comparison of your organization with others who have taken the challenge. Once the fundamental questions about your organizational description and organizational challenges are clear, your organization will be ready to proceed to evaluating and improving its performance.

The Baldrige scoring criteria (*Figure 2*) give leaders a vision of typical landmarks that organizations achieve as they mature in development of their knowledge manage-

Figure 2: Scoring Guidelines[4]

0%	• no systematic approach evident; information is anecdotal
10% to 20%	• beginning of a systematic approach to the primary purposes of the criteria item • major gaps exist in deployment that would inhibit progress in achieving the primary purposes of the item • early stages of a transition from reacting to problems to a general improvement orientation
30% to 40%	• an effective, systematic approach, responsive to the primary purposes of the item, is evident • the approach is deployed, although some areas or work units are in early stages of deployment • beginning of a systematic approach to evaluation and improvement of key processes is evident
50% to 60%	• an effective, systematic approach, responsive to the overall requirements of the item and your key organizational requirements, is evident • approach is well-deployed, although deployment may vary in some areas or work units • a fact-based, systematic evaluation and improvement process is in place for improving the efficiency and effectiveness of key processes • approach is aligned with your basic organizational needs
70% to 80%	• an effective, systematic approach, responsive to multiple requirements of the item and your current and changing health care needs, is evident • the approach is well deployed, with no significant gaps • a fact-based, systematic evaluation and improvement process and organizational learning/sharing are key management tools; there is clear evidence of refinement, innovation, and improved integration as a result of organizational-level analysis and sharing
90% to 100%	• an effective, systematic approach, fully responsive to all the requirements of the item and all your current and changing health care needs, is evident • approach is fully deployed without any significant weaknesses or gaps in any areas or units • a very strong, fact-based, systematic evaluation and improvement process and extensive organizational learning/sharing are key management tools; strong refinement, innovation, and integration, backed by excellent organizational-level analysis and sharing, are evident • approach is fully integrated with your organizational needs

ment systems and organizational performance results. Award recipients generally score above 60%. As you can see from the scoring guidelines, this means "organizational learning/sharing are key management tools; there is clear evidence of refinement, innovation, and improved integration as a result of organizational-level analysis and sharing."

Where do you think your organization would fall in these scoring guidelines? As *Figure 2* indicates, at 30 points, the organization is beginning to show evidence of a "systematic approach to evaluation and improvement of key processes." The 30% to 40% range represents organizations that are beginning to show cycles of learning which result from the application of knowledge management to key processes. A scoring range of 10% to 20% indicates an organization that is still more prone to react to problems than to proactively manage potential problems; these organizations would have limited application of knowledge management concepts and techniques. According to the Institute of Medicine (2001) and Davies and Nutley (2000), most healthcare organizations have not moved beyond detection and correction of errors to using performance measures to redesign and continually improve their work. This would imply a large proportion of healthcare organizations would score in the 10% to 20% range. As they begin to develop a more systematic approach to the generation, analysis, synthesis, communication, and use of knowledge from inside and outside the organization, they would begin to move along the scoring guidelines continuum.

CONCLUSIONS

The Baldrige Healthcare Criteria for Performance Excellence offer a useful framework for developing a knowledge management system at the organizational level in an increasingly complex environment. Organizations use the criteria for self-assessment in order to achieve high levels of quality and organizational effectiveness, and one healthcare organization has received the Baldrige National Quality Award.

The Baldrige National Quality Program offers several tools that healthcare institutions can use at various levels of organizational development. These range from the E-assessment that takes minutes to a full application that provides the benefit of self-assessment during preparation and concludes with invaluable feedback from a team of experts in the field of performance excellence. Information about these documents and other information can be found on the Baldrige web site at www.quality.nist.gov.

Use of the Baldrige Criteria will enhance the knowledge assets of your organization. The Baldrige Criteria define knowledge assets as, "the accumulated intellectual resources of your organization. It is the knowledge possessed by your organization and its staff in the form of information, ideas, learning, understanding, memory, insights, cognitive and technical skills, and capabilities ... Building and managing its knowledge assets are key components for the organization to create value to its stakeholders" (2003 Healthcare Criteria for Performance Excellence, p. 37).

Using the Baldrige Criteria will enable your organization to deliver more value to patients and other customers and improve organizational efficiency and effectiveness through the management of individual, team, and organizational knowledge.

REFERENCES

Baldrige National Quality Program, National Institute of Standards and Technology, U.S. Department of Commerce. (2003). *2003 Health Care Criteria for Performance Excellence.* Gaithersburg, MD: National Institute of Standards and Technology.

Berwick, D. M. (2003). Disseminating innovations in health care. *JAMA,* 289, 1969-1975.

Davies, H. T. O. & Nutley, S. M. (2003). Developing learning organisations in the new NHS. *British Medical Journal,* 320, 998-1001.

Goldstein, S. M. & Schweikhart, S. B. (2002). Empirical support for the Baldrige Award framework in U.S. hospitals. *Health Care Management Review,* 27, 62-75.

Hofer, T. P., Hayward, R. A., Greenfield, S., Wagner, E. H., Kaplan, S. H. & Manning, W. G. (1999). The unreliability of individual physician "report cards" for assessing the costs and quality of care of a chronic disease. *JAMA,* 281, 2098-2105.

Institute of Medicine. (2000). *To Err Is Human: Building a Safer Health System.* L. T. Kohn, J. M. Corrigan, & M. S. Donaldson (eds.). Washington, DC: National Academy Press.

Institute of Medicine. (2001). *Crossing the Quality Chasm: A New Health System for the 21st Century.* Washington, DC: National Academy Press.

McGlynn et al. (2003). The quality of health care delivered to adults in the United States. *New England Journal of Medicine,* 348, 2635-2645.

Nelson et al. (2003). Microsystems in health care: Part 2. Creating a rich information environment. *Joint Commission Journal on Quality and Safety,* 29, 5-15.

Peleg et al. (2003). Comparing computerinterpretable guideline models: A case-study approach. *Journal of the American Medical Informatics Association,* 10, 52-68.

Prybutok, V. R. & Spink, A. (1997). Transforming a health care information management system. *Top Health Information Management,* 18, 1-11.

Shirks, A., Weeks, W. B. & Sein, A. (2002). Baldrige-based quality awards: Veterans Health Administration's 3-year experience. *Quality Management in Health Care,* 10, 47-54.

Stefanelli, M. (2002). Knowledge management to support performance-based medicine. *Methods Information Med,* 41, 36-43.

Weeks, W. B., Hamby, L., Stein, A. & Batalden, P. B. (2000). Using the Baldrige management system framework in health care: the Veterans Health Administration experience. *Joint Commission Journal on Quality Improvement,* 26, 379-387.

ENDNOTES

[1]   *2003 Health Care Criteria for Performance Excellence,* p. 5. Baldrige National Quality Program, Gaithersburg, MD. http://www.quality.nist.gov (accessed February 13, 2004).

[2]   *2003 Health Care Criteria for Performance Excellence,* pp. 1-4. Baldrige National Quality Program, Gaithersburg, MD. http://www.quality.nist.gov (accessed February 13, 2004).

[3]   Baldrige Award Recipient Profile: SSM Health Care. Baldrige National Quality Program, Gaithersburg, MD. http://www.quality.nist.gov/Award_Recipients.htm (accessed February 13, 2004).

4   Baldrige National Quality Program, *2003 Health Care Criteria for Performance Excellence*, p. 59.

Chapter XIII

Realizing Knowledge Assets in the Medical Sciences with Data Mining:
An Overview

Adam Fadlalla, Cleveland State University, USA

Nilmini Wickramasinghe, Cleveland State University, USA

ABSTRACT

This chapter provides insight into various areas within the medical field that strive to take advantage of different data mining techniques in order to realize the full potential of their knowledge assets. Specifically, this is done by discussing many of the limitations associated with conventional methods of diagnosis and showing how data mining can be used to improve these methods. Comparative analyses of different techniques associated with various areas within the medical field are outlined in order to identify the right technique for particular medical specialties. Furthermore, suggestions are provided to appropriately utilize the various data mining techniques thereby leading to effective and efficient knowledge management and knowledge utilization. In this chapter we highlight the potential of data mining in improving the exploratory as well as the predictive capabilities of conventional diagnostic methods in medical science.

INTRODUCTION

Knowledge management is an emerging business approach aimed at solving current business challenges to increase efficiency and effectiveness of core business processes while simultaneously fostering continuous creativity and innovation. Specifically, knowledge management through the use of various tools, processes and techniques combines germane organizational data, information and knowledge to create business value and enable an organization to capitalize on its intangible (e.g., knowledge) and intellectual assets so that it can effectively achieve its primary business goals as well as maximize its core business competencies (Swan et al., 1999; Davenport & Prusak, 1998). The need for knowledge management is based on a paradigm shift in the business environment where knowledge is central to organizational performance (Drucker, 1993).

Knowledge management offers organizations many tools, techniques and strategies to apply to their existing business processes. In essence then, knowledge management not only involves the production of information but also the capture of data at the source, the transmission and analysis of this data as well as the communication of information based on or derived from the data to those who can act on it (Swan et al., 1999). Fundamental to knowledge management is effectively integrating people, processes and technologies.

A pivotal technique in knowledge management is data mining which is used to discover new knowledge from existing data and information and thus grow the extant knowledge asset of the organization. This is particularly relevant to health care because not only is health care a knowledge-based industry, but it is also currently experiencing exponential growth in the collection of data and information primarily due to new legislative initiatives such as Managed Care and HIPAA (Health Information Portability and Accountability Act) in the US. This then makes it imperative for medical science to incorporate the benefits of this technique. We address this imperative by first discussing basic concepts of data mining and how they relate to the medical sciences. Next we elaborate upon key data mining techniques as well as their advantages and disadvantages and how they contribute to the building of important knowledge assets within health care.

BACKGROUND TO DATA MINING

In the literature, data mining is generally described at two levels: a broad perspective and a narrow perspective. While the broader perspective equates data mining to the process of Knowledge Discovery in Databases (KDD), the narrow perspective sees data mining as a step within this KDD process. In either case data mining can be defined as, *"The nontrivial extraction of implicit, previously unknown, and potentially useful information from data"* (Frawley et al., 1992). Data mining uses machine learning, as well as statistical and visualization techniques to discover and present knowledge in a form that is easily comprehensible to humans. Data mining involves sifting through huge amounts of data and extracting the relevant pieces of data for the particular analysis of a problem. More than just conventional data analysis (such as basic statistical methods), the technique makes heavy use of artificial intelligence. Often the emphasis is not as much on the extracting of data but more on the generating of a hypothesis, as in the case of exploratory data mining. Data mining also uses sophisticated statistical analysis and modeling techniques, which allow users to find useful information such as trends and patterns hidden in their business data. Data mining is one of the latest technologies to assist users deal with the abundance of data that they have collected over time. For example, this technique will help optimize business decisions, increase the value of each customer, enhance communication, and improve customer satisfaction. The retail industry has been using data mining technology to understand customer buying patterns, product warranty management, detection of fraud, and identification of good credit risks. Data Mining has become more popular over time due to the following reasons:

1.   The main reason for the popularity of various data mining techniques is due to the large amount of data already collected and newly appearing data that requires processing beyond traditional approaches. The amount of data collected by various businesses, scientific, medical and governmental organizations around the world is enormous. It is impossible for human analysts to cope with the ever-growing and overwhelming amounts of data.

2.   When a person analyses the data, he/she is liable to make errors due to the inadequacy of the human brain (i.e., the bounded rationality problem) to solve complex multifactor dependencies in the data and sometimes a lack of objectiveness in such an analysis. A human always tries to derive results based upon previous experiments and experiences gained from investigating other systems, unlike data mining which simply reflects what the data is conveying without preconceived hypotheses.

3.   One more advantage of data mining is that, particularly in the case of large amounts of data, this process involves a much lower cost than hiring a team of experts. Although this technique does not discard the human involvement, it significantly simplifies the job and allows an analyst who is not proficient in statistics or programming to manage the process of extracting knowledge from data (Mega Computer Intelligence).

DATA MINING IN MEDICAL SCIENCES

The medical sciences offer a unique opportunity to apply the many techniques of data mining. This is because health care generates mountains of administrative data about patients, hospitals, utilization, claims, etc. In addition, clinical trials, electronic patient records and computer supported disease management increasingly produce large amounts of clinical data. This data, both the administrative and clinical, is a strategic resource for health care institutions since it represents a raw form of their knowledge

Data mining discovers the patterns and correlations hidden within this raw knowledge, i.e., the data repository. Furthermore, it enables health care professionals to use these patterns to aid in decision making and the establishment of revised and improved treatment protocols, and thereby enhance organizational performance.

Previous studies (Maria-Luiza et al., 2001) in various areas of the medical sciences have revealed that conventional methods of detecting symptoms or other health-related problems have been very costly and error prone. Due to the complexities and inconsistencies in these detection methods, the diagnoses which are based on the information gained from these methods can lead to outcomes that are sometimes dangerous and even could lead to a person's death. For example, during the prognosis of breast cancer, the main detection method available is mammography. Due to the high volume and variation in the stage of potential malignancy of tumors from mammograms that need to be read by physicians, the accuracy rate tends to decrease, and methods that focus on automatic reading of digital mammograms become highly desirable. It has been proven that double reading (by two different experts) of mammograms increases the accuracy but also naturally increases the costs. Thus, making it even more imperative to incorporate computer-aided diagnosis systems to assist medical professionals in achieving cost efficiency and diagnostic effectiveness and thereby enabling more appropriate and timely treatment.

In more litigious environments, the increasing risk to health care organizations and providers due to error in detection and interpretations has become extremely costly. Therefore, it is becoming a necessity to adopt new methods to facilitate not only more accurate detection and then treatment but also better preventative measures. Health care organizations have already accumulated large raw knowledge assets in the form of administrative and clinical data. What is now important for them to do is to maximize the potential of this strategic asset, hence the need for embracing data mining.

DATA MINING TECHNIQUES AND THEIR ROLE IN HEALTHCARE

Data mining techniques are not only used in the detection of diseases but they also are beneficial in helping to compare the different procedures required for a prognosis. For example, a physician who has newly started in practice can learn from the association of different procedures to certain diagnoses, which is the result of exploratory data mining and thus can take advantage of these findings to more effectively treat their patients, rather than depending more on the prolonged "trial and error" diagnostic path which is both more time consuming and a lower quality of care approach. The following data mining techniques are recognized for being of great benefit to many areas in business, engineering, as well as other industries. Health care should not be an exception in the application of these techniques:

- Association Rules
- Clustering
- Neural Networks
- Decision Trees

While we acknowledge that there are numerous data mining techniques, we focus on these techniques since they are some of the major techniques that are most suitable in our opinion to the medical sciences. The first two techniques are used for exploratory data mining, the latter two techniques are used for predictive data mining. We will first outline the major steps involved in data mining in order to achieve the final goal of knowledge creation before we describe each of the above data mining techniques.

Knowledge Discovery Process

Figure 1 shows the knowledge discovery process, the evolution of knowledge from data through information to knowledge (Fayyad et al., 1996) and the types of data mining (exploratory and predictive) and their interrelationships. It is essential to emphasize here the importance of the interaction with the medical professionals and administrators who should always play a crucial and indispensable role in a knowledge discovery process, as depicted in *Figure 1* in the interpretation step. This is particularly true when we take into consideration features that are specific to the medical databases. For example, more and more medical procedures employ imaging as a preferred diagnosing tool. Thus, there is a need to develop methods for efficient mining in databases of images, which is inherently more difficult than mining in numerical databases. Other significant features include but are not limited to security and confidentiality concerns and the fact that the physician's interpretation of images, signals, or other clinical data, is written in unstructured English, which is also very difficult to mine (McGee, 1997). Some important data issues that data mining is most useful in helping organizations wrestle with include: huge volumes of data, dynamic data, incomplete data, imprecise data, noisy data, missing attribute values, redundant data, and inconsistent data.

Figure 1 also shows how data goes through the following process steps before being used for any decision-making:

- Selection: selecting the data according to some criteria, e.g., all those people who are suffering from or at risk of cardiac complications.
- Preprocessing: this is the data cleansing stage where certain unwanted information which may not be relevant or useful to the analysis is removed.
- Transformation: the data is not merely transferred but also changed using various mathematical manipulations (such as logarithmic transformations).
- Data mining: this stage is concerned with the extraction of patterns from the data. It includes choosing a data-mining algorithm, which is appropriate to discover a particular pattern in the data.
- Interpretation and evaluation: this is where human interaction and intervention is essential, specifically the patterns identified by the system are interpreted into knowledge by humans and thereby redundant or irrelevant patterns are removed while patterns deemed useful are translated into potential treatment decisions.

Association Rule Mining

Association rules are used to discover relationships between attribute sets for a given input pattern. Such relationships do not necessarily imply causation, they are only associations. For example, an association rule that can be derived from medical data could be that 80% of the cases that display a given symptom are diagnosed with a similar condition and hence improves diagnostic capabilities. These patterns (associations) are not easily discovered using other data mining techniques. The support of an association rule is the percentage of cases which include the antecedent of the rule, while the confidence of the association rule is the percentage of cases where both the antecedent and the consequence of the rule are displayed. Only rules whose support and confidence exceed predetermined thresholds are considered useful. The classic algorithm used to generate these rules is the Apriori *algorithm* (Laura, 1990).

Figure 1: Overview of the Knowledge Discovery Process

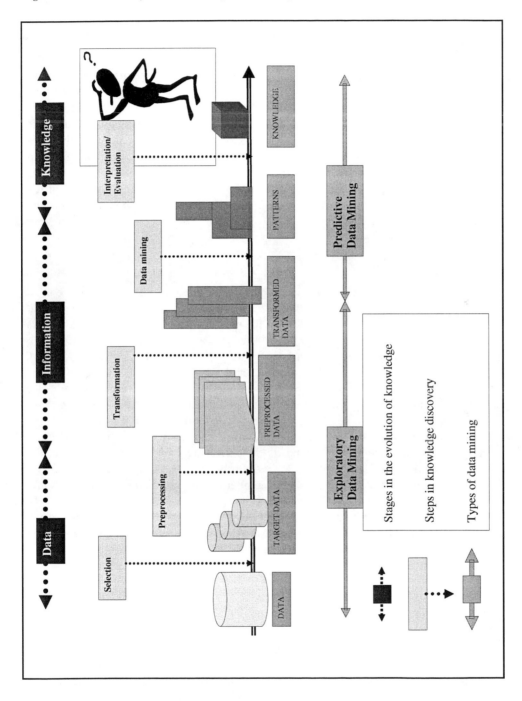

Advantages of Association Rule
- Association rules are readily understandable.
- Association rules are best suited for categorical data analysis
- It is widely used in hospitals to maintain patient's records.
- The outcomes are easy to interpret and explain and thus easy to use in the aiding of decision making.

Disadvantages of Association Rule Mining
- Generate too many rules and sometimes these are even trivial rules.
- The association rules are not expressions of cause and effect, rather they are descriptive relationships in particular databases, so there is no formal testing to increase the predictive power of these rules.
- Insight, analysis and explanation by health care professionals are usually required to identify the new and useful rules and thereby achieve the full benefits from such association rules.

Clustering

In clustering we are trying to develop groupings that are internally homogenous, mutually exclusive and collectively exhaustive. For example, in the study and treatment of chromosomal and DNA-related problems the clustering technique is important. This technique is an exploratory data mining technique. The outcome from the clustering process can then be used as input into a decision tree or neural network (Berkhin, 2002).

The most frequently used clustering method is k-means. This is a geometrical method, which uses the distance from the average location of all the members of a particular cluster to place a specific data point. The whole data field is divided into numbers and then these numbers are normalized. The value of each field is interpreted as the distance from the origin along corresponding axes. The initial clusters are randomly defined and computationally refined during the clustering process. The working of the clustering technique is dependent on two main criteria: (1) the members of a cluster should be most similar to each other, and (2) members of any two different clusters should be most dissimilar.

In most cases clusters are usually mutually exclusive but in some instances they may be overlapping, probabilistic or have hierarchical structures. In k-means a data point is assigned to the cluster which has the nearest centroid (i.e., the nearest mean). Clustering requires the data in numeric form since it works by assigning the cluster points accordingly. This process of assigning points to clusters continues until points stop changing positions (i.e., cluster hopping).

Advantages of Clustering
- The main strength of clustering is that it is an undirected knowledge discovery technique.
- The clustering can be used as a preparatory technique for other data mining techniques such as decision trees or neural networks.
- The outcome of clustering can be visually represented and hence easily understood.

- Creating clusters reduces the complexity of the problem by subdividing the problem space into more manageable partitions.
- The more separable the data points the more effective clustering is.

Disadvantages of Using Clustering
- Clustering represents a snap shot of the data at a certain point in time and thus may not be as useful in highly dynamic situations.
- Sometimes the clusters generated may not even have a practical meaning.
- Sometimes it is possible not to spot the cluster since you do not know what you are looking for.
- Clustering can be computationally expensive.

Neural Networks

The technique of neural networks is modeled after the human brain and normally consists of many input nodes, one or more hidden (middle) layer nodes and one or more output nodes. The input and output nodes relate to each other through the hidden layer. The input layer represents the raw information that is fed into the network. The hidden layer represents a computational layer that transforms the inputs coming from the input layer into inputs to the output layer. The behavior of the output layer depends on the activity of the hidden layer where the weights between the hidden and output layers are used as a reconciliation mechanism to help minimize the difference between the actual and desired outputs.

The outcome of a neural network is improved through the minimization of an error function, i.e., namely the difference between a desired output and an actual output value. The most widely used algorithm used to minimize this error function is known as backpropagation. Each input pattern is evaluated individually and if its value exceeds a predetermined threshold, then a pre-specified rule fires (i.e., is activated) whereby its outcome is fed forward to the next layer. The firing rule is an important concept in neural networks and accounts for their high flexibility since it determines how one calculates whether a subsequent neuron (node) should fire for any given input pattern.

The most important application of neural networks is pattern recognition. The network is trained to associate specific output patterns with input patterns. The power of neural networks comes into play in its predictive abilities, i.e., associating an input pattern that has not previously been classified with a specific output pattern. In such cases, the network will most likely give the output that corresponds to a pre-classified input pattern that is least different from the new input pattern.

Neural networks are mainly used in the medical sciences in recognizing disease types from various scans such as MRI or CT scans. The neural networks learn by example and therefore the more examples we feed into the neural network the more accurate its predictive capabilities become. Neural networks can process a large number of medical records, each of which includes information on symptoms, diagnoses, and treatments for a particular case. The use of neural network as a potential tool in medical science is exemplified by its use in the study of mammograms. In breast cancer detection the primary task is detection of a tumorous cell in the early stages. The best probability for a successful cure of this disease is in its early detection. Therefore, the power of neural networks lies in that they could be used to detect minute changes in tissue patterns (a key indicator of the existence of malignant cells) that are often difficult to detect with the human eye.

Advantages of Neural Networks

- Neural networks are good classification and prediction techniques when the results of the model are more important than the understanding of how the model works.
- Neural networks are very robust in that they can be used to model any type of relationship implied by the input patterns.
- Neural networks can easily be implemented to take advantage of the power of parallel computers with each processor simultaneously doing its own calculations.
- Neural networks are also very robust in situations where the data is noisy.

Disadvantages of Neural Networks

- The key problem with neural networks is the difficulty to explain its outcome. Unlike decision trees, neural networks use complex nonlinear modeling that does not produce rules and hence it is hard to justify one's decision.
- Significant preprocessing and preparation of the data is required.
- Neural networks will tend to over-fit the data unless implemented carefully. This is due to the fact that the neural networks have a large number of parameters which can fit any data set arbitrarily well.
- Neural networks require extensive training time unless the problem is small.

Decision Trees

In critical decision situations, mistakes could be costly and have far reaching impacts. Thus data mining techniques are adopted in an attempt to minimize such mistakes. Decision trees split the available information in a treelike form and then arrive at a final decision by continuously refining the decision choices. The decision is usually made based on the choice between binary outcomes. For example, consider the binary decision of choosing between two methods—surgery and radiation—in the case of cancer treatments.

Decision making permeates health care but is of particular significance in the treatment of life-threatening diseases such as cancer. The decision tree then becomes a particularly powerful tool in such circumstances. Particularly in the case of cancer, early detection is critical since the disease grows rapidly and secondaries are more likely to develop in the meantime. A principal decision-making aspect is to decide quickly upon the specific treatment technique and then administer it and proceed with the delivery of care. For example, in *Figure 2* we can see a simple decision tree that tries to model the underlying decision problem of which drug to administer under which circumstances/conditions. At the root (the top node), the data is split into two partitions with respect to this decision problem, where one partition reflects cases where the Na/K ratio is less than or equal to 14.6 and it is not clear which drug should be administered, while the other partition represents the cases where the Na/K ratio is greater than 14.6 and it is clear that Drug Y is the drug of choice. Partition 1 therefore needs to be further subdivided into three sub-partitions; namely high (partition 1.1), low (partition 1.2) or normal (partition

Figure 2: Data Mining Resulting in the Decision Tree —Each Path from the Tree Root Down Represents a Rule (i.e., a Type of Pattern)

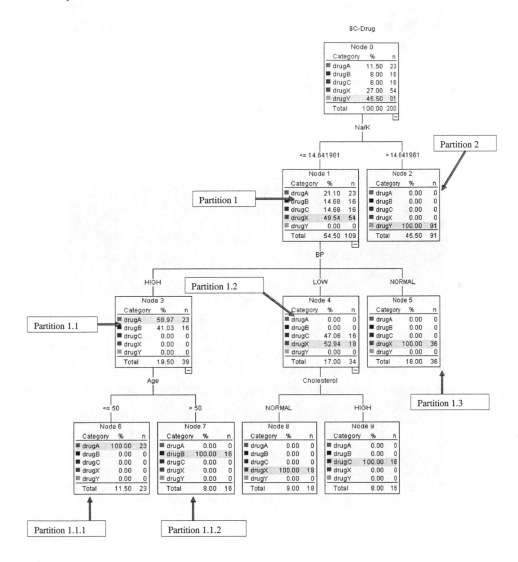

Knowledge stage: Knowledge
Type of data mining: Predictive

1.3) blood pressure cases. In the case of partition 1.1 we can see that the choice is narrowed to Drug A or Drug B, so further sub-partitioning is required (namely, partition 1.1.1 and partition 1.1.2) and is performed on age in order to get clear decisions. It then becomes clear that age is a deciding factor between administering Drug A or Drug B— something that could not be seen from partition 1.1 or even less obvious from partition 1.

Advantages Of Decision Tree:

- The graphical representation of a decision tree makes it a convenient and user-friendly modeling technique since it becomes very easy to visually follow the appropriate decision path and thereby facilitate accurate decision making.
- The decision tree algorithms are not only very fast and efficient to implement but the results are also unambiguous and thus easy to interpret. This feature of easy interpretability becomes of even greater significance in the medical sciences because often times doctors must justify their treatment decisions, such as in litigation instances.
- Decision trees can handle categorical (non-numeric) decision variables which are common in the medical sciences such as in *Figure 2* where the decision variable is the drug to be administered.
- Decision trees can handle modeling situations where there is missing data, a situation that better mirrors practice.
- Decision trees prioritize the variables, using those with the most predictive power early in the partitioning process, hence using the most informative data first.

Disadvantages of Decision Trees

- When a decision variable is continuous, a categorization scheme needs to be developed first before applying the decision tree. Any weaknesses in this categorization scheme will be reflected in the outcome of the decision tree technique.
- There are dependencies between generations of splits (i.e., partition 1 impacts partitions 1.1, 1.2, etc.).
- The way in which decision trees handle numeric variables sometimes leads to loss of information due to loss of detail.

CONTRIBUTION TO KNOWLEDGE ASSETS

Irrespective of the specific data mining technique adopted, the significant common outcome of the application of all of these techniques is the generation of new knowledge. This newly created knowledge grows the extant knowledge base of the organization and thus not only adds value to its intangible assets but also increases its overall organizational value as new management techniques, such as the balanced scorecard, have demonstrated (Kaplan & Norton, 1996). In today's knowledge-based economy sustainable strategic advantages are gained more from an organization's knowledge assets than from its more traditional types of assets. Therefore, processes, tools and techniques that serve to grow the knowledge assets of an organization and thereby increase their value are strategic necessities to effectively compete in today's economy.

Healthcare is noted for using leading edge medical technologies and embracing new scientific discoveries to enable better cures for diseases and better means to enable early detection of most life threatening diseases. However, the healthcare industry globally, and in the US specifically, has been extremely slow to adopt key business processes (such as knowledge management) and techniques (such as data mining) (Wickramasinghe et al., 2003; Wickramasinghe & Mills, 2001). "Despite its information-intensive nature, the healthcare industry invests only 2% of gross revenues in information technology, compared with 10% for other information-intensive industries" (Bates et al., 2003). Furthermore, "[e]ven though US medical care is the world's most costly, its outcomes are mediocre compared with other industrial nations" (Bates et al., 2003). Therefore, making more of an investment in key business processes and techniques is a strategic imperative for the US healthcare industry if it is to achieve a premier standing with respect to high value, high quality and high accessibility of its healthcare delivery system.

In the final report compiled by the Committee on the Quality of Healthcare in America (Crossing the Quality Chasm, 2001), it was noted that improving patient care is integrally linked to providing high quality healthcare. Furthermore, in order to achieve a high quality of healthcare the committee identified six key aims — namely that healthcare should be: (1) safe: avoiding injuries to patients from the care that is intended to help them, (2) effective: providing services based on scientific knowledge to all who could benefit and refraining from providing services to those who will not benefit (i.e., avoiding under-use and overuse), (3) patient-centered: providing care that is respectful of and responsive to individual patient preferences, needs, and values and ensuring that patient values guide all clinical decisions, (4) timely: reducing waiting and sometimes harmful delays for both those receiving care and those who give care, (5) efficient: avoiding waste and (6) equitable: providing care that does not vary in quality based on personal characteristics.

Most of the poor quality connected with healthcare is related to a highly fragmented delivery system that lacks even rudimentary clinical information capabilities resulting in poorly designed care processes characterized by unnecessary duplication of services and long waiting times and delays (ibid). The development and application of sophisticated information systems is essential to address these quality issues and improve efficiency, yet healthcare delivery has been relatively untouched by the revolution of information technology, new business management processes such as knowledge management or new techniques such as data mining that are transforming so many areas of business today (Wickramasinghe et al., 2003; Wickramasinghe & Mills, 2001; Bates et al., 2003; Crossing the Quality Chasm, 2001; Wickramasinghe, 2000; Stegwee & Spil, 2001; Wickramasinghe & Silvers, 2002).

CONCLUSIONS

This chapter attempted to provide a survey of the four major data mining techniques and their application to the medical science field in order to realize the full potential of the knowledge assets in healthcare. We also presented an enhanced framework of the knowledge discovery process to highlight the interrelationships between data, information and knowledge as well as between knowledge creation and the key steps in data mining. There is no single data mining technique that will be best under all circumstances in healthcare as well as other industries. However, a comparative analysis of the various techniques as they are used in medical science suggests the following:

1. Neural networks are general and flexible thus can model situations with either numeric or non-numeric data. Further, they can handle noisy data effectively. However, their major limitation is that it is difficult to understand the reasoning behind their outcomes.

2. Decision trees on the other hand are very intuitive to understand but are not as flexible, nor as tolerant with noisy data.

3. Clustering provides a powerful exploratory data mining technique, however it can also be very computationally expensive. Further, it could sometimes generate clusters that are difficult to justify in practice. Clustering can be used as a first step for either decision trees or neural networks.

4. Association rules are very general in nature and their outcomes are very easy to understand, since these outcomes are made up of nested if-then rules. However, they require human insights to identify which rules are significant and useful and which are trivial.

Finally, we discussed the importance of data mining to the growing of the organizational knowledge assets and argued why this is of such significance in today's knowledge-based economy for healthcare. Clearly, as much as there is a need for such techniques in creating knowledge-based organizations in healthcare, there is still much to be done before knowledge management enabled through the adoption of these data mining techniques is diffused en mass throughout healthcare organizations and thereby enabling these organizations to realize the full benefits of their knowledge assets. This chapter then has served as an overview of how to realize the full potential of knowledge assets in the medical sciences using various key data mining techniques. There is naturally scope for future research to take a more detailed view of these techniques within the medical sciences.

REFERENCES

Antonie, M. L., Zaiane, O. R., & Coman, A. (2001, August). *Application of Data Mining Techniques for Medical Image Classification*. DataBase Laboraratory, Department of Computing Science, University of Alberta, Canada.

Bates, D., Ebell, M., Gotlieb, E., Zapp, J., & Mullins, H. (2003, Jan/Feb). A proposal for Electronic Records in U.S. *Primary Care JAMIA*, 10(1), 1-9.

Berkhin, P. (2002). *Survey of Clustering Data Mining Techniques*. Accrue Software, Inc.

Crossing the Quality Chasm - a New Health System for the 21st Century. (2001). Committee on Quality of Health Care in America Institute of Medicine. Washington, D.C.: National Academy Press.

Davenport, T. & Prusak, L. (1998). *Working Knowledge*. Boston, MA: Harvard Business School Press.

Drucker, P. (1993). *Post-Capitalist Society*. New York: Harper Collins.

Fayyad, Piatetsky-Shapiro, & Smyth (1996). From data mining to knowledge discovery: An overview. In Fayyad, Piatetsky-Shapiro, Smyth, & Uthurusamy, *Advances in Knowledge Discovery and Data Mining*. Menlo Park, CA: AAAI Press/The MIT Press.

Frawley, W., Piatetsky-Shapiro, G., & Matheus, C. (1992, Fall). Knowledge discovery in databases: An overview. *AI Magazine*, 213-228.

Kaplan, R. & Norton, D. (1996). *The Balanced Scorecard: Translating Strategy into Action*. Boston, MA: Harvard Business School Press.

Kolbasuk McGee, M. (1997, September). High-tech healing. *Information Week*.

Laura, Lanzarini, Ing. A. De Giusti, (1990). *Pattern Recognition in Medical Images using Neural Networks*.

Mega Computer Intelligence. Data Mining 101. Retrieved from the World Wide Web: http://www.megaputer.com/dm/dm101.php3.

Stegwee, R. & Spil, T. (2001). *Strategies for Healthcare Information Systems*. Hershey, PA: Idea Group Inc.

Swan, J., Scarbrough, H. & Preston, J. (1999). Knowledge management – The next fad to forget people? *Proceedings of the 7ᵗʰ European Conference in Information Systems*.

Wickramasinghe, N. (2000). IS/IT as a Tool to Achieve Goal Alignment: A theoretical Framework. *International J. Healthcare Technology Management*, 2(1/2/3/4), 163-180.

Wickramasinghe, N. & Mills, G. (2001). MARS: The electronic medical record system the core of the kaiser galaxy. *International Journal Healthcare Technology Management*, 3(5/6), 406-423.

Wickramasinghe, N. & Silvers, J. B. (2003). IS/IT the Prescription To Enable Medical Group Practices Attain Their Goals. Healthcare Management Science, 6, 75-86.

Wickramasinghe, N., Fadlalla, A., Geisler, E. & Schaffer, J. (2003). Knowledge Management and Data Mining Strategic Imperatives for Health Care. *Proceedings of the 3rd Hospital of the Future conference*, Warwick.

Section III

Key Issues and Concerns of Various Knowledge Management Implementations: Evidence from Practice

Chapter XIV

Organizational Control Mode, Cognitive Activity & Performance Reliability:
The Case of a National Hospital in Japan

M. Saito, Waseda University, Japan

T. Inoue, Waseda University, Japan

H. Seki, Ryutsu Keizai University, Japan

ABSTRACT

Objectives: Improvement of service quality and security is required in any business area in society. The purposes of this chapter are to identify and to verify our study hypotheses that cognitive activities, work environment and organizational climate/culture are highly related with human performance reliability and that human performance reliability was predicted by organizational control mode. This chapter will also emphasize that it is important to focus on the implication of latent variables perceived for tacit knowledge as well as articulate knowledge in knowledge management. Methods: The subjects surveyed in the case study are 356 clinical nurses and healthcare providers working in a national hospital in Japan. The questionnaires used were prepared by referring to the methodologies developed by Hollnagel et al. for assessing human reliability. Results: The score of improved reliability in strategic organizational control mode was the highest, while the one in scrambled mode was the lowest among four control modes of organization. Performance reliability was significantly influenced by organizational climate and work environment as well as cognitive activities of the participants. This was the similar trend observed in industry. In concluding, the latent factors, i.e., the variables in the genotype embedded deep in a complex organization, were the determinants for predicting human performance reliability in this case study. These results suggested that the variables in the genotype representing cognitive activities, nursing work environment and organizational safety climate were important factors as well as the variables in the phenotype which were observable.

INTRODUCTION

Organizational performance may be shaped by multi-factorial causes emerging in the synergetic process of individual, organization and technology. Improvement of healthcare performance is required for providing appropriate quality of care and security for clients/customers who have a large variety of needs, some of which require a long term of continuous healthcare. Our major concern in this chapter is on the quality of healthcare in terms of security which is delivered in a hospital under the external and internal pressures of diversity and uncertainty in financial, technical and organizational environments. Risk assessments carried out in the hospitals in Japan are not adequately programmed. Some trends in the occurrence of individual erroneous action were reported in Japan (Japanese Ministry of Health, Labor & Welfare, 2003; Tokyo Women's Medical University, 2003), in Europe and the US (WHO, 2000; WHO, 2001), but adequate countermeasures against organizational behavior have not yet developed because of the complex and uncertain structure of the problems (Mckee & Healy, 2002). The contextuality of individual erroneous action is to be disclosed and to be asked the reason why she/ he has to take such an action. Focuses were placed on organizational management design for the identification of the relation between performance reliability and organizational control mode and for enhancing healthcare quality and security as one of the solutions in hospitals changing for coping with problematic situations of organizational management. This chapter is organized into two parts. First, we explain key concepts in this chapter, i.e., organizational control mode and cognitive activity in the relation with performance reliability. Second, we summarize the case study carried out in a national hospital in Japan by illustrating the linkages among cognitive activity of clinical demands, work environment and organizational climate. Finally, we emphasize the importance of the latent variables embedded in the organizational environment and the assessment of performance reliability influenced by the organizational control mode as mentioned in the case study.

PERFORMANCE RELIABILITY AND ORGANIZATIONAL CONTROL MODES

Most of the erroneous actions and inefficient actions in social services cause the organizational situation insufficiently supported for service/care-providers to take action. Higher job-competency of an individual is primarily required in any job areas in society and care-providers, like other professional workers, are continuously required to develop their professional knowledge and to enhance their practical skills in the course

Figure 1: Contextual Control Mode of Cognition (Hollnage, 1993)

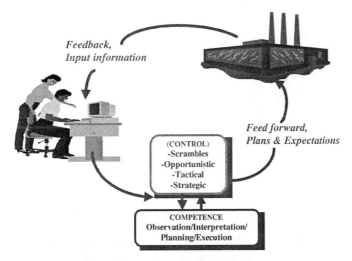

of professional experience. As in the theory of the contextual control model of cognition (Hollnagel, 1993), reliability of work performance is predicted by an individual provider's cognitive competency (observation, interpretation, planning, execution) related with the organizational control modes (scrambled, opportunistic, tactical and strategic) of the enterprise where they work (*Figure 1*). Human performance reliability is tantamount to cognitive reliability in information processing while working. The essential elements of cognition adopted in The Simple Model of Cognition (Hollnagel, 1991), such as observation, interpretation, planning/choice and action/execution are considered to be main action steps in cognitive information processing work. Incidental and erroneous actions in a hospital may occur in any steps of cognition related with any type of organizational control modes.

FOUR TYPES OF ORGANIZATIONAL CONTROL MODE AND OCCURRENCE PREDICTION OF ERRONEOUS BEHAVIOR

There is a large difference in work performance reliability between in the organization adequately controlled and in the organization inadequately controlled. Organizational control is classified into four types of control mode: scrambled, opportunistic, tactical and strategic by common performance conditions (CPC's) consisting of nine working conditions which were developed by Hollnagel (1998). We will mention about the CPC's hereinafter in the method of case study. The mode of scrambled is a disorganized situation in which erroneous behaviors and failures occur very likely. The mode of opportunistic is loosely organized, with no planning and with limited chance of success. The tactical is well-organized, but limited planning with good reliability. The strategic is the state of being highly organized with high reliability. Performance reliability intervals in each mode of organizational control were also determined by Hollnagel for predicting action failure (Hollnagel, 1998). Predicting models of human erroneous action which have been popularly used in the industrial field are developed by the relation with generic tasks and associated error probabilities (Reason, 1997; Rasmussen et al., 1994). It is our thought that the methodology developed by Hollnagel is effective to identify human erroneous actions reported in the field of medical and healthcare for predicting performance reliability of care-providers engaging in hospital work and for forecasting health-care quality and security which people require.

PERFORMANCE RELIABILITY AND COGNITIVE ACTIVITY OF CLINICAL DEMANDS

Cognition-action coupling is formed both in the feedback process and in the feed-forward process in information processing work. It is in the feed-forward process for actors to interpret the information and to make judgments to decide for selecting final action. This means that latent failures resulted in feed-forward process are the main causation of erroneous behaviors and failures in the real field. It is our study hypothesis that care-providers take action in the relationship among cognitive activity of clinical demands, nursing work environment and organizational safety climate/culture in the feed-forward process. Articulate knowledge of the observed variables in the feedback

Figure 2: Cognition-Action Coupling Process in the Relation Among Nursing Activity Perceived, Work Environment and Organizational Safety Climate (Saito, 2002)

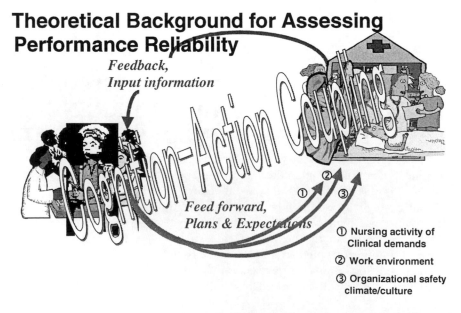

process and tacit knowledge of perceived nursing activity, perceived work environment and perceived organizational safety climate in the feed-forward process work together in the cognition-action coupling process as shown in *Figure 2*. Scenario or narrative analysis on the causal relationship among latent variables representing these three components is needed for redesigning the organization to attain its goal.

CASE STUDY IN JAPANESE NATIONAL HOSPITAL

Study Purposes

The purposes of the case study are: (1) to identify organizational control mode evaluated by nine conditions of the common performance conditions (CPC's) and cognitive function types which may give an effect on performance reliability, and to clarify the relationship between organizational control modes and the types of cognitive function; (2) to identify the latent factors on organizational safety climate, on nursing work environment and on cognitive activity of nursing demands, and to clarify the relationship among these variables; and (3) to propose the most stable covariance structure model representing the reality in the workplace, i.e., the model consisted of the construct variables of performance reliability as an endogenous variable and of organizational safety climate as an exogenous variable with the intervening variable of work environment.

Study Hypotheses

Performance reliability is perceived in relation to cognitive resources of the individuals with workplace conditions and their organizational climate. Human knowledge representing cognitive resources is formulated in the recursive process of information processing of both articulate knowledge and tacit knowledge. Cognition-action coupling emerges in the recursive process in the perceptual world. Human action is formed in the perpetual step forward and step back process in the actual field, not in the single and particular process, nor in the predetermined process. As shown in *Figure 3*, our study hypothesis is that performance reliability perceived by care-providers is highly related with nursing activity of clinical demands, nursing work environment and organizational safety climate where they work. It is not independently determined by the individual resources, nor by technology. In this case study, performance reliability perceived is dealt with for predicting occurrence of erroneous behaviors in the real, working field.

Methods

1. Subjects surveyed are 356 registered nurses (average age ± SD, 35.7 ± 10.7) engaging in a national hospital providing approximately 700 beds and affiliated with a national university in Japan.
2. Self-administered questionnaire forms on organizational control and cognitive types developed by Hollnagel (1998) were applied for this study by revising and adding a few question items for the hospital surveyed. The modality of organiza-

Figure 3: Study Hypothesis in Perceptual World and Real World

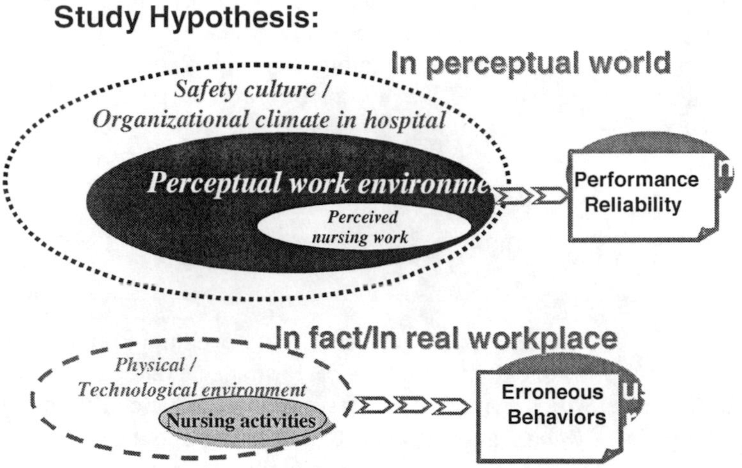

Study Hypothesis:

tional control was assessed by the scores of the CPCs composed by nine condi-tions, such as: (1) adequacy of organization, (2) working conditions, (3) adequacy of MMI (= Man-Machine Interface) and operational support, (4) adequacy of procedure, (5) number of simultaneous goals, (6) available time, (7) time of day, (8) adequacy of training and experience, and (9) crew collaboration quality, with a three to four point-scale in each condition. The other forms of the questionnaire on nursing work environment consisting of 34 question items with a four-point scale and nursing activity of clinical demands consisting of 35 question items with a four-point scale were prepared for this case study. The questionnaire on organizational safety climate/culture was prepared for this study by referring the questionnaire items on safety culture developed by Hosoda et al. (2000).

3.   The subjects were asked to report incident experience during their working days for three weeks by using the incident checklist prepared for this survey. This checklist form consisting of a total of 45 items was made by preparing several question items in each process of cognitive function in appreciation, judgment and execution.

Results and Discussion

1.   *Performance reliability by organizational control:* Reduced reliability and im-proved reliability were compared among four organizational control modes. As shown in *Figure 4*, average scores of reduced reliability were increased by organizational control mode, the highest score was in scrambled mode, while the lowest was in strategic mode. In improved reliability, the highest was in strategic mode, while the lowest was in scrambled as shown in *Figure 5*.

2.   *Cognitive activity types clustered and performance reliability:* Two asymmetric types of cognitive activity were obtained by clustering as shown in *Figure 6*. The higher factor loadings in observation and interpretation and the lower factor loadings in planning and execution of cognitive activity were obtained as the one type of cognition which was treated as Group 1 (N=191). The other type was treated

Figure 4: Average Score of Reduced Reliability by Organizational Control Mode

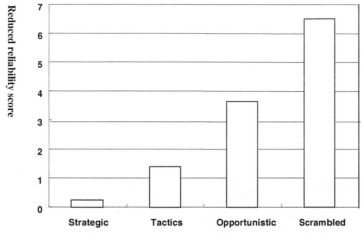

Performance reliability by organizational control

as Group 2 (N=170), where the lower factor loadings in observation and interpretation and the higher factor loadings in planning and execution were obtained. Significant difference in performance reliability was scarcely observed between these two groups.

3.   *Incident rates by organizational control and by cognitive activity type:* The subject numbers of the nurses who responded to the checklist were limited to 24 nurses in Group 1 and 74 nurses in Group 2. The incident experience was compared among four modes of organizational control. It was found that the incident rate (number of incident experiences/number of nurses) in tactical mode was so high that it exceeded the dotted line of the prediction curve of performance reliability,

Figure 5: Average Score of Improved Reliability by Organizational Control Mode

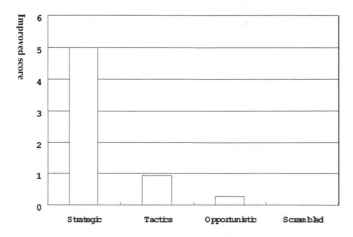

Figure 6: Two Assymetric Groups by Clustering Cognitive Behavior

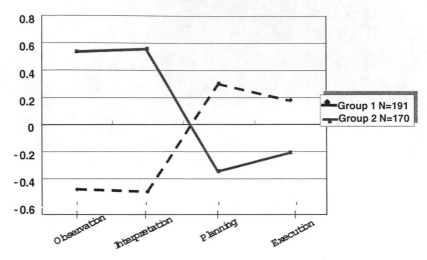

Figure 7: Incident Rate by Organizational Control Mode and by Work Competency Representing Cognitive Function During Providing Nursing Care

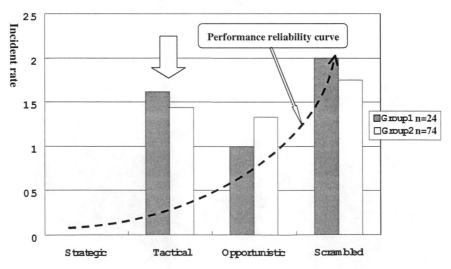

as shown in *Figure 7*. This result suggested that some problematic situations may exist in tactical mode and some counter measures should be taken.

4.   *Incident rates by time series in the day:* By comparing the occurrence of the number of incidents reported in every 30 minutes from 8:30 in the morning to 8:00 the next morning between tactical and opportunistic control modes, some problematic situations were disclosed as shown in *Figure 8* and *Figure 9*. The number of incidents reported in tactical mode were extremely high in the particular time at 10:00 in the morning when the nursing team was changing shifts with the next nursing team as shown in *Figure 8*, while in opportunistic control mode, dangerous spots appeared in any time of the day as shown in *Figure 9*. This particular time of the day, around 10:00 a.m. shown in *Figure 8*, was found out to be the spot for nurses to pay careful attention and to take action for harnessing the supporting systems

Figure 8: Incident Number Every 30 Minutes in Tactical Mode

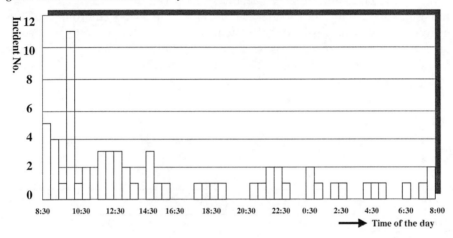

Figure 9: Incident Number Every 30 Minutes in Opportunistic Mode

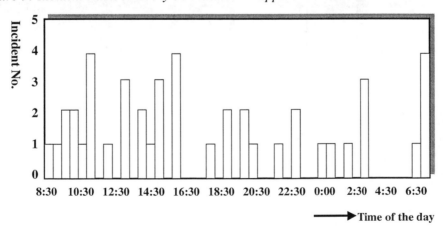

to cope with the high level of incidents and overcome the weak spot this in time series of the day. Fundamental counter measures must be taken in opportunistic mode of organizational control to cope with the random occurrence of incidents during the course of the day.

5.   *Correlation among the latent variables:* Nursing clinical demands, such as direct patient care and care planning extracted by Factor Analysis, are significantly related with cognitive function or activity. Job discretion as one of the latent factors of nursing work environment was significantly related with all the variables of cognitive activity and nursing clinical demands. Nursing work environment was also highly related with the latent factors of information feedback representing organizational safety culture. Two types of cognitive activity mentioned above were shown to have a higher relationship between observation and interpretation and between planning and execution. As correlation coefficients among all the variables in the case study are shown in *Table 1*, the antecedents in both reduced and improved reliability were embedded deep in the situations of the real field represented by organizational safety culture and nursing work environment. These analytical results suggested that the latent variables, i.e., the genotype of action are virtually related to appear as behavior in real field. This means that articulate knowledge is closely accompanied by tacit knowledge and works together in information processing.

Table 1: Correlation Coefficient Among the Variables Measured and Figures in Parentheses are Alpha Reliability Coefficients

	Human Reliability		CognitiveActivity				ClinicalDemands			Nurse Work Environment					Safety Culture		
	IMPROVED	REDUCED	Observation	Interpretation	Planning	Execution	CD1	CD2	CD3	NWE1	NWE2	NWE3	NWE4	NWE5	SC1	SC2	SC3
IMPROVED	□																
REDUCED	-0.297**	□															
Observation	0.113*		□														
Interpretation	0.153**	-0.160**	0.356**	(0.74)													
Planning					□												
Execution				0.147**	0.615**	(0.76)											
CD1 Direct pt. care			0.212**	0.196**	0.156**	0.247**	(0.83)										
CD2 Pt.care plan	0.105*		0.133**	0.262**	0.147**	0.185**		(0.76)									
CD3 Clinical tools	0.176**		0.107*						(0.70)								
NWE1 Team work	0.199**						0.160**		0.147**	(0.82)							
NWE2 Shared org.	0.265**	-0.177**					0.148**	0.125**	0.129*		(0.78)						
NWE3 Communication	0.148**	-0.254**	0.130**	0.183**			0.169**					(0.75)					
NWE4 Job discretion	0.128*		0.227**	0.233**	0.202**	0.245**	0.190**	0.415**	0.335**				(0.75)				
NWE5 Trad.nursing		0.120*	-0.205**	-0.240**										(0.44)			
SC1 Safety training	0.198**	-0.132*					0.199**	0.279**	0.160**	0.207**	0.151**	0.120*			(0.87)		
SC2 Information feedback	0.268**	-0.298**					0.136**	0.122*	0.247**	0.149*	0.462**	0.175**				(0.85)	
SC3 Safety documentation			0.113*	0.164**	0.255**		0.124*	0.245**	0.117*	0.164**		0.230**					(0.84)

$** p < 0.01$

$* p < 0.05$

6. *Cause-effect relationship among the latent variables:* Covariance structure models measured and selected are shown in *Table 2*. Among six trimmed models, two of them, M3-2 and M4-3I, were shown respectively in *Figures 10* and *11*. In the Model of M3-2 shown in *Figure 10*, information feedback (ξ^1) representing organizational safety climate gave significant direct effect ($\gamma = 0.47$, p < 0.01) on performance reliability (η^2) formed by two observed variables, X8 and X9 and also

Figure 10: Covariance Structure Model 3-2

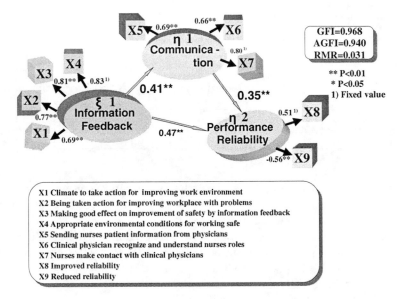

X1 Climate to take action for improving work environment
X2 Being taken action for improving workplace with problems
X3 Making good effect on improvement of safety by information feedback
X4 Appropriate environmental conditions for working safe
X5 Sending nurses patient information from physicians
X6 Clinical physician recognize and understand nurses roles
X7 Nurses make contact with clinical physicians
X8 Improved reliability
X9 Reduced reliability

Figure 11: Covariance Structure Model 4-3i

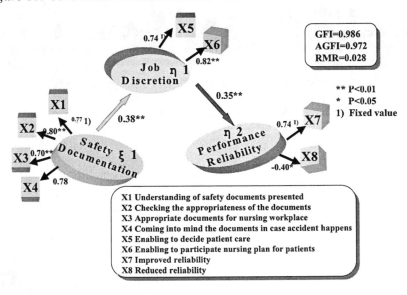

X1 Understanding of safety documents presented
X2 Checking the appropriateness of the documents
X3 Appropriate documents for nursing workplace
X4 Coming into mind the documents in case accident happens
X5 Enabling to decide patient care
X6 Enabling to participate nursing plan for patients
X7 Improved reliability
X8 Reduced reliability

Table 2: Covariance Structure Analysis Goodness-of-Fit Measurement for Each Model

	χ^2	p	GFI	AGFI	NFI	RMR	CFI	AIC
M3-2 *Communication-Feedback control*	52.956	0.001	0.968	0.940	0.952	0.031	0.973	94.956
M4-2 *Job discretion-Feedback control*	37.233	0.003	0.974	0.946	0.962	0.030	0.979	75.233
M3-3 *Communication-Safety documentation*	33.693	0.090	0.980	0.962	0.965	0.030	0.989	75.693
M3-3 i *Communication-Safety documentation*	35.458	0.080	0.979	0.962	0.963	0.033	0.989	75.458
M4-3 *Job discretion-Safety documentation*	18.293	0.371	0.987	0.973	0.978	0.021	0.998	56.293
M4-3 i *Job discretion-Safety documentation*	20.882	0.285	0.986	0.972	0.975	0.028	0.996	56.882

indirect effect ($\beta = 0.14$, p < 0.01) in the path of information feedback (ξ^1) through communication (η^1)) representing nursing work environment, and total effect ($\beta = 0.61$, p < 0.01) on performance reliability (η^2).

In the model of M4-3i shown in *Figure 11*, work discretion (η^1) representing nursing work environment gave significant effect ($\beta = 0.35$, P < 0.01) on performance reliability (η^2) formed by X7 and X8, and indirect effect ($\beta = 0.13$, P < 0.01) as the exogenous variable (ξ^1) of safety documentation representing organizational safety climate on performance reliability (η^2).

General Discussion

1. Performance reliability in hospital nurses was identified by applying human reliability analysis methods developed by Hollnagel. Nursing work environment was divided into four modes of organizational control (strategic, tactical, opportunistic and scrambled) as being similarly observed in industrial organizations. The highest reliability was in strategic control mode, while on the whole the lowest was in scrambled. Although performance reliability scores were scarcely related with the types of cognition, due to insufficient data collected in the case study, cognitive functions (observation, interpretation, planning, execution) in information processing are to be analyzed in the relation with performance reliability and organizational control.

2. Significant interrelation was observed between the latent variables extracted by FA, such as information feedback representing organizational safety climate and communication and shared organization representing nursing work environment with performance reliability. Work discretion representing nursing work environment was significantly related with all the latent factors of cognitive activity and nursing clinical demands. This result suggested that clarification of interaction

among the latent variables and narratives of the situation were of importance for service quality management and for improvement of performance reliability.

3.   The cause-effect models measured by Covariance Structure Analysis and selected were representative and accountable of reality in the nursing workplace. The structure of these models were formed in the relationship among organizational safety culture as exogenous variable, nursing work environment and performance reliability as endogenous variables. This result suggests that the states of organizational safety culture and nursing work environment have significant direct and indirect effects on performance reliability.

4.   The occurrence of incident experience could be decreased and avoided in the higher control of organizational environment, that is, in the strategic management harnessed by leadership and creative actions. This trend was observed in the hospital surveyed, as well as in the other fields we have so far conducted research (Saito et al., 2000, 2001, 2002). The authors would like to emphasize the importance of managing the latent factors in organizational and technological environments for improving human performance reliability which, we believe, brings along continuous quality of care and harnessing security in hospital nursing services. It is required to redesign the working environment to make it more flexible, adaptive for the nurses to behave in a discretionary manner and to enable to nurses to take strategic actions in the place where they work.

Limitations of this Study

1.   A larger number of subjects sampled than our samples in this case study are required to introduce a general model. The classification of cognitive function type that we have found in the case study will have to be confirmed in a future study.

2.   Private and other community hospitals may be placed in different situations, and nurses' roles and responsibilities, especially job discretion freedom for a professional care-provider are to be surveyed for organizational management to improve the quality of care and security.

FUTURE DIRECTIONS OF HEALTHCARE RESEARCH

1.   Job discretion, communication representing work environment and information feedback and safety documentation representing organizational safety climate are important factors as the determinants of human performance reliability. The trends in this case study of a national hospital are similar to the industrial fields we have so far observed. Future research on organizational environment is of importance to develop the management methodologies based on action research for improving human performance reliability. In so doing, it is inevitable to elaborate upon the analysis method to extract latent variables existing deep in their internal world, i.e., genotypes of the observing variables existing in the context of organization in parallel with articulate knowledge-based variables which are the phenotypes of the observed variables existing in the external universe.

2.   Study subjects to be included should not only be clients but also the other stakeholders with the same goal in the healthcare fields, so that team performance and organizational performance might be measured and assessed. Healthcare providing models in which both needs of care-providers and care-receivers are adequately supplied and the models which enable both to change in response to any transformation of organizational goals are required in order to be a participative type of organization.

REFERENCES

Hollnagel, E. (1993). *Human Reliability Analysis: Context and Control.* London: Academic Press.

Hollnagel, E. (1998). Search for causes: Retrospective analysis. *CREAM: Cognitive Reliability and Error Analysis Method,* Elsevier, 191-215.

Hollnagel, E. (1998). The Quantification of Prediction. *CREAM: Cognitive Reliability and Error Analysis Method,* Elsevier, 234-261.

Hollnagel, E. & Cacciabue, P. C. (1991, September). Cognitive modeling in system simulation. *Proceedings of Third European Conference on Cognitive Science Approaches to Process Control,* (September 2-6).

Hosoda et al. (2000). On human behavior under emergency. *Journal of Science of Labor,* 76, 519-538.

Japanese Ministry of Health, Labor & Welfare (n.d.). Retrieved from the World Wide Web: http://www.mhlw.go.jp/houdou.

Mckee, M. & Healy, J. (2002). *Hospitals in a Changing Europe.* Open University Press.

Rasmussen, J., Pejtersen, A. M. & Goodsterin, L. P. (1994). *Cognitive Systems Engineering.* London: John Wiley and Sons.

Reason, J. (1997). *Managing the Risks of Organizational Accidents.* Ashgate Publishing.

Saito, M., Ikeda, M. & Seki, H. (2000). A study on adaptive action development: Interference of mood states with perceived performance and perceived efficacy. *Proceeding of the 14th International Congress of Ergonomics,* San Diego, (vol. 5, pp. 48-51).

Saito, M., Inoue, T. & Seki, H. (2002). Organizational control and erroneous behavior in hospital nurses. *Proceedings of the 2nd International Conference on Management of Healthcare and Medical Technology,* IIT in Chicago (July 28-30).

Saito, M., Inoue, T., Seki, H. & Ikeda, M. (2001). *The Effect of Mood States on Perceived Performance and on Perceived Health.* International Congress on Work Life in the 21st Century, Oct 15-17, Helsinki.

Tokyo Women's Medical University (n.d.). Retrieved from the World Wide Web: http://www.twmu.ac.jp/.

WHO. (2000). *The World Health Report 2000. Health Systems: Improving Performance.* Geneva: WHO.

WHO. (2001). *WHO European Health for All Databases.* Copenhagen: WHO Regional Office for Europe.

Chapter XV

Tele-Medicine:
Building Knowledge-Based Tele-Health Capability in New Zealand

Nabeel A. Y. Al-Qirim, Auckland University of Technology, New Zealand

ABSTRACT

This chapter reviews the strategic planning of health information systems in New Zealand. This step is deemed necessary to identify the main accelerators and/or impediments that influence technology adoption and diffusion in health organisations in New Zealand. This research introduces the tele-medicine technology as one possible solution to provide continuous, quality, and immediate medical care to rural patients and to encourage networking among the different hospitals in New Zealand. This research suggests that in order to realise tele-medicine benefits in health care delivery in New Zealand, certain issues need to be addressed such as implementing comprehensive cost-benefit analysis and identifying the benefits sought from adopting the tele-medicine technology. The New Zealand context is unique and this perspective with respect to tele-medicine adoption and success is addressed in this research.

INTRODUCTION

Information systems (NZHIS, 1995a; NZHIS, 1995b; NZHIS, 1996; Neame, 1995; Austin, Trim & Sobczak, 1995; Conrad & Shorttel, 1996), information technology (IT) (Bomba, Cooper & Miller, 1995) and technology (Little & Carland, 1991) have been emphasised as strategic tools for enhancing health care delivery and for improving performance, leading to optimised services and efficiencies. However, the New Zealand studies (NZHIS, 1995a; NZHIS, 1995b; NZHIS, 1996; Neame, 1995) indicate that the sector is "relatively devolved," with purchasing contracts being the main mechanisms to drive sector-wide change at the provider level. Much of the information needed is unavailable in the form needed or at the time that it is needed most. This in part is related to gaps in the conceptual understanding of service delivery, which is in this sector is a very complex business, spanning what has been an extensive range of relatively autonomous functional areas. But it is also due to a lack of reliable information about outcomes, effectiveness and actual costs on which improvements can be based. Because of this lack of empirical data, the tools for dealing with this complexity, and understanding what happens and why, are deficient (NZHIS, 1996). Various organisational issues and the lack of coordination at the national level were also identified. Expertise in health information management and systems is limited. Currently few health and disability sector personnel have the knowledge and skills to understand the issues or to make informed judgements about the validity of the advice they obtain.

New Zealand is not alone in this situation and different countries are facing similar difficulties although the severity of this situation varies from one country to another (Austin, 1992; Bakos & Tracy, 1986; Shortell, Morrison & Friedman, 1990; Topping & Hernandez, 1991; Conrad & Shortell, 1996). This literature points to different organisational, technological, and environmental impediments in adopting and in making use of IS/IT in organisations (Austin, 1992; Austin, Trimm & Sobczak, 1995; Ward, Griffiths & Whitmore, 1990). The 23 Health and Hospital Services (HHSs)[1] that exist all over New Zealand are no longer in competition with each other or paid in principal according to the number of people they care for. The competition from the few private hospitals has no effect on them. Ever-lacking government funds (Neame, 1995) are faced with further reduction on the medical portfolio by reducing or eliminating less priority and less life threatening services for the sake of introducing important new ones. The various gaps that exist between the various stakeholders and the lack of a leader (e.g., the government) to coordinate between the different HHSs result in having 23 different information systems that eventually do not interact with one another.

Diminishing funds from the government and cost control mechanisms have led to the need for alternative and more cost-effective means of providing care (Edelstein, 1999; Neame, 1995). In many cases, this has become necessary for survival (Edelstein, 1999) in order to sustain the increased competition among health care providers. The business of health care has become so competitive in different countries that many small rural hospitals are trying to align themselves with larger tertiary care centres in a community health-information network, a tele-medicine network, or some other type of partnership in order to survive and to retain their local patients (Huston & Huston, 2000). Within these challenges, tele-medicine emerge as one possible solution to New Zealand health providers in reaching out to rural patients (Charles, 2000; Harris, Donaldson & Campbell, 2001), to areas where patient volumes for certain services are limited (Edelstein, 1999), to conduct administrative and clinical meetings, and to conduct different training courses to patients (smoke treatment centres), doctors, nurses, and other medical staffs (Perednia & Allen, 1995; Wayman, 1994).

Tele-medicine means medicine from a distance where distant and dispersed patients are brought closer to their medical providers through the means of telecommunication technologies (Charles, 2000; OTA, 1995; Noring, 2000; Perednia & Allen, 1995; Wayman, 1994). Noring (2000) provided an interesting comparison between the former definition for tele-medicine and tele-health. This researcher defined the term tele-health as expanding the capacity of tele-medicine to provide the full continuum of care, from health promotion and disease prevention through curative treatment and terminal care. This term also implies including non-physician-based health care providers.

Tele-medicine covers a wide spectrum of benefits through the use of video conferencing (VC) technology in areas such as consultations, diagnostics, therapeutic, transfer of patient-related records, case management, training, and meetings. Researchers envision tele-medicine to be an important building block in the strategic plan of many health care organizations (Charles, 2000). In a rural setting, tele-medicine could help New Zealand health providers in supplying quality, fast, and economical medical services to rural patients and hence save doctors and patients valuable time wasted in commuting long distances. Specialists could utilise this extra time in seeing more patients at the main hospital.

Thus, this research is interested in introducing the tele-medicine technology as one of the strategic building blocks of Health and Disability Information Systems (HDISs) integration across the different health care providers in New Zealand. This research is interested in achieving the following objectives:

1.   Highlight the status of tele-medicine in New Zealand.
2.   Highlight the importance of tele-medicine to health care providers in New Zealand and elsewhere. Identifying the accelerators and/or the impediments that influence tele-medicine success could assist health care providers in New Zealand and elsewhere in planning their adoption and use of tele-medicine. This research utilises the technological innovation literature as a guiding theoretical framework in highlighting these factors.

Before expanding on the potential benefits of tele-medicine to health care providers, the following section examines the status of tele-medicine in New Zealand.

TELE-MEDICINE IN NEW ZEALAND

One of the early initiatives that emerged in 1993 within Northland HHS was transmitting radiology images between two hospitals using leased telephone lines. Tele-medicine has been investigated by most of the health providers in New Zealand. The entire crown-owned hospitals in New Zealand are managed by regional organisations known as Health and Hospital Services (HHS)[2]. Some HHS regions have one hospital and others have more than one. In the North Island, Waitemata Health has three video teleconferencing systems. Two of those systems are used in psychiatry and the third one is used in administrative and training purposes (ADMN). Health Waikato has two VC systems. Two of these systems are used in dermatology and the third one is used in ADMN. Northland Health Ltd (Whangarei) has two VC systems and another two PC-based VC. These systems are used in psychiatry and ADMN. Starship Children's Hospital (part of Auckland Healthcare Services) is in the process of establishing a national tele-paediatric network across the 23 HHSs and already started with a pilot project. Middlemore Hospital (South Auckland Health) has one group VC system for

ADMN. Auckland University School of Medicine has one group VC system for training purposes and for conducting regular clinical meetings with other CHEs in New Zealand. Lakeland Health, LTD has two group video-teleconferencing systems for ADMN purposes.

In the South Island, Coast Health Care, LTD has three VC systems used in paediatrics, psychiatry, and ADMN.—HYPERLINK "canterburyhlth.html"—Canterbury Health, Ltd (Christchurch) has one video-conferencing system for paediatrics and for ADMN purposes. Healthlink South, LTD (Christchurch) has two group systems for psychiatry and ADMN. –HYPERLINK "hlthsthcant.html"—Health South Canterbury, Ltd (Timaru), Healthcare Otago, LTD, –HYPERLINK "nelsonmarlboro.html"—Nelson-Marlborough Health Services, LTD, and Southern Health, LTD each have one group system. Otago University in Dunedin is using it for training in their school of medicine. It is interesting to know that there is a level of cooperation among CHEs in the South Island in the areas of psychiatry and paediatrics.

A stock-take of the VC technology in these hospitals reveals that medical schools in New Zealand were among the early adopters and users of the technology. Out of the 23 HHSs in New Zealand, only 12 have actively adopted tele-medicine. The adopted systems ranged between one and four tele-medicine systems with the majority of HHSs adopting one system only. Those HHSs that adopted one tele-medicine system use it mostly for general purposes such as managerial meetings, case discussions and occasionally for clinical training. Such initiatives were described as being initial and experimental. Where an HHS owned more than one tele-medicine system, it was oriented for clinical purposes such as psychiatry, paediatric, and dermatology areas. Hence, an attempt is being made to adopt tele-medicine to provide prompt, inexpensive, and quality medical care to geographically dispersed patients, which was otherwise not possible.

TELE-MEDICINE: A BACKGROUND

The first tele-medicine initiative employing interactive television sessions for medical purposes emerged in 1959 by using a microwave link for tele-psychiatry consultations between the Nebraska Psychiatric Institute in Omaha and the state mental hospital 112 miles away (Perednia & Allen, 1995). In the late 1980s tele-medicine was being used routinely to deliver general health services to remote regions of Norway (Noring, 2000). In the US, interest in tele-medicine was initially focused on use in the military, in space programs, on off-shore oil rigs, in prisons, and in rural areas (Noring, 2000). It seems the opportunities provided by tele-medicine inspired many innovative ideas. For example, BMI British Midland has become the first airline to install tele-medical technology on planes making long-haul flights to the US Virgin Atlantic has also purchased the system and will start installing it in long-haul aircraft this year. The device monitors blood pressure via a wrist cuff, pulse rate, temperature via an ear probe, electrocardiogram, blood oxygen and carbon dioxide levels. Using a modem, this data is sent to physicians who can advise the crew on what action to take (Anonymous, 2002).

Since tele-medicine's inception in the 1950s, Perednia and Allen (1995) reported limited growth and pointed to the fact that only few tele-medicine projects were instituted in the 1970s and 1980s at several sites in North America and Australia. They confirmed that none of the programs begun before 1986 has survived. Although data is limited, the early reviews and evaluations of these programs suggest that the equipment was reasonably effective at transmitting the information needed for most clinical uses and that users were for the most part satisfied. However, when external sources of funding were withdrawn, the programs disappeared, indicating that the single most important cause of their failure was the inability to justify these programs on a cost-benefit basis. Other issues, such as limited physician acceptance, played a less significant role in their downfall (Perednia & Allen, 1995).

The views about tele-medicine effectiveness in the medical area vary from one adopter to another. Depending on one's viewpoint, tele-medicine can be seen as a valuable tool for providing immediate specialty care services to rural areas, a more efficient use of existing medical resources, a way to attract patients living outside a hospital's normal service area, a way of bringing international health care dollars. On the other hand, others could see it as a serious misallocation of increasingly scarce health care dollars (Perednia & Allen, 1995). This challenge needs to be resolved by highlighting the importance of the tele-medicine technology in a rural setting specifically.

In review of the literature it was observed that despite the rapid growth and high visibility of tele-medicine projects in health care (Grigsby & Allen, 1997), few patients are actually being seen through tele-medicine for medical purposes. In almost every tele-medicine project, tele-consultation accounts for less than 25% of the use of the system (Perednia & Allen, 1995). The majority of the online time is used for medical education and administration (Wayman, 1994; Perednia & Allen, 1995; Hassol, 1996). The low level of usage can be explained in part by the federal government's position on reimbursement for tele-medicine consultations (Hassol, 1996). However, this author did not find any association between reimbursement and tele-medicine utilisation in this research. Other issues need to be resolved first before the different benefits of tele-medicine can be realised. These unresolved important issues revolve around how successful tele-medicine can be in providing quality health care at an affordable cost and whether it is possible to develop a sustainable business model that could maintain profitability over time. This depends on (Perednia & Allen, 1995): (1) clinical expectations, (2) matching technology to medical needs, (3) economic factors like reimbursement, (4) legal (e.g., restrictions of medical practices across state lines (licensure) and issues of liabilities), and social (e.g., changing physician behaviours and traditional practices and workflow) issues (Anderson, 1997), and (5) organisational factors. These issues are discussed in the following sections.

TELE-MEDICINE ADOPTION: A THEORETICAL FRAMEWORK

Larsen (1998) states that information systems innovations are considered key enablers for business innovativeness. On the other hand, he asserted that the increased rate of failure among IS projects within organisations calls for an increased understanding about IS innovations (Moore & Benbasat, 1991). Innovation can be defined as an idea, practice or product that is perceived as new by the potential adopters even if it had existed earlier elsewhere (Rogers, 1995). The recent success and emergence of tele-medicine using the video conferencing (VC) technology in the early 1990s is an innovative

Table 1: Innovation Characteristics

Innovation Characteristics
1. *Relative advantage:* the degree to which using technology is perceived as being better than using its precursor of practices.
2. *Complexity:* the degree to which technology is perceived as being easy to use.
3. *Compatibility:* the degree to which using technology is perceived as being consistent with the existing values, and past experiences of the potential adopter.
4. *Trialability:* the degree to which technology may be experimented with on a limited basis before adoption.
5. *Observability:* the degree to which the results of using technology are observable to others.
6. *Cost:* the degree to which technology is perceived as cost effective.

approach of its adoption for medical purposes. In search for models that would explain technologies adopted by organizations, Rogers' (Rogers, 1983, 1995) model appeared to be the most widely accepted model by researchers in identifying critical characteristics for innovations (Moore & Benbasat, 1991, 1996; Premkumar & Roberts, 1999; Thong, 1999). Rogers classical adoption model is made up of the following factors: relative advantage, complexity, compatibility, observability, and trialability (*Table 1*). The results of using tele-medicine (observability) are quite observable to the different hospitals and have been highly publicised by the literature (Al-Qirim, 2002; Grigsby & Allen, 1997). Cost has been outlined as an important determinant of adoption by Rogers (1995) and other researchers (Bacon, 1992; Elliot, 1996; Tornatzky & Klein, 1982) (*Figure 1*).

In the following, the different factors that influence tele-medicine success are reviewed in the light of the technological innovation literature. Further identification of these factors that facilitate and/or hinder adoption and diffusion of tele-medicine could help HHSs and policymakers in New Zealand and elsewhere in adopting tele-medicine and in overcoming different barriers that could hinder its adoption.

Relative Advantage

Table 2 identifies some of the stakeholders involved in tele-medicine adoption and depicts their perception about tele-medicine advantages in comparison with their earlier practices (Al-Qirim, 2002; Perednia & Allen, 1995; Wayman, 1994).

1.   issues concerning patient's privacy;
2.   specialists may reject extending their knowledge to rural doctors (profession protection) (Gammon, 1994);
3.   some physicians prefer ambulatory services as a way to break a way from the hospital's stressful environment; and
4.   some busy doctors tend to see tele-medicine as an extra burden (Gammon, 1994).

The most extensive use of tele-medicine has been to support continuing education over VC. Many more doctors and nurses are now able to attend conferences or classes because the direct (travel) and indirect (out-of-office) costs are decreased (Wayman, 1994). This raises concerns about the main objective(s) of tele-medicine and how it is perceived in the minds of the adopters. Is it a teaching utility or a patient care utility?

Table 2: Tele-Medicine Advantage

Stake Holder	Practices with tele-medicine	Earlier practices	Remarks
Specialists	Seeing patients one-on-one through poor clarity video screen, ISDN connection keeps disconnecting.	One-on-one, in person	Disadvantage
	Studio scheduling and moving to studio	No need, regular appointments in physician's office.	Disadvantage
	Second opinion from expert	No or not easy or cheap option Off-line, local	Advantage
	Case discussion and management		Advantage
	Immediate reporting from video	Immediate and accurate from the patient	Disadvantage
	Could record session (legal & judicial reviews)	Difficult	Advantage (1)
	Meeting rural doctors	Difficult	Advantage (2)
	Training rural doctors	Longer time	Advantage (2)
	Time optimisation (reduced ambulatory)	Longer waiting time	Advantage (3,4)
	Less waiting time for rural patients	More referrals	Advantage
	Fewer referrals to specialists	Increased	Advantage
	Reduced turnover of medical staff at rural areas – they feel less isolated from the outside world		Advantage
	Logistics: Seeing rural patients over video reducing waste (time, traveling, lodging, etc.).	Travel to patient	Advantage (3)
	Lost supplementary income	Supplementary income	Disadvantage
Management	Meeting rural managerial staff, managerial training	Difficult	Advantage
Patients	See specialist over the video with the presence of rural medical staff	Commute to central specialist or wait for specialist to come to rural	Advantage

Although the former leads eventually to better care and stable physicians at rural areas, the latter is envisioned to be the ultimate goal.

Cost Effectiveness

There will be no advantage in adopting tele-medicine if the investment is not justifiable in terms of its acceptable financial returns. On the other hand, healthcare providers in general, including New Zealand, emphasise the importance of providing quality care and preserving human's well-being. Thus, making the cost element one factor in the adoption decision of tele-medicine, but not the most important one. On the other hand, hospitals have limited resources and hence, it is feared that hospitals would assess the tele-medicine technology as a non-priority medical technology (Al-Qirim, 2002), which emphasises the need to strike a balance between its financial feasibility and its advantages. Let us not forget that tele-medicine is an ideal technology in a rural setting, which makes the cost element insignificant to a certain degree for various reasons. Rural areas typically experience a severe shortage in specialist staff. This is due to vast rural areas to service, poor payment levels for this specialty, significant difficulty in recruitment and retention, and the professional isolation specialists experience in rural areas are some of the reasons (Al-Qirim, 2002; Charles, 2000; Harris et al., 2001).

The potential importance of tele-medicine in impacting the health and the welfare of rural communities is tremendous. The estimates of the percentage of tele-medicine patient candidates who can be retained by the rural hospital vary between 50% and 80% (Wayman, 19945). This patient retention not only has a direct, positive effect on the rural hospital and rural physician, but also on the area economy. The average dollar in a rural community circulates seven times; each patient trip to receive speciality consultation encounters costs in gas, lodging, and food, not to mention lost wages for the patient and assisting family/friends (Wayman, 1994). Early intervention has often proved to be less expensive in the long run, so access to specialty care via tele-medicine can ultimately result in decreased healthcare costs to rural areas (Huston & Huston, 2000).

Despite the ongoing evaluations of tele-medicine feasibility in healthcare and the different attempts to measure the costs and benefits of using the tele-medicine technology, there are still not enough data to provide accurate estimates of tele-medicine costs (Huston & Huston, 2000). Another important point to indicate here is that sometimes and according to the internal policy of certain hospitals the financial benefits are hidden or intangibles and difficult to calculate. Direct costs such as the cost of equipment, training, maintenance and ongoing support, upgrades, and ongoing telecommunications are quite obvious and indeed resemble the major costs involved in any tele-medicine project. In a recent research study in the US it was suggested that reimbursement and the cost of telecommunications were identified as the most important barriers of tele-medicine adoption (Grigsby & Allen, 1997).

Perednia and Allen (1995) indicate that current literature tackling tele-medicine has failed in addressing its cost-effectiveness on the basis of its use: as a diagnostic tool and/ or as a therapeutic tool and/or case management tool. This further complicates the cost/ benefit formula. The concern would be whether tele-medicine is used in the correct place initially and whether it is being used effectively in any of the above three areas. It is essential in the process of adopting certain tele-medicine technology to choose the right one that matches the hospital needs. Using tele-medicine to transmit video when the case necessitates that (i.e., psychiatry, physical and occupational therapy, orthopedics, some neurology applications, etc.), text when appropriate (i.e., lab reports, patient histories and physicals, dietary evaluations, insurance information, medication histories, etc.) using email, still images (i.e., X-rays, pathology slides, lab specimen slides, CTs, MRIs, lung scans and ultra sounds) using scanners or still digital camera or fax machines, and audio (i.e., electronic stethoscope) using telephone or email. It is of utmost importance to remember that most diseases do not move and hence, there is no need for real time and full motion VC equipment (Perednia & Allen, 1995; Wayman, 1994).

Resources available for medical care are limited and the use of expensive tele-medicine technologies will reduce the total number of tele-medicine sites that can be installed regionally or nationally. While use of the latest and most powerful equipment may seem logical, the early adoption of two-way, full-motion video may be unrealistic for many rural and under-served areas (Perednia & Allen, 1995). This is due to logistical reasons concerning the quality of telecommunication lines provided to rural areas (Charles, 2000).

Evidence suggests that other forms of cost control initiatives in the US such as the establishment of health maintenance organisations (HMO) and managed care have a significant effect in the adoption of more technologies and systems than others (Baker & Wheeler, 1998). In the US, most cost-effective applications are those that are paid for by insurers, such as the use of tele-medicine for radiology, prisoner healthcare[3], psychiatry, and home healthcare. Other applications enhance access to care but are not cost effective because third-party payers (e.g., HMO) do not pay for related costs for professional fees or the implementation of the technology (Charles, 2000; Huston & Huston, 2000). However, this situation does not apply to New Zealand because healthcare providers are paid ultimately by the government to provide healthcare services to patients in the regions they serve.

There are different ways to reduce the huge expenses in setting and running the tele-medicine sites and recent research suggests that some hospitals tend to promote other services through their tele-medicine network (i.e., like renting the facility to private entities and offices in rural areas to connect to their central offices) or encourage other health providers within and outside the hospital to join them and share the facility (Al-Qirim, 2002; Perednia & Allen, 1995).

Compatibility

Perhaps the greatest dilemma associated with all these changes is how to ensure that innovations in the process of delivering care are not achieved at the expense of sacrificing widely accepted values of what constitutes the humanity of care (Noring, 2000).

Tornatzky and Klein (1982) in their meta-analysis found compatibility features to be an important determinant of adoption. Rogers' (1995) compatibility characteristic is highly stressed here because past research in healthcare (Austin, 1992; Austin, Trimm & Sobczak, 1995) considered the problem relating to physicians accepting IS for clinical purposes. The use of computers and cameras suggests a shift away from the one-on-one personal interaction now viewed as essential and desirable in healthcare delivery (*Table 2*). Issues such as "Surgeon syndrome" which is conservatism towards all other technologies than one's own was highlighted as an impediment to the adoption of tele-medicine (Gammon, 1994). Some view it as an alternative to lack of care or treatment altogether; others view it as a dramatic quality and efficiency improvement to current levels of care (Wayman, 1994). On the other hand, these significant changes to the physician's and patient's treatment environment (i.e., one-to-one through the VC *Vs*. one-on-one and in person) are expected to create resistance for the tele-medicine technology (Al-Qirim, 2002). For example, recent research found that in an extreme case, one of the clinical staff in the rural area almost fainted when she saw herself in the television screen of the VC equipment (Al-Qirim, 2002). It is important that the changes introduced by tele-medicine be compatible with the hospital's value, practice, and experience to ensure its successful adoption. Issues such as gradual introduction and motivation are highly envisaged here.

The concern is that physicians are reluctant to accept the technology. Gammon (1994) suggested that doctors in general and specialists, specifically, would be the single most influential group affecting the diffusion process of tele-medicine. Gammon (1994) distinguished between two groups of physicians: expertise delivering physicians and expertise receiving physicians. The first group consists primarily of specialists at central hospitals who either, have ambulated (conducted outside treatment visits or operations) visits and enjoyed supplementary income[4] or have contributed significantly to hospital income by treating guest patients from neighboring municipalities. By carrying out distant consultations, they experience a reduction in income both for themselves and for their hospital. Furthermore, some physicians have shown a negative attitude toward allowing receiving (primarily rural) hospitals to participate (via VC) in medical meetings, while they are positive towards participating in similar meetings when they themselves are recipients. Physicians working in environments characterised by overload and stress will most likely perceive implementation of tele-medicine as an additional burden. This, coupled with tele-medicine's replacement of ambulatory, as well as a possible fall in income will muster their resistance to tele-medicine, if not absolute sabotage towards the implementation of tele-medicine (Gammon, 1994). Development of reasonable incentives as well as measures for integrating tele-medicine into the working environment will be an important step.

Security and legal issues are some of the impediments to the success of tele-medicine in New Zealand (*Table 2*). The security of patient's data and VC encounters are important issues and need to be addressed. Legal issues relating to operating a tele-medicine network including corporate practice of medicine, patient confidentiality and privacy, malpractice, informed consent, licensure and credentialing, intellectual property, funder's (Medicare and Medicaid) payment, fraud and abuse, medical device regulation, and antitrust (price fixing) (Edelstein, 1999) are some of the major issues, which could bring any tele-medicine project to a complete halt. However, countries such as the US are well ahead in addressing these issues (Edelstein, 1999). Edelstein (1999) reports that in one session of the American Congress, 22 pieces of legislation relating to tele-medicine were introduced. Four tele-medicine-related bills have been introduced in the 106th Congress.

Complexity

Complexity in the case of tele-medicine could be divided into two parts: Firstly, complexity relating to technical limitations in the VC equipment and bandwidth. Buying the wrong or ill-specified technology such as not presenting clear picture and voice or the different components in the VC equipment are not fully compatible with each other may result in frustrating the users. Selecting the right communication technology and bandwidth such as ISDN, ADSL, and Bridges is essential in order to have clear images and voice, file download/upload, and a valid and reliable connection, respectively. It should be noted here that installing the VC equipment needs a special room with specialised lighting and acoustic system. Secondly, user's complexity is related to the ease-of-use and to the simplicity of the VC equipment. Providing appropriate training courses earlier on could assist in removing lots of the misperceptions about the complexity of the equipment. This part should not be confused with the compatibility characteristic above, such as convincing the specialists moving from their offices or clinicians to the VC theatre. It could be argued here that the perceived complexity of the VC equipment could lead to incompatible perceptions amongst clinicians. Recent research examining the acceptance of the tele-medicine technology amongst physicians suggests that perceived usefulness was found to be a significant determinant of attitude and intention to adopting tele-medicine. However, the perceived ease of use was not significant (Hu, Chau, Sheng & Tam, 1999).

Trialability

Another important point here is the issue of trying and experimenting with the tele-medicine system before adopting it. Tele-medicine involves a considerable investment in buying the equipment and the training to know how to use it. Most importantly, it should be integrated into the hospital environment in general and in the clinical area specifically to witness its effectiveness. According to the reported challenges above, trying the system in the intended real setting could provide initial and vital signs, which could assist decision-makers in making accurate decisions concerning adopting or rejecting the technology. This makes the limited trialing of the system not sufficient to yield useful results. The issue here is whether the different HHSs are willing to make this involving step or whether the suppliers will accept lending their equipment for a considerable time to HHS to trial their system — and hence remains unanswered.

DISCUSSION AND CONCLUSIONS

If tele-health services are properly introduced and based on evidence of effectiveness, *"... telehealth has the capacity to improve the quality of healthcare, provide equity of access to healthcare services, and reduce the cost of delivering healthcare"* (Noring, 2000).

This research introduced the importance of adopting the tele-medicine technology by healthcare providers in New Zealand specifically. Tele-medicine represents a great opportunity for healthcare providers in New Zealand to network and to provide integrated healthcare and administrative services to rural areas specifically. This could provide important surrogates to the different gaps existing in the HDIS of the different HHSs in New Zealand. The lack of coordination and cooperation between the different HHSs in New Zealand needs to be resolved in order for this integration to succeed.

This research relied on the technological innovation literature to guide the development of the different factors that could accelerate or impede tele-medicine adoption. These factors are important to the strategic adoption and use of tele-medicine by the different HHSs in New Zealand and elsewhere. Tele-medicine introduces various clinical and administrative advantages as highlighted in this research and these advantages could be focused in delivering quality care and services to rural patients and physicians. However, as a precursor to adoption, it is important to identify the particular advantages sought from tele-medicine, taking into consideration the adoption context and the actual needs of the different HHSs. In a worst-case scenario, tele-medicine enables specialists in the main hospital give second opinions or allow for efficient follow-up and case management. If the costs involved in adopting and running the tele-medicine project were not planned well, the whole project could be brought to a complete standstill. Considering issues such as running costs and hidden costs needs to be identified earlier on. Issues pertaining to the complexity of the technology and to its compatibility with the physician's working environment needs to be addressed with more emphasis put on the latter as it could prove detrimental to the whole success of the tele-medicine project. Therefore, providing a framework where physicians are encouraged to accept and use the technology in providing healthcare services to patients and to other rural physicians is highly stressed here.

New Zealand's small area and population (3.82 million) (NZStat, 2001) could lessen the impact of many of the big challenges that hinder tele-medicine adoption in countries such as the US. Issues like licensure and reimbursement are major impediments in the US but not in New Zealand. There is one legal system in New Zealand and hence, interstate legalities and boundaries are large issues in the US but not in New Zealand. New Zealand has a sophisticated telecommunication (networks, mobile) infrastructure, which could serve the large-scale diffusion of tele-medicine across the different HHSs. This research demonstrated that tele-medicine provides various advantages and its potential in reducing costs at different levels has been established. It is important to further assess the strategic importance of tele-medicine within the different HHSs and at the national level in New Zealand. This task is quite achievable and requires the involvement of the different stakeholders highlighted in this research. Creating a national strategic plan aiming at identifying opportunities with respect to speciality-care, rural coverage and medical needs, and other administrative objectives could assist in driving the health sector forward and in providing fast and quality care to rural patients in the first place and to all New Zealanders eventually. Creating this integrated tele-medicine network amongst the different HHSs could prove viable to healthcare delivery in New Zealand.

REFERENCES

Al-Qirim, N. (2002). Enabling electronic medicine in New Zealand: The case of video conferencing adoption in KiwiCare. In F. Tan (Ed.), *Cases on Global IT Applications and Management,* (pp. 186-203). Hershey, PA: Idea Group Inc.

Anderson, J. (1997). Clearing the way for physicians: Use of clinical information systems. *Communication of the ACM, 40*(8), 83-90.

Anonymous. (2002). Telemedicine flying high. *Professional Engineering, 15*(9), 47.

Austin, C. (1992). *Information Systems for Health Services Administration.* Michigan: AUPHA Press/Health Administration Press.

Austin, C., Trimm, J. & Sobczak, P. (1995). Information systems and strategic management. *Healthcare Management Review, 20*(3), 26-33.

Bacon, C. (1992, September). The use of decision criteria in selecting information systems/technology investments. *MIS Quarterly,* 369-386.

Bakos, J. & Treacy, M. (1986). Information technology and corporate strategy: A research perspective. *MIS Quarterly, 10*(2), 107-126.

Charles, B. (2000). Telemedicine can lower costs and improve access. *Healthcare Financial Management Association, 54*(4), 66-69.

Edelstein, S. (1999). Careful telemedicine planning limits costly liability exposure; *Healthcare Financial Management, 53*(12), 63-69.

Elliot, S. (1996). Adoption and implementation of IT: An evaluation of the applicability of Western strategic models to Chinese firms. In K. Kautz & J. Pries-Heje (Eds.), *Diffusion and Adoption of Information Technology* (pp. 15-31). London: Chapman & Hall.

Harris, K., Donaldson, J. & Campbell, J. (2001). Introducing computer-based telemedicine in three rural Missouri countries. *Journal of End User Computing, 13*(4), 26-35.

Hu, P., Chau, P., Sheng, O. & Tam, K. (1999). Examining the technology acceptance model using physician acceptance of telemedicine technology. *Journal of Management Information Systems, 16*(2), 91-112.

Huston, T. & Huston, J. (2000). Is telemedicine a practical reality? *Association for Computing Machinery. Communications of the ACM, 43*(6), 91-95.

Josey, P. & Gustke, S. (1999). How to merge telemedicine with traditional clinical practice. *Nursing Management, 30*(4), 33-36.

Kwon, T. & Zmud, R. (1987). Unifying the fragmented models of information systems implementation. In R. Borland & R. Hirschheim (Eds.), *Critical Issues in Information System Research* (pp. 252-257). New York: John Wiley.

Larsen, T. (1998). Information systems innovation: A framework for research and practice. In T. Larsen & E. McGuire (Eds.), *Information Systems Innovation and Diffusion: Issues and Directions* (pp. 411-434). Hershey, PA: Idea Group Inc.

Little, D. & Carland, J. (1991). Bedside nursing information system: A competitive advantage. *Business Forum Winter,* 44-46.

Mathews, J. (2000). Satellites Filling Telemedicine Niche. *Aviation Week & Space Technology, 153*(18), 10.

Moore, G. & Benbasat, I. (1991). Development of an instrument to measure the perceptions of adopting an information technology innovation. *Information Systems Research, 2*(3), 192-221.

Moore, G. & Benbasat, I. (1995). Integrating diffusion of innovations and theory of reasoned action models to predict utilisation of information technology by end-users. In K. Kautz & J. Pries-Heje (Eds.), *Diffusion and Adoption of Information Technology* (pp. 132-146). London: Chapman & Hall.

Neame, R. (1995). *Issues in Developing and Implementing a Health Information System.* Wellington: Ministry of Health.

Noring, S. (2000). Telemedicine and telehealth: Principles, policies, performance, and pitfalls. *American Journal of Public Health, 90*(8), 1322.

(NZHIS) New Zealand Health Information Service. (1995a). *Health Information Strategy for the Year 2000: Stocktake of Current Position and Future Plans.* Wellington: Ministry of Health.

(NZHIS) New Zealand Health Information Service. (1995b). *Health Information Strategy for the Year 2000: Gaps, Overlaps, and Issues Report.* Wellington: Ministry of Health.

(NZHIS) New Zealand Health Information Service. (1996). *Health Information Strategy for the Year 2000.* Wellington: Ministry of Health.

(NZStat) Statitics New Zealand. (2001). *A report on the Post-enumeration survey 2001.* Retrieved November 9, 2002 from the World Wide Web: www.stats.govt.nz/domino/external/pasfull/.

Office of Technology Assessment U.S Congress (OTA). (1995). *Bringing Health Care On Line: The Role of Information Technologies,* OTA-ITC-624. Washington, D.C: US Government Printing Office.

Perednia, D. & Allen, A. (1995, February). Telemedicine technology and clinical applications. *The Journal of the American Medical Association (JAMA), 273*(6), 483-488.

Premkumar, G. & Roberts, M. (1999). Adoption of new information technologies in rural small businesses. *The International Journal of Management Science (OMEGA), 27,* 467-484.

Rogers, E. (1995). *Diffusion of Innovation.* New York: The Free Press.

Shortell, S., Morrison, E. & Friedman, B. (1990). *Strategic Choices for America's Hospitals*. San Francisco, CA: Jossey-Bass.

Thong, J. (1999). An integrated model of information systems adoption in small businesses. *Journal of Management Information Systems, 15*(4), 187-214.

Topping, S. & Hernandez, S. (1991). Health care strategy research, 1985-1990: A critical review. *Medical Care Review, 48*(1), 47-98.

Tornatzky, L. & Klein, K. (1982). Innovation characteristics and innovation adoption implementation: A meta-analysis of findings. *IEEE Transactions on Engineering Management, 29*(11), 28-45.

Ward, J., Griffiths, P. & Whitmore, P. (1990). *Strategic Planning for Information Systems*. London: John Wiley & Sons.

Wayman, G. (1994). The maturing of telemedicine technology Part I. *Health Systems Review, 27*(5), 57-62.

ENDNOTES

[1]   Recently, hospitals are now the provider arm of the District Health Boards, e.g., Waikato District Health Board (W-DHB).

[2]   Recently, hospitals are now the provider arm of the District Health Boards, e.g., Waikato District Health Board (W-DHB).

[3]   Avoiding the costs of transportation and additional security measures.

[4]   However, it seems this has no adverse effect on New Zealand doctors as rural trips are considered part of their activities and hence, not paid any extra wage (Oakley et al., 2000).

Chapter XVI

Aligning Multiple Knowledge Perspectives in a Health Services System:
A Case Study

Tanya Castleman, Deakin University, Australia

Paul Swatman, University of South Australia, Australia

Danielle Fowler, University of Baltimore, USA

ABSTRACT

This chapter reports the results of a feasibility study into electronic collection of service data at "point of delivery" for disability programs. The investigation revealed that while the proposed system would have produced more fine-grained data, it would not have improved any actor's knowledge of service delivery. The study illustrated the importance of context in the transition from data to knowledge; the diffused and fragmented organisational structure of social service administration was shown to be a major barrier to effective building and sharing of knowledge. There was some value in the collection of detailed service data but this would have damaged the web of relationships which underpinned the system of service delivery and on which the smooth functioning of that system depended. The study recommended an approach to managing the informal and tacit knowledge distributed among many stakeholders, which was not especially technologically advanced but which supported, in a highly situated manner, the various stakeholders in this multi-organisational context.

INTRODUCTION

The provision of human (health and social) services by the State is necessarily a geographically and organisationally distributed activity. Such an activity sets a range of interest groups with a variety of requirements within a single problem context. Government-run healthcare systems are large-scale and include many divisions and linked organisations. They must manage varied (and sometimes contradictory) interests of the parties involved. In many ways it is difficult to align the goals and perceptions of participants into a coherent and effective knowledge management system. Information can become knowledge only if the context in which it exists is understood. Coming to an understanding of this rich context is a key challenge for government.

There are many stakeholder groups in these systems, each with their own interests and goals and while these are usually not irreconcilable, they are not always in harmony. This may involve different views about both the level of service, as well as individual choice of service options. There are potential conflicts among stakeholders over balancing accountability and organisational information needs with the privacy and dignity of the individual. The context of service provision is complex as is the relationship between the service providers and their clients, which is often a long-term relationship. An effective KM system for such an organisation would need to manage the informal and tacit knowledge that is distributed among many stakeholders and is highly contextual. In an area where there is such sensitivity and the personal and interpersonal issues are so central to the well-being of the clients, KM initiatives have the potential to be positive but may also have negative consequences for vulnerable clients.

In this chapter, we discuss a study which we and a number of colleagues undertook for a government department responsible for the provision of services to people receiving **disability** benefits. In assessing a proposed **electronic data collection** and payment system for disability services, we gained insight into the nature and importance of knowledge management for health and **social services**. Contrary to our expectations, we concluded that the most significant impediment to the effective creation and sharing of knowledge was the highly diffused, fragmented, interlocking organisational structure of the social service administration itself. Our investigation raised few issues about the technicalities of information collection and explicit knowledge management, but it did raise many issues about the design of the underlying organisational system for service provision, the level of detail required in the service data and the locus of decision-making power among the stakeholders. All of these issues bear directly on the system's effectiveness in providing appropriate services to disabled clients.

Governments have shown a keen interest in the use of information technology in healthcare delivery as a mechanism to improve quality, access and efficiency. Improved information systems and technology are essential components of managed healthcare (Shortell et al., 1994; Cave, 1995), which focuses on increased cost consciousness and a more market-driven industry with increased competition. To some extent Australia has followed the US shift to managed care, although the reaction has not been entirely positive (Stoelwinder, 1990).

The use of technology and innovation in restructuring healthcare delivery (Geisler, 2001; More & McGrath, 2002) has been indispensable, particularly in its ability to support explicit knowledge capture and transfer (Fedorowicz & Kim, 1995; Detmer & Shortliffe,

1997), but it also raises cultural and ethical issues associated with patient care (Menzel, 1992; Moore, 1994).

SOCIAL SERVICES PROVISION IN A DISPERSED NETWORK: A CASE STUDY

In 1998 our team was engaged to conduct a feasibility study for one section of an Australian government department which provided health and related social services. We were asked to assess whether an advanced IT solution (*viz.*, the use of electronic recording devices to document those services as they were provided to the clients) could provide better quality data and more effective reporting than the existing system. We were asked to advise whether the replacement of the existing paper-based system by an electronic system would help those agencies which delivered the services to report against their obligations under their service contracts. This was driven by government concerns about system inefficiency, inaccuracy, financial accountability and the need for service planning. From a KM perspective the department was looking for improved knowledge capture and transfer at the same time as delivering an improved level of service. They hoped these information system changes might help them improve their performance in the areas of procedures, rules, daily management of the system and their decision-making ability: the "managerial aspect" of their organisational knowledge (Gao et al., 2002). Identifying and capturing knowledge, connecting people to people through electronic means, and sustaining an organisation's growth and learning ability are common themes in most KM projects (Chong et al., 2000). This project focused on the first of these goals, building an electronic repository for organisation knowledge captured.

There were three major stakeholder groups in this context:

- The government Department of State Services ("The Bureau") included a centrally-located head office and a number of regional offices. It assessed applicants for care and determined the level of their care entitlement. It was responsible to the Minister for State Social Services and accountable through her for appropriate support to people needing disability care. Prudent and economical expenditure of public funds to achieve these aims was a prime **political** goal of the Government.
- Independent (non-government) **agencies** were contracted to provide care to the recipients. They were paid in advance for services to be provided and the accounts were subsequently reconciled on the receipt of delivery data. The agencies employed staff (often non-skilled and hourly-paid) to deliver the services either in a care centre or in the homes of the recipients.
- The **clients** were people with a range of disabilities from motor-muscular impairment to severe intellectual disability. Most were reported to have multiple disabilities. The majority of clients required family care-givers to manage for them as a result of their intellectual disability. Several welfare and advocacy groups provided support and advice to the clients and represented them in political forums.

Our investigative approach was broadly guided by the conceptual foundations of **Soft Systems Methodology** (SSM) (Checkland 1981; Checkland & Scholes, 1990; Checkland

& Holwell, 1998). We chose an SSM-style approach to analyse this context because the issues of health and human service provision were the subject of public controversy and SSM is well suited for dealing with **multiple perspectives** and conflicts. It provides a means of examining real world problems and accommodating diverse interests. As a cyclic learning process, knowledge management can be examined through the SSM lens, which offers insight into how an organisation learns (Gao et al., 2002).

STAKEHOLDER ANALYSIS

The team held a series of consultations with Bureau staff in the service management and IT areas (11), agency managers (nine), direct care providers employed by one of the agencies (five), clients (five) and representatives of client advocacy groups (three). Members of four other provider organisations were also interviewed. All information collected during the consultations was treated confidentially by the team and the participants were candid and informative as a result. In the consultations we asked about current practices including technology use, information needs, organisational relationships and any difficulties with service provision or its management. The line of questioning varied depending on the stakeholder group interviewed. This dialogic approach yielded a thorough understanding of the range of practices and solid insights into the various perspectives and interests of the groups. They also provided much material on the contextual issues, reflected in *Figure 1* as a Rich Picture[2].

In this multi-organisational context, overall responsibility was held by the Bureau which:

- evaluated individuals' eligibility to receive services;
- contracted with provider agencies (often charities) to supply services to those people with disabilities who had been evaluated and allocated a benefit; and
- maintained a waiting list of eligible individuals and allocated them to a suitable place as they became available within the system.

The existing administrative practices involved paper-based capture of service data at the point of delivery by the agencies which provided electronic summaries of services on a six-monthly basis. This system was acknowledged to be laborious and inaccurate with considerable problems of interoperability between agency systems and a variety of systems used by Bureau branches. It was not easy to use and often the data that were submitted did not conform to the required format, were unreadable and could not be amalgamated for analysis and storage.

The care system was extensive and even the two programs we were asked to examine served 5,500 clients through over 300 outlets. The two programs were designed to provide support for people who suffered disabilities which made it difficult to manage daily life. One program, Day and Respite Care (DARC), provided activities, training and a safe environment for clients during the day, usually in a centre but activities were often conducted elsewhere. Clients commonly attended programs with the same organisation for years on end. Most DARC users were intellectually disabled and many had multiple disabilities and behavioural problems. Contracts between the Bureau and a DARC agency were not written with respect to individual clients. Instead, blanket contracts were written to provide care places for a specified number of people for a specified number

Figure 1: Rich Picture of Benefit Allocation and Service Management

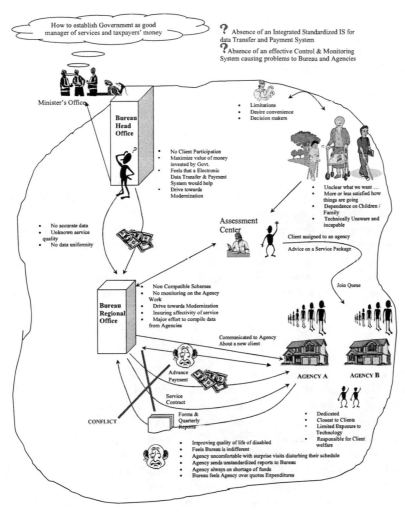

of months. A client was listed as a recipient of care by a particular agency, often one which specialised in his type of disability and, were he to leave this agency, he would go back on the waiting list. This was a major barrier preventing people from "shopping around" or changing agencies and the Bureau was concerned that clients should have more choice and flexibility in their service providers.

The second program, Home Based Support (HBS), was typically accessed by people with mobility problems (such as paraplegia or muscular dystrophy). Many HBS clients had no intellectual disabilities although all were seriously and irreversibly disabled. Care was provided at designated times during the day (such as help with bathing and dressing). HBS care could also be provided outside the home, such as help with shopping. Because this type of support was provided flexibly, clients could choose which agency supplied their care. Some did "shop around," but in many areas there were few agencies and thus, not much effective choice.

A number of attempts had been made earlier to bring together a coherent system of data reporting across programs, but there was still concern by members of the Bureau that they received incomplete and inaccurate data from the agencies on service provision and that they might be paying for services that had not, in fact, been delivered. In a system where there was pressure on funding (and waiting lists for services), any such inefficiency would have a negative effect on the delivery of care. In line with government policy and legislation, the Bureau wished to move to quality service provision centred on the recipients and to empower them to find services from the providers that best met their needs. Thus, rather than being obliged to access their care services from a designated provider agency, clients would increasingly choose both services and service providers to suit their needs, a situation that would require more effective management of knowledge both about a client's needs, but also about a complex and changing array of services used.

The KM system envisaged by the Bureau would enable improved client care supported by accurate collection of service data. It sought distributed access to knowledge about clients for the various regional Bureaus (sometimes clients accessed services through more than one region) and support for their planning, performance monitoring, administration and management of contracts with the agencies. The system would also need to be affordable, easy to use and reliable. The Bureau sought more control over a large and diverse sector by gaining more accurate and timely data on service provision. This, they hoped, would enable better allocation of resources, cost saving and greater accountability from agencies.

The perspective of the agencies was very different. The funding they received from the Bureau was often barely sufficient to cover the demand for their services, so they had little margin in budgetary matters. They experienced considerable difficulties with the reporting structure and several complained about errors and malfunctions in the lodging of reports because of the Bureau's format. The lag time between data reporting and reconciliation of accounts was also problematic for their planning. The agencies we consulted (six in total) reported few difficulties in maintaining data on service provision but many difficulties in reporting this on to the Bureau.

The agency managers' response to the proposal for an electronic data collection system was cool (and in some cases strongly opposed). They objected to the mismatch between the highly specified conceptualisation of service delivery and the real-life context in which service was delivered. In one DARC agency this problem was vividly described[3] by a long-standing member of its staff.

Although a service is defined as "attendance," this may not reflect the real costs of providing that service, especially if it is disrupted and extra work or financial outlay is required to deal with the disruption. For example, many of our clients' disabilities mean that they have behavioural problems and can become violent. So, say we're getting a group ready to get onto a bus for an outing. One person has a behavioural incident. He hits another client and breaks a bus window. We have to send him home (he obviously can't continue on the excursion in that condition). We have to get the person he hit to a doctor, which requires getting an extra staff member called in. We also have to get the window fixed. It's not out of the question that this incident may trigger other behaviours among the others who are waiting, some of whom may also have to be sent home. In the scenario you're painting [of the single data entry for a service], we're trying, in the middle of this chaos, to manage swiping everyone's smartcards. The Centre has, maybe, three cancellations plus several extra costs. How does that help us deliver service or our clients to get better service?

This raised the question of what data to collect in an electronically-based system. Service provision was not well categorised and did not relate closely to the actual activities that were performed at the DARC centres. Capturing the knowledge about attendance at DARC facilities on a daily basis was seen as trivial since clients enrolled for a series of sessions over several weeks. There were rules about attendance levels and if a client was absent for more than a few sessions, they risked forfeiting their place, which would then be allocated to another person on the waiting list. These Bureau rules, designed to keep the system operating at or near capacity, presented some difficulties for the DARC agencies. A client might decide to discontinue attendance for a time, either unaware of the longer-term consequences, or because their decisions were shaped by extraneous factors. Several agency staff reported cases like the following:

We had a young intellectually-disabled man who was quite happy at the Centre. But his father wasn't too happy about that and this got worse as the kid got older. I do not know what the father's problems might have been, but he absolutely insisted that his son leave the Centre and "grow up." We had known the son for years and we knew it would not work for long — he required just too much care and he could not become what his father hoped. We told his father that he'd need a place again soon and that taking him out would put him back on the waiting list and all. But the father could not be persuaded. What could we do? Well, we didn't notify a vacancy and in the meantime we were able to include a person travelling from interstate — we identified them through contacts with colleagues. Of course, within a few months the young man did return as we knew he had to, but he would have forfeited his place had we strictly adhered to the rules.

The professional staff in the agencies had to manage these absences knowing that the client would need and want to return later, but not within the time stipulated by Bureau regulations. Conversely, clients often arrived at the DARC on days they weren't scheduled to attend, because they were confused about the day or simply wanted to be there. Because of their dependency, agency staff rarely turned them away but the agency incurred some additional costs in providing for these unanticipated attendees. Agency managers juggled these contingencies in order to satisfy the care needs of their clients, the demanding budgetary constraints and the employment needs of the staff they relied on. Their solutions were sometimes creative but, in our view, always oriented to the goal of providing appropriate care for as many clients as possible.

The HBS program had few problems with clients' behaviour. Its clients usually could competently conduct their own care management. Many planned ahead and saved some of their service allocation for times when they anticipated greater need. The HBS agencies typically provided them with monthly accounts. On the face of it, the HBS program seemed well suited to electronic data capture and management. However, when we asked about an electronic data recording system, both direct care providers and HBS clients were vociferous in their opposition. They both saw this as an undesirable attempt to monitor the care providers more closely by getting them to "clock in."

In the HBS program (as with DARC) there was evidence of considerable unofficial flexibility to meet the clients' needs. Direct care providers reported that they would provide additional, uncharged services to clients when circumstances required this. Agency managers frowned on this practice and Bureau staff seemed largely unaware of it, but the relationships between care providers and care recipients were often valued by both of them and a degree of give-and-take seemed to suit both. There were a number of other programs in the social services area that had implemented electronic systems for keeping track of service (the measure was minutes of service provision). These programs provided domiciliary support to a broader clientele and were reported to work well. But the HBS care providers we spoke with found this system offensive and one told us she would not work in such a system, even though the pay was higher, because she did not want to forfeit the degree of autonomy she had in her job. Some clients also rejected this technique as inconsistent with the relationships of trust that had developed between them and their care providers. The system depended to a significant extent on the dedication and sense of vocation of the direct care providers. An intrusive, disciplinary data collection system could damage that dedication and the agencies were well aware of this.

Our care-givers are chosen for their professionalism. The HBS focus is about assisting people whose daily living is compromised and it is especially important to maintain the individual's dignity. If such staff are not treated with respect by the agency, they will not continue the work. It takes a very special person to get up at 6 a.m., drive for an half and hour in the dark to wipe someone's bum for a modest wage. If they are given decent wages and trust and their professionalism is recognised, they will provide good service and deal with the agency honestly. There is a difference from other home-help schemes which provide short pieces of assistance such as those run by local government.

Both DARC and HBS agencies feared that a more fine-grained data collection system would have the effect of reducing the level of service to clients. DARC centres could only lose (when clients did not attend), while additional services (to those who attended for extra sessions) could not be recognised as it would exceed their allocated benefit. Importantly, it would erode the agencies' ability to manage the complexities involved in providing care to people whose lives cannot easily fit into the logic of bureaucratic order.

In addition to the data collection issues, there were significant usability issues in the proposed electronic data collection systems, especially for intellectually disabled clients. One of the mooted solutions was the use of Smartcards to collect and store service data. As a technology, a smartcard has much to recommend it. As a device to be understood, remembered, carried and used by clients, it presented an unmanageable challenge. We discovered that many direct care providers (often not highly educated) and very many clients (usually intellectually disabled) did not understand or use such common devices as magnetic strip cards or credit cards. At that time, at least, the training costs for introducing such a system would have been high. Further, one DARC centre reported that the daily loss rate of (nonelectronic) ID cards issued to clients attending a program outside the centre approached 100%. Replacement costs for electronic devices at even a fraction of that rate would have been prohibitive. Alternative devices (such as chips embedded in jewelry) were seen as socially stigmatising. In any case, the current system of paper-based data on service provision was judged to be sufficiently accurate, usable and flexible between direct care-givers and the agencies.

It was not possible (for ethical and practical reasons) for us to consult with a broad range of clients. The clients and their care-givers with whom we spoke were very satisfied with the agencies and the individuals who provided their care. They reported few problems in keeping track of their service allocations or receiving appropriate care. But they were largely unaware of the services they might be able to access or the rules governing their access to care. This information was often provided by agency staff, but as it was not officially part of their role, it was a matter of luck whether clients were fully informed. The knowledge requirements of a client were not fixed and a change in their circumstances for any reason meant that new issues would arise and they would need to access other sources of support.

The Bureau was aware of these needs and was working towards a person-based system of service provision. The transition to this approach was hampered by the lack of a universal case management system for clients. Some clients managed their own cases or had family members who could do this. Some had a Bureau-appointed case manager and some received assistance from an agency, but this did not cover all clients by any means. Another factor which hampered the accessibility of information was the complexity of the system of service provision. This was structured into a series of support programs which were not unified into seamless service provision. Some of the Bureau and agency people we consulted claimed that this was partly the result of the political pressure on Ministers and governments to produce initiatives to demonstrate government action in social service provision. A new program could be launched with considerable fanfare, whereas incremental improvements were far less newsworthy. They argued that this had resulted in the unintegrated and changing system of care which was opaque to many of the recipients. It was problematic for knowledge management focused on care provision to the individual rather than a program or agency basis. We found no evidence that agencies were abusing the system by providing lower service than stipulated in their contracts, although it was not impossible for an agency to do so given the problems of the reporting and data management system. If a case of agency mismanagement of funds had arisen and been made public, this would have been embarrassing for the Bureau and the Minister and detrimental to the whole system. Thus, the goal of the Bureau to have an accurate system of service data reporting and management was a reasonable one, even if the proposed solution was not feasible.

Our account here illustrates the existence of multiple, incommensurate, but valid perceptions of human service provision. Our analysis of this context is primarily in terms of decision-making, and highlights three important issues:

- *The Silo Effect:* Multiple and separate programs, developed to meet diverse needs, can lead to fragmentation and can undermine the ability of the system to provide the requisite information to the people who need it. Lack of a comprehensive view of such a system undermines informed decision-making.
- *The Granularity Problem:* Common sense would suggest that the more detailed the information is that is made available, the greater the ability to understand it and thus manage a system. However, if the level of detail is not appropriate to the

context, it can detract from knowledge creation and distort the system itself. Finely grained information (even if "accurate" at one level) does not add to knowledge. The challenge is to strike the right level of granularity of data collection and management for the context to which it applies.

- *Locus of control and decision-making:* Data and the associated knowledge system are relevant primarily to improve decision-making of all the stakeholders. The locus of control for various types of decisions is important. Knowledge quality and availability need to align to the relevant decision-maker. With multiple stakeholders, the issue of control will be an important issue for a system. The challenge here is to design a system with the potential to deliver the appropriate type and level of control to each stakeholder group.

These three elements are interrelated. The existence of silos influences granularity questions and shapes the decision-making processes. The granularity of data collection is intimately connected with the issue of which stakeholders can access information, how relevant it is to their concerns and how they can use it to make decisions. The locus of control will influence the way each of the other elements operates and is a fundamental aspect of the balance of power within the system.

The information granularity issue presented significant problems. Much of the service information provided to the Bureau was extremely coarse-grained (e.g., some providers were required to acquit their entire budgets on a biannual cycle) while other parts of the system were very fine-grained (e.g., other providers were expected to provide data on service provision in small, specific time chunks). In general, the Bureau wanted finer levels of granularity of service data collection in all cases, whereas the agencies preferred a more coarse grained focus that would give them greater management flexibility. The clients' focus, in contrast, was on gaining access to services that could support their lives in the community. The granularity issue for them was important only insofar as they could get adequate support; otherwise, it was irrelevant at best and intrusive at worst.

While defining, collecting and analysing data at a fine degree of granularity can be a benefit in a highly-defined, predictable context where the environmental variables are well known, in this complex human services context, more precise data would have produced few benefits (in terms of better system understanding and better management tools) and would have been counterproductive to understanding the needs of the service recipients and attaining the ultimate goals of the system. Coarse levels of granularity are important where the services delivered involve holistic care and where the recipients are highly dependent. Finer granularity is appropriate where the end-users have greater power, where the delivered service is routine and defined and where the service context is relatively independent (e.g., routine domiciliary services), though even these systems may be deceptive and incorporate a higher degree of flexibility and negotiation than their designers and managers are aware.

Silo structures obscured information from the clients whose needs were highly individualistic and changing. A multitude of separate and overlapping schemes of service provision, each with its own administrative structure, rendered the system as a whole unintelligible to all but those expert in its mysteries. These schemes were designed to provide specific services (for example, a scheme to provide cleaning and home maintenance, another to provide assistance with personal care, another for home refitting and mobility aids, etc.). The schemes were based on a variety of crosscutting principles (e.g., schemes to assist people with particular disabilities, schemes for people whose disabilities had been acquired through accidents at work, schemes for young people).

While the Bureau seemed to be getting the "right story for the wrong reasons," given the inadequacy of the information system, many clients experienced a serious lack of information about the system as a whole and what they might reasonably request in the way of support. Access to this knowledge was far from universal and needed to be better provided in a more open, integrated and transparent system.

- Clients and their representatives need knowledge that will help them formulate their service requests and manage the use of their service quantum.
- Agencies need knowledge to manage their client mix, their staffing levels and their service provision profiles over time.
- The Bureau needed knowledge to ensure the integrity of the whole system, to plan future provision arrangements and to identify non-performing providers, overlaps and gaps in service provision, inequities emerging in the system and inefficiencies in service provision arrangements.

A KM approach was needed to support individuals making decisions at a level in the system where they are most in touch with the complex, non-routine and even chaotic events that affect the people who suffer illness or incapacity. In trying to improve explicit knowledge capture and transfer, the Bureau's approach failed to capture essential aspects of the context of that knowledge. It was trying to capture and institutionalise knowledge that resided in separate organisations, those agencies that supplied the client services. The key task of knowledge management is to connect people to each other to enable them to share what expertise and knowledge they have at the moment (Lang, 2001). The proposed system to collect service data would not have achieved that aim. More troublesome, it would have prevented the rich knowledge that existed at the agency level from informing decisions about client care.

Control, in a complex social system, is always difficult. Rarely are control strategies entirely satisfactory. Traditionally, governments (like many other organisations) have adopted a bureaucratic management strategy and, with damage limitation in mind, develop ever more elaborate sets of rules and regulations to limit discretionary decision-making which may result in potentially hard-to-justify decisions made low within the hierarchy. The approach to data collection suggested by the Bureau aimed, consistent with this strategy, to increase centralised control. The conflict here, common to healthcare institutions such as hospitals, is that strategic fit must be achieved: a balance must be found between a professional focus on quality of care, and an administrative/ bureaucratic focus on cost efficiencies. The trend seems to have been toward greater and more mechanistic bureaucratic control to meet budgetary goals (Yetton & Johnson, 2001; Pettigrew et al., 1992; Loveridge & Starkey, 1992; Strong & Robinson, 1990).

The weakness of such a system of control in a social situation is the difficulty of predicting (and therefore covering within the set of rules and regulations) all the decisions which might be necessary. It is clear that in many instances associated with the provision of disability services effective decisions require specific but potentially unpredictable case information and must be made promptly. Whereas bureaucratic rule-following and fine-grained data management serve the needs of those organisationally and politically accountable for an efficient system, the people at the care delivery end require the flexibility of a system that allows them to exercise judgment on their own or others' behalf. "On the ground" rather than "head-office" control (though transparent and auditable) is essential in order to ensure the system meets the needs of those it was designed to serve.

The difficulty of making informed decisions within the system of human service provision was, in our view, the key problem. A resolution of this problem is possible through knowledge management — an approach which can, by effectively supporting distributed but transparent decision-making throughout the system, combine flexibility of action with control and accountability.

TOWARD EFFECTIVE DISPERSED DECISION MAKING

Once we had rejected the option of instituting a more detailed level of data collection and rule enforcement as an effective solution to the perceived problem, we had, in effect, rejected increased centralisation of control. We were, then, drawn to consider whether we could find an accommodation acceptable to all parties through an approach based on a form of managed delegation of responsibility. Such a strategy might be effective if decisions were made by individuals who had the necessary knowledge (including explicit knowledge of the rules and regulations, as well as tacit knowledge of the specific case) and were accountable.

Consistently good decisions require a thorough knowledge of the problem itself and the possibilities for its solution. Decision-makers must be accountable and their decisions must be open to scrutiny. While it is clear that the availability of information low down in the bureaucracy can enable effective decision-making in a highly variable and sensitive social context, two associated aspects, accountability and knowledge collection, deserve some attention.

The Bureau, reasonably, was concerned to minimise the possibility of being required to answer for "bad" decisions. But how great is this danger in practice? Exposure falls into two categories:

- A single bad decision may be made which has the effect of causing immediate and acute disadvantage to a client.
- A single bad decision, or a series of bad decisions, may be made which results in invalid expenditure.

The first form of exposure can, of course, be minimised by denying the right for such decisions to be made on-the-spot — in essence, through the simple expedient of an overarching "Golden Rule" that the immediate well-being of the client always takes priority. Having applied first-aid, responsibility for a sensitive decision may be passed up the hierarchy.

The second form of exposure is less immediate, more diffuse and, in the current situation very difficult to detect — indeed, it was this exposure which led to the proposed data collection system. This exposure, as the Bureau clearly saw, may be minimised by monitoring behaviour within the system. Such behaviour can only be effectively monitored to the extent that a body of reliable, accessible and analysable data exists. The law of diminishing returns suggests that the analysis undertaken by the Bureau should be automated where possible and that human intervention within the process should be based on "exceptions." In essence, one can mine a database seeking patterns and anomalies.

BUILDING A KNOWLEDGE SYSTEM

We recommended the development of a database which would support decision-making by all actors in the system. The design of such a database is, in no sense, conceptually or technically novel. It may readily be built following the principles of Object Oriented or Relational Database design. In this instance we recommended a relational approach based primarily upon the existing systems infrastructure and skills and experience base of the IT Branch of the Bureau. Formally designed databases support both pre-specified and ad-hoc extraction, structuring and analysis suitable to support decision-making by many actors in a broad range of contexts. This would allow the Bureau to break the constraints of the "silo structure" and build a cross-scheme picture of the range of support being provided to one or more individuals and to a (potential) client to identify the range of support services that might be available to him or her.

We sought a solution to collect the necessary data (information, to be accurate, must be placed in context and actionable) while minimising its impact on the work practices of the ultimate care-givers and making the least possible demands on the technological infrastructure. Service delivery data may be captured either directly (at the point of the transaction) or indirectly. Service delivery data was already being collected, though not in a form satisfactory for monitoring by the Bureau.

Monitoring the hours of service provided to each client is central to the satisfactory operation of the HBS. Typically, each care-provider is given a scheduled time sheet, nominating for each visit: client, start and finish time, and duties. At the end of the prescribed period, the time sheet, adjusted from "scheduled" to "actual" is submitted by the care-provider to the agency to form the basis of both pay for the care-giver and adjustment of the clients' records. We suggested that the time sheets form the basis of data input for the proposed KM system. This meant little or no disruption to existing work practices for HBS. In contrast, there is little intrinsic motivation for accurately recording DARC attendance. Nonetheless, the Bureau already requires accurate recording of attendance. We suggested an approach to reporting, based around a simple attendance register. Capturing register information and submitting it, on a regular basis, to the Bureau in computer-readable form is not a particularly onerous task, especially since it replaces the previous data collection mechanisms.

The mode of data transmission could be via the Internet, by direct telephone connection to the Department's system, physical transfer of data on floppy disk or by paper report (least satisfactory since the Bureau must then key the data into the system). At that time electronic transmission was problematic because of many agencies' lack of IT capability or poor regional telecommunications infrastructure. Over time, we expect electronic transmission to become standard.

CONCLUSIONS

In this chapter, we have considered how a KM-based approach can:

- support the various actors in human services systems by offering appropriate and timely information, which together with guidelines (as opposed to rules) support effective, distributed decision-making
- help to unify the various perspectives from which the actors view human service provision
- allow both decisions and service provision to be monitored centrally, both on an *ad hoc* and on an exception reporting basis, in a timely and effective manner.

The key finding of the study was that the highly diffused and fragmented organisational structure of social service administration was the major impediment to the effective building and sharing of knowledge. Outsourcing and instability added to these difficulties. Many of these impediments were the result of political, administrative and organisational practices which were difficult to overcome. But, what was more significant was that meaningful and important knowledge was not simply reducible to descriptions of service allocation and service provision. The context of service provision is as complex as is the (often long-term) relationship between the service providers and their clients. Consequently, we argued that an effective KM system for this organisational network would manage the informal and tacit knowledge which is both distributed among many stakeholders and highly contextual. This is more effective than a response based on control through structured feedback. In an area where there is such sensitivity and the personal and interpersonal issues are so central to the well-being of the clients, KM initiatives have the potential to be integrative or disruptive, with either positive or negative consequences for vulnerable clients and the organisational network as a whole.

The use of SSM and stakeholder analysis as an investigatory tool proved to be a useful lens in examining this highly complex environment, and we argue it will be appropriate in any knowledge management system, particular those spanning organisational, cultural, and geographical boundaries.

REFERENCES

Cave, D. (1995). Vertical integration models to prepare health systems for capitation. *Health Care Management Review*, 20(1), 26-39.

Checkland, P. (1981). *Systems Thinking, Systems Practice*. Chichester, UK: John Wiley & Sons.

Checkland, P. & Holwell, S. (1998). *Information, Systems and Information Systems Making Sense of the Field*. New York: John Wiley & Sons.

Checkland, P. & Scholes, J. (1990). *Soft Systems Methodology in Practice*. Chichester, UK: John Wiley & Sons.

Chong, C. W., Holden, T., Wilhelmij, P. & Schmidt, R. A. (2000). Where does knowledge management add value? *Journal of Intellectual Capital*, 1(4), 366-80.

Detmer, W. & Shortliffe, E. (1997). Using the Internet to improve knowledge diffusion in medicine. *Communications of the ACM*, 40(8), 101-108.

Fedorowicz, J.& Kim, C. (1995). Information technology: Managed care's critical tool. *International Journal of Technology Management.* Special Publication on the Role of Management of Technology in Clinical and Administrative Health Care Delivery, pp. 175-185.

Gao, F., Li, M. & Nakamori, Y. (2002). Systems thinking on knowledge and its management: Systems methodology for knowledge management. *Journal of Knowledge Management,* 6(1), 7-17.

Geisler, E. (2001). Technology and innovation in the restructuring of healthcare delivery. *International Journal Healthcare Technology and Management,* 3(2/3/4), 111-22.

Lang, J. (2001). Managerial concerns in knowledge management. *Journal of Knowledge Management,* 5(1), 43-57.

Loveridge, R. & Starkey, K. (eds). (1992). *Continuity and Crisis in the NHS.* Buckingham: Open University Press.

Menzel, P. (1992). Some ethical costs of rationing. *Law, Medicine, and Health Care,* 20(1/2), 57–66.

Moore, S. (1994). Understanding innovation in social service delivery systems. *Health Marketing Quarterly,* 11(3), 61-73.

More, E. & McGrath, M. (2002). An Australian case in e-health communication and change. *The Journal of Management Development,* 21(8), 621-632.

Pettigrew, A., Ferlie, E. & McKee, L. (1992). *Shaping Strategic Change.* London: Sage.

Shortell, S., Gillies, R. & Anderson, D. (1994). The new world of managed care: Creating organized delivery systems. *Health Affairs,* 13(5), 46-64.

Stoelwinder, J. (1990). Dear Minister, please save me from case-mix funding. *Australian Health Review,* 13(4), 318-325.

Strong, P. & Robinson, J. (1990). *The NHS: Under New Management.* Buckingham: Open University Press.

Yetton, P. W. & Johnston, K. D. (2001). Competing forms of fit in a professional bureaucracy: IT management dilemmas. *International Journal of Healthcare Technology and Management,* 3(2/3/4), 142-159.

ENDNOTES

[1] The writing for this chapter was conducted while Paul Swatman was employed by the Stuttgart Institute for Management and Technology, Stuttgart, Germany.

[2] We would like to thank Aashish Joshi, Shashank Jindal and Alpaslan Acka, MBA students at SIMT, for the artwork presented in *Figure 1.*

[3] All the quotations provided here have been constructed from handwritten notes of one or more team members taken during the interviews. They do not have the accuracy of a verbatim transcription but are correct in both content (what they describe) and in flavour (the speakers' emotive emphasis).

Chapter XVII

Knowing How Intranets Enable Knowledge Work:
An Exploratory Study in Public Health

Martin Hughes, National University of Ireland, Galway, Ireland

William Golden, National University of Ireland, Galway, Ireland

ABSTRACT

This chapter explores the role of intranet technology as an enabling technology for supporting the knowledge worker, knowledge work and various forms of knowledge management. The Earl-Hopwood model is utilized to map the intranet enabled knowledge management practices to the work patterns of the knowledge worker. This mapping process yields a greater understanding of the likely impacts of IS developments on the activities of knowledge workers. The research consisted of longitudinal case studies conducted in two Irish public sector hospitals. A wide diversity of knowledge management utilization patterns was found to exist in both organizations with, training, the presence of critical information and ease of use positively influencing the use of the Intranet as a knowledge management tool. Inhibiting factors identified include lack of recognition of the intranet as a knowledge management system, the absence of a knowledge management champion and the lack of strategic intent. Cumulatively, these factors resulted in suboptimal knowledge management usage patterns.

INTRODUCTION

Knowledge management has been identified as a core competency for building and maintaining a competitive advantage (Stonehouse, Pemberton & Barbor, 2001; Teece, 1998). Knowledge management is also recognised as a change management process which involves changing organizational information technology to support knowledge management but more importantly, it changes company culture to achieve a collaborative environment (Lewis, 2002). Knowledge management has been broken down into a three step process of knowledge acquisition, knowledge production and knowledge integration (Weidner, 2002).

Drucker (1993) asserts that the knowledge-based economy has superseded post-industrial society and consequently knowledge has become the main competitive tool of this new economy. Sustainable competitive advantage will be enhanced by knowledge that is irreplaceable, difficult to imitate and easily transferable within the firm (Lubit, 2001). However, our understanding of knowledge worker productivity is wholly under-developed (Davenport, Thomas & Cantrell, 2002; Drucker, Dyson, Handy, Saffo & Senge, 1997).

The term knowledge worker describes members of the workforce who possess competencies, knowledge and skills in an organization (Lee & Yang, 2000). The ability to increase the productivity of knowledge workers would significantly enhance innovation, long-term organizational sustainability and growth (Davenport et al., 2002). Finding ways to increase the productivity of knowledge workers is thus imperative for any company seeking to sharpen its competitive edge (Wang, 2000). The objective of this chapter is to explore how Intranet technology supports knowledge work by mapping the Intranet enabled knowledge management processes to the work patterns of the knowledge worker.

THE NATURE OF KNOWLEDGE

A common distinction drawn in knowledge management literature is the distinction between explicit (codified) and tacit knowledge (Nonaka & Konno, 1998; Nonaka & Takeuchi, 1995; Polanyi, 1958; Smith, 2001; Teece, 1998). Explicit or codified knowledge is equated with knowledge that can be expressed in words, numbers, and formulae and is often technical, scientific or academic in nature (Nonaka & Konno, 1998; Smith, 2001; Tuomi, 1999). The formalized nature of explicit knowledge facilitates easy transmission between individuals and groups (Nonaka & Takeuchi, 1995). Conversely, tacit knowledge is knowledge that is not easily codified. Tacit knowledge is often explained by the dictum "we know more than we can tell" (Teece, 1998). Some authors further divide tacit knowledge into technical, as in the sense of a skill or craft, and cognitive, which includes beliefs, values, schemas, and mental models (Nonaka & Konno, 1998; Smith, 2001).

Knowledge in the Organization

Exploring the concept of knowledge in the organization has lead to the identification of individual knowledge and organizational knowledge as being distinct, yet interrelated concepts (Bhatt, 2000, 2002). Organizational knowledge is dependant on individual knowledge. However, its value is more than the sum total of all the individual knowledge within the organization (Bhatt, 2000). The formation of organizational knowledge is the product of a complex process involving interactions between technologies, techniques and people (Bhatt, 2001).

Knowledge Management

Smith (2001) presents four definitions of knowledge management which emphasize the procedural nature of knowledge management (Bonner, 2000; Chait, 1998; Liss, 1999; McClune, 1999). The complex interaction between technologies, techniques and people has profound ramifications for the knowledge management process (Bhatt, 2001). In addition, Binney (2001) suggests that knowledge management is best viewed as a spectrum ranging from transactional knowledge management to innovation and creation knowledge management. Specific knowledge management applications can then be mapped to the elements of the spectrum as depicted in *Figure 1*.

Recognising the highly complex nature of the knowledge management process, many authors have argued for the need for devising and pursuing knowledge management strategies in order to achieve successful knowledge management implementations (Armistead & Meakins, 2002; Bhatt, 2002; Binney, 2001; Birkinshaw & Sheehan, 2002; Choi & Lee, 2002; Teece, 1998).

Figure 1: KM Applications Mapped to the Elements of the KM Spectrum

	Transactional	Analytical	Asset Management	Process	Developmental	Innovation & Creation
Knowledge Management Applications	Case Based Reasoning (CBR) Help Desk Applications Customer Service Applications Order Entry Applications Service Agent Support Applications	Data Warehousing Data Mining Business Intelligence Management Information Systems Decision Support Systems Customer Relationship Management (CRM) Competitive Intelligence	Intellectual Property Document Management Knowledge Valuation Knowledge Repositories Content Management	TQM Benchmarking Best Practices Quality Management Business Process (Re)Engineering Process Improvement Process Automation Lessons Learned Methodology SEI/CMM, ISO9XXX, Six Sigma	Skills Development Staff Competencies Learning Teaching Training	Communities Collaboration Discussion Forums Networking Virtual Teams Research & Development Multi-disciplined Teams

Source: Binney (2001)

The Enabling Role of Technology

Information technology offers many potential value-creating opportunities in the knowledge management domain (Walsham, 2001) with new technologies enabling the capture and sharing of knowledge within applications and across organizations (Teece, 1998). In fact, many recently developed technological tools are aimed specifically at effectively supporting knowledge management within organizations (Johannessen, Olaisen & Olsen, 2001). The benefits of information technology include faster, cheaper, and broader sources of data and means of communication which enable the generation and sharing of knowledge (Walsham, 2001). The advent of web related tools such as intranets, extranets and intelligent agents have contributed significantly to the technological capabilities of knowledge management systems (Carayannis, 1998; Chou & Binshan, 2002; Scott, 1998).

Wang (2002) identifies the development of competent human-centred web-based support systems beyond databases, information repositories and groupware systems as the key to effective knowledge management. From the IS perspective, Web technologies, in particular Intranets, offer formidable advantages over traditional technologies which tend only to support well defined tasks (Damsgaard & Scheepers, 1999). These include: rapid scalable development across a range of platforms (Betts, 1997), access to corporate legacy systems and data warehousing capabilities (Scott, 1998), and development on existing networks with lower implementation costs compared to traditional client/server solutions (Sprout, 1995).

Since its introduction, Intranet Technology has been applied in four distinct waves: Information Publishing; Information Collaboration; Transaction Oriented Applications; and Formal Collaborative Applications. Thus, as the technology matured, IS professionals became aware of the potential of Intranets as a strategic tool (Curry & Stancich, 2000). Intranets are highly suited to use as a strategic tool in knowledge management due to their ability to support distribution, connectivity and publishing (Tiwana & Ramesh, 2001) as well as access to legacy systems and integration of incompatible systems (Scott, 1998). In addition, Intranets are suited to the deployment of XML-based systems which provide advanced technological capabilities for developing knowledge management systems (Cook, 2000). Finally, Intranets have the advantage of being acceptable to end users due to the ease of use and proliferation of the Internet (Stanton, 1995).

Understanding Knowledge Work

While an immense body of literature now exists on knowledge management, there is a dearth of frameworks, which seek to explain the complex tasks of knowledge work and the modes of operation of the knowledge worker. This is consistent with the findings of Davenport (2002), who claims that knowledge work has no Frederick Taylor or Henry Ford and that no one seems to own the problem of knowledge worker performance.

Earl and Hopwood (1980) developed a model (*Figure 2*) in order to understand how managers acquire the information necessary to perform their managerial functions. As the model indicates, managers typically utilize a wide variety of resources that are not limited to the formal processes. More important to our understanding of knowledge work, however, are the dimensions of the model. The authors divide the activity of managers (knowledge workers) into tasks and modes of operation. Tasks are divided into routine and non-routine, while modes of operation are divided into official and unofficial.

Figure 2: Earl-Hopwood Model

Mode/Task	Routine	Non-Routine
Official	MIS Management accounting systems Production control systems	Access facilities Task forces Liaison roles
Unofficial	Black books Just in case files	The grapevine Lunch table chats

Source: Earl and Hopwood (1980)

This framework can be utilized to increase our understanding of contemporary knowledge workers and how they interact with specific technologies in the performance of knowledge work.

RESEARCH METHOD

This research examines the role of intranet technology as an enabler of knowledge management and a supporter of knowledge work in two public sector hospitals. Due to the complex nature of knowledge work, substantial in-depth analysis was required within the participating organizations. As a consequence, it was decided to adopt longitudinal exploratory research methods and the case study method of research was selected as the most suitable method of research for the completion of this study.

Two Irish public sector hospitals were selected. Data collection consisted of interviews with the IS Managers and Assistants in both organizations. The interviews were initially conducted in 1997, with repeat interviews in 2000 and 2003. IS personnel, as opposed to end users, were purposefully selected. As the research was exploratory in nature, it was deemed necessary to interview personnel who would have a broad overview of the system, and its usage patterns across a wide variety of users, and functional areas. Onsite visits and a review of internal documentation were also conducted. The interviews were conducted according to a preformatted questionnaire, supported by technical demonstrations, and supplemented by access to internal documentation. Records were kept of the content of all interviews. Further clarifications and updates were obtained by email and telephone contact.

Case Studies: Organization Comparison

The organizations under study were Beaumont Hospital, Dublin and St. James Hospital, Dublin. Both organizations operate in the public sector under the same regional health authority. Both organizations are of approximately the same size and operated with

Table 1: Organizational Comparison

	Beaumont	St. James's
Activity		
Inpatients	21,600	21,000
Outpatients	110,000	140,000
Day patients	20,000	25,000
Accident &	56,000	54,000
Emergency		
Resources		
Beds	720	760
Specialities	48	46
Annual Budget	€130m	€142m
Staff	2,200	2,500

similar levels of resources. Furthermore, both organizations began the planning and implementation stages of their respective Intranets within months of each other.

When measured by their key activities and resources (*Table 1*) both hospitals are approximately equivalent.

Overview of the Cases

Each hospital began to implement web technologies in 1996 and have had a dedicated Intranet in place for an almost identical time period. *Table 2* summarises the initial utilization patterns in each organization. Both identified the similar need for change in their systems. Inefficient processes were hindering the performance of key functions, resulting in delays for the patient and inefficient use of resources.

Beaumont Hospital

The driving force behind the implementation of the intranet in Beaumont was the IS department. The motivation behind the introduction of the intranet was to improve communication and deal more efficiently and effectively with the vast amounts of paper,

Table 2: Utilization Patterns 1997-2000

	Beaumont	St. James's
Initial Conception	October 1996	February 1997
Pilot Project	Yes: Publishing and Distribution	No
Early Utilization Patterns	Staff Locator	HIV Unit
	Newsletter	Cancer Unit
	Theatre List	
	On Call List	
	Email	

which accumulates, in the hospital's various departments. The IS department operates primarily as a support function with very stringent budgetary constraints. In 1996, they identified intranet technology as a powerful new technology and believed that it could be leveraged in the hospital. Three factors supported this belief: the low cost of initial implementation, ease of use, and the range of processes that Intranets could be used to support.

A pilot project was initiated in October 1996 with the purpose of implementing the technology and gathering initial end user feedback. The pilot was to consist of the publication of policy and procedure documents for the pharmacy, nursing administration and infection control departments. Although the pilot project yielded mixed results, it was decided to continue with a further expansion of the intranet. Reviewing the pilot project, the IS department felt that it would take at least a year before an intranet would have any significant impact on the organization. By June 2000, the Intranet manager felt that the Intranet had reached a critical mass, as it was now accessible by all staff from over 400 terminals dispersed throughout the organization. However, it had taken longer, than the predicted one year, to reach maturity. During the 2000-2003 period, the IS department became more ambitious and purposefully strove to leverage the capabilities beyond document distribution. They identified a number of paper-based, cross-departmental processes: theatre lists, on-call lists, and holiday schedules, as "missionary" processes that would prove the capabilities of the technology to improve inefficient processes, and deliver tangible benefits without exposing the organization to risk. By successfully transferring these processes to the Intranet and the subsequent removal of the paper-based equivalents, the IS department demonstrably proved the potential value of the Intranet, in terms of efficiency and effectiveness improvements, to the hospital. In addition, the Intranet became central to the day-to-day work patterns of staff, as it became the sole source of critical pieces of information.

St. James's Hospital

In contrast to the IS lead development at Beaumont, St. James's formed a multi-discipline team, consisting of members from administrative, clinical, management and IS departments, that was to devise a web strategy. This team identified four customer groups: patients; general practitioners; healthcare professionals and hospital administrators whose needs were to be addressed by the overall web strategy. By modeling the patient care process against Porters value chain, through contact with international peer groups and through consultation with their clinical colleagues within the hospital, web technology in the form of the Internet, Intranets and Extranets were identified as having enormous potential for improving the level of patient care and for addressing the information dissemination requirements of the hospital. As such, the Intranet in St. James' was viewed as a logical extension to the hospital web site and not an individual project.

As a result, during 1997, the intranet development was slower and less focused than the Beaumont Intranet. Content development encountered more difficulties than anticipated with the main problems identified as: users unfamiliar with publishing methods, the already heavy workloads of potential content managers and concerns relating to the ownership of content. This initial lack of development resulted in delays in achieving a critical mass of content and users. Initially, only two clinical disciplines, HIV and cancer made use of the Intranet to support best practices in clinical care. By 2000, these end user concerns had been addressed by training liaison people in each department. Hospital management reacted swiftly, utilizing the Intranet for dissemination of information on healthcare issues. The Intranet began to expand more rapidly. In order to manage this expansion, a content management system was implemented and the Intranet was redesigned to facilitate greater usability. The most recent development has been the procurement of Intranet booths that are strategically positioned around the hospital to increase the number of multiple user access points.

Supporting the Knowledge Worker

The traditional focus of IS support in each organization was to support hospital functions, such as administration, which was done largely on an individual departmental basis. Support for collaborative information sharing consisted primarily of using bar code systems to share minimal patient data for processes like admissions. More recently, there has been an increased awareness of the need to support the knowledge work of medical staff, as this is typically the biggest cost in the treatment process. However, this has been recognised by both IS departments as a difficult and complex task as the following problems were identified with knowledge work in the healthcare industry.

- The knowledge worker owns the process.
- Processes are difficult to define. "How do you define the process for cardiology?"
- The more complex the knowledge, the more difficult it is to support.

Faced with these realities, it was felt that IS developments to date within the organizations have had little direct impact on supporting knowledge work.

Intranet Utilization Patterns

However, a clearer interpretation of support for knowledge work can be achieved by mapping the actual Intranet utilization patterns to the knowledge management spectrum and subsequently to the Earl-Hopwood Model. At this juncture it is worth recalling that the Intranets, in these organizations, were not actually implemented as part of a knowledge management strategy. *Table 3* maps the Intranet utilization patterns found in the research to the six segments of the knowledge management spectrum as identified by Binney (2001).

Table 3 illustrates some evidence of knowledge management utilizations under the first two segments, transactional and analytical, and no evidence of asset management utilizations. However, rich tapestries of utilization patterns were found to be evident in the process, developmental, and innovation and creation segments. Both Intranets are quite extensively utilized to promote and support best practices in clinical care. The HIV and cancer units of St. James' were found to be particularly active in leveraging the advantages of the Intranet to support best practices in clinical care. Evidence of quality management practices, in various forms, including clinical guidelines and quality suggestion schemes, are also supported by both Intranets. Strong evidence of process improvements were found in both hospitals as the Intranet has enabled the removal of paper-based Theatre and On Call lists and replaced them with electronic equivalents. This has achieved significant improvement in the timeliness and certainty of delivery as well as the accuracy of the content, resulting in better utilization of human and physical

Table 3: Intranet Facilitated KM Applications

KM Application	Beaumont	St. James's
Transactional		
Online Forms		Yes
Analytical		
Business Intelligence		Yes
Asset Management		
Process		
Best practices	Yes	Yes
Quality Management	Yes	Yes
Process Improvement	Yes	Yes
Process Automation		
Lessons Learnt		Yes
Developmental		
Skill Development		Yes
Staff Competencies		Yes
Learning		Yes
Teaching		Yes
Training		Yes
Innovation and Creation		
Communities	Yes	Yes
Collaboration	Yes	Yes
Discussion Forums		

resources. The improved process has also resulted in additional security, as access to the Theatre list is now password controlled, which helps to protect patient privacy.

The St. James' Intranet is widely utilized under the developmental segment of the knowledge management spectrum with clear evidence of usage in each of the knowledge management application areas as identified in the Binney (2001) framework. Specific examples include interactive teaching modules delivered via the Intranet and dedicated training sections which offer access to a variety of training resources.

Innovation and creation usage pattern were also evident with community and collaboration practices well utilized on both Intranets. Both Intranets also serve as repositories of organization documentation and as a key communications channel with their respective organizations.

UNDERSTANDING THE IMPACT OF THE INTRANET ON KNOWLEDGE WORK

Utilizing the Earl-Hopwood model, it is possible to further map the various knowledge utilization patterns that were found on the hospital Intranets to the operational dimensions of the knowledge worker. As the model indicates, knowledge-based work can be divided into routine and non-routine tacks or activities that are performed through

Figure 3: Mapping Usage Patterns

Mode/Task	Routine	Non-Routine
Official	Best Practices Document Mangement Process Improvement Process Automation Lessons Learnt	Skill Development Staff Competencies Learning; Teaching; Training
Unofficial		Communities Collaboration Discussion Fora

official and unofficial means or modes. *Figure 3* maps the specific knowledge management applications as identified in the Binney (2001) spectrum that were found to be evident in the cases to the Earl-Hopwood model. This mapping process results in a richer understanding of how the organizational intranets impact on the individual in these knowledge-intensive working environments. As *Figure 3* illustrates, the intranets in these organizations richly support the knowledge-intensive workers in terms of the official/routine, official/non-routine, and unofficial/non-routine dimensions of their work.

Factors Influencing the Development of KM Practices

The factors that influenced the utilization of the Intranet as a knowledge management tool are identified as: the provision of training and IS support; the redesign of the intranets to ensure ease of use; the development of content, both information and processes, that is directly relevant to daily work activities; the provision of resources relevant to career enhancement; and the provision of facilities which promote a sense of inclusion.

The factors that inhibited the use of the Intranet as a knowledge management resource are identified as: the defined or assumed scope, that is, neither Intranet was actually implemented as a knowledge management system; absence of a knowledge management champion; lack of recognition of the Intranet as a knowledge management tool; and the absence of knowledge management practices as a strategic intent.

Organizational Comparison

Initially, both intranets were implemented essentially as publishing and distribution tools and similar issues relating to poor initial adoption by both content creators and end users was evident in both organizations. Continued development, awareness programmes and staff training were utilized to overcome these early problems. The Beaumont Intranet developed at a faster pace, primarily due to the focus placed on it by the IS team with specific processes quickly targeted and implemented to build critical mass. In comparison, the evolution of the St. James' Intranet occurred more slowly as it did not initially enjoy a privileged status. Evidence from the cases suggests that the evolution into a knowledge management tool was for the most part an unintended occurrence in both hospitals. More recently, greater attention has been paid to the support of knowledge work via intranets within both organizations. While the specific utilization patterns differed within both organizations, the only discernable factor identified in this research to explain these differences was the number of services actually available via the organizations' intranets.

CONCLUSIONS

The intranets of the organizations in this study, despite having not been implemented as knowledge management tools, clearly supported a wide diversity of the day-to-day activities of knowledge workers and knowledge-based work. This support is provided across the majority of the segments of the knowledge management spectrum and is manifested in three dimensions of the knowledge worker's activities. While neither organization purposefully set out to implement an intranet as a knowledge management system, knowledge management practices emerged nonetheless. These knowledge management utilization patterns evolved even in the absence of a corporate knowledge management champion - albeit as islands of utilization driven by localized Intranet champions. This illustrates the core strength of an Intranet as a powerful knowledge management tool, as knowledge management practices emerged in both organizations even in the absence of a strategic influence. This also highlights the capability of Intranets as a tool that can be managed by the owner of the process, which in this instance was the actual knowledge workers themselves.

However, the initial focus of the Intranets on lower order capabilities such as publishing and distribution, the lack of awareness of the knowledge management capabilities and the absence of a strategic intent has resulted in a suboptimal utilization of the technology as a knowledge management tool. This is further illustrated by the absence of measures of performance, such as reduced costs or service improvements.

The cases do, however, provide strong evidence to support the use of Intranet technology as a knowledge management tool. The positive and diverse utilization of the technology as a facilitator of knowledge work proves its knowledge management capabilities and acceptability to knowledge workers. Even greater success could be achieved by universally recognising the Intranet as a knowledge management system and by having organizational level and local level knowledge champions to actively promote knowledge management activities.

The findings of this research also indicate the value in utilizing the Earl-Hopwood model to increase our understanding of the dynamics of the knowledge worker. This model segments the activities and modes of operation of knowledge workers thereby giving a richer insight into the complex nature of knowledge worker activities and how they can be supported. More specifically, the Earl-Hopwood model can illuminate how information systems are likely to impact on the effectiveness of the knowledge worker by clarifying the segments of knowledge worker activities that specific applications can support.

While this research has provided strong evidence for the use of intranets as a knowledge management tool, further research conducted within individual user group settings could provide a greater insight into and a more quantitative analysis of Intranet-facilitated knowledge work patterns.

REFERENCES

Armistead, C. & Meakins, M. (2002). A framework for practising knowledge management. *Long Range Planning, 35*, 49-71.

Betts, B. (1997). Intranets: Let's see what it can do. *Computer Weekly, 16(1)*.

Bhatt, G. D. (2000). A resourced-based perspective of developing organisational capabilities for business transformation. *Knowledge and Process Management, 7*(2), 119-129.

Bhatt, G. D. (2001). Knowledge management in organistions: Examining the interaction between technologies, techniques, and people. *Journal of Knowledge Management, 5*(1), 68-75.

Bhatt, G. D. (2002). Management strategies for individual knowledge and organisational knowledge. *Journal of Knowledge Management, 6*(1), 31-39.

Binney, D. (2001). The KM Spectrum: Understanding the KM landscape. *Journal of Knowledge Management, 5*(1), 33-42.

Birkinshaw, J. & Sheehan, T. (2002, Fall). Managing the knowledge life cycle. *MIT Sloan Management Review*, 75-83.

Bonner, D. (2000). The knowledge management challenge: New roles and responsibilities for chief knowledge officers and chief learning officers. In J. J. Phillips & D. Bonner (Eds.), *Leading Knowledge Management and Learning*. Alexandria, VA: American Society for Training and Development.

Carayannis, E. (1998). The strategic management of technological learning in project/program management: The role of extranets, intranets and intelligent agents in knowledge generation, diffusion and leveraging. *Technovation, 18*(11).

Chait, L. (1998). Creating successful knowledge management systems. *Prism, Second Quarter*.

Choi, B. & Lee, H. (2002). Knowledge management strategy and its link to knowledge creation process. *Expert Systems with Applications, 23*, 173-187.

Chou, D. C. & Binshan, L. (2002). Development of web-based knowledge management systems. *Human Systems Management, 21*, 153-158.

Cook, J. H. (2000, May/June). XML sets the stage for effective knowledge management. *IT Pro*.

Curry, A. & Stancich, L. (2000). The intranet — an intrinsic component of strategic information management? *International Journal of Information Management, 20*(4), 249-268.

Damsgaard, J. & Scheepers, R. (1999). Power, influence and intranet implementation. *Information Technology & People, 12*(4), 333-358.

Davenport, T., Thomas, R. J. & Cantrell, S. (2002, Fall). The mysterious art and science of knowledge-worker performance. *MIT Sloan Management Review*, 23-30.

Drucker, P. F., Dyson, E., Handy, C., Saffo, P. & Senge, P. M. (1997). Looking ahead: Implications of the present. *Harvard Business Review, 75*(5), 18.

Earl, M. J. & Hopwood, A. G. (1980). From management information to information management. In H. C. Lucas, F. F. Land & T. Lincoln (Eds.), *The Information Systems Environment*. Amsterdam: North-Holland.

Johannessen, J., Olaisen, J. & Olsen, B. (2001). Mismanagement of tacit knowledge: The importance of tacit knowledge, the danger of information technology, and what to do about it. *International Journal of Information Management.*

Lee, C. C. & Yang, J. (2000). Knowledge value chain. *Journal of Management Development, 19*(9), 783-793.

Lewis, B. (2002, January/February). On-Demand KN: A two tier architecture. *IT Pro.*

Liss, K. (1999, February). Do we know how to do that? Understanding knowledge management. *Harvard Business Update,* 1-4.

Lubit, R. (2001). Tacit knowledge and knowledge management: The keys to sustainable competitive advantage. *Organizational Dynamics, 29*(4), 164-178.

McClune, J. C. (1999, April). Thirst for knowledge. *Management Review,* 10-12.

Nonaka, I. & Konno, N. (1998). The concept of "Ba": Building a foundation for knowledge creation. *California Management Review, 40*(3), 40-54.

Nonaka, I. & Takeuchi, H. (1995). *The Knowledge Creating Company: How Japanese Companies Create the Dynamics of Innovation*: Oxford: University Press.

Polanyi, M. (1958). *Personal Knowledge*. London: Routledge.

Scott, J. E. (1998). Organizational knowledge and the intranet. *Decision Support Systems, 23*(1), 3-17.

Smith, E. (2001). The role of tacit and explicit knowledge in the workplace. *Journal of Knowledge Management, 5*(4), 311-321.

Sprout, A. (1995). The Internet inside your company. *Fortune, 27(11).*

Stanton, S. (1995). In search of 60-day wonders. *Datamation, 1(7).*

Stonehouse, G. H., Pemberton, J. D. & Barbor, C. E. (2001). The role of knowledge facilitators and inhibitors: Lessons from airline reservations systems. *Long Range Planning, 34,* 115-138.

Teece, D. J. (1998). Capturing value from knowledge assets: The New Economy, markets for know-how, and intangible assets. *California Management Review, 40*(3), 55-79.

Tiwana, A. & Ramesh, B. (2001). Integrating knowledge on the Web. *IEEE Internet Computing, 5*(3), 32-39.

Tuomi, I. (1999). Data is more than knowledge: Implications of the reserved knowledge hierarchy for knowledge management and organisational memory. *Journal of Management Information Systems, 16*(13), 107-121.

Walsham, G. (2001). Knowledge management: The benefits and limitations of computer systems. *European Management Journal, 19*(6), 599-608.

Wang, F. K. (2000). Designing a case-based e-learning system: What, how and why. *Journal of Workplace Learning, 14*(1).

Wang, S. (2002). Knowledge maps for Web-based business. *Industrial Management and Data Systems, 102*(7), 357-364.

Weidner, D. (2002, January/February). Using connect and collect to achieve the KM endgame. *IT Pro.*

Chapter XVIII

Knowledge Management in Indian Companies:
Benchmarking the Pharmaceutical Industry

John Gammack, Griffith University, Australia

Pranay Desai, Griffith University, Australia

Kuldeep Sandhu, Griffith University, Australia

Heidi Winklhofer, Griffith University, Australia

ABSTRACT

In this chapter we look at knowledge management in India with particular regard to the pharmaceutical industry. In India, changes in government policy linked to global factors are bringing about increased pressures to strategically manage knowledge effectively. At the same time, significant knowledge management initiatives are already underway in other industry sectors. We outline some of the changes affecting the pharmaceutical industry globally, and consider India on some relevant activities. The development of IT solutions is seen as enabling effective knowledge management. We look at a range of knowledge management technologies and their existing or planned use in industry. The IT however merely underpins the knowledge management philosophy, which must be incorporated into processes, strategies and organisational culture for successful adoption. India and its indigenous organisations may be characterised by some specific cultural factors. Effective implementation of KM will depend on a conducive cultural climate, both organisationally and nationally. We also therefore examine the extent of the perceived benefits, that shape the cultural shift from understanding knowledge management as simply an IT problem to recognition of knowledge management as a strategic process as seen by CEOs and top managers in indigenous Indian Fortune 100 companies. We look at how the pharmaceutical industry compares to other organizations of significant size in India across a range of factors concerned with knowledge management activity, using survey and interview techniques. We conclude that while only a few significant sectoral differences are evident, there is generally a heavy orientation towards IT-based conceptions of KM, which may be incompatible with the requirements for future success in the pharmaceutical industry globally.

INTRODUCTION

In this chapter we consider knowledge management initiatives with particular regard to the example of the Indian pharmaceutical industry. This industry exemplifies a knowledge-intensive industry area with an uncertain future due to a required change in practices in the context of international developments. Regulatory compliance, new knowledge creation, patent application and protection, sharing knowledge in partnerships and alliances, and widespread and timely access to information are all indicated areas of knowledge-based activity. The management of these processes entails their embedding into cultural and organisational practice, and this moderates the effectiveness of knowledge management tools. Many organisations face analogous issues of implementing KM strategies, despite sectoral differences, and we contextualise the Indian pharmaceutical industry both in its Indian and in its industry context. Lessons learned by benchmarking it in these contexts allow insights applicable to other healthcare industries. The chapter is organised as follows: first we review the global state of play in KM in large industries, concentrating on their strategic directions in KM, and highlight some issues applicable in specific countries and industries of concern here. Then we examine the particular industry environment surrounding pharmaceuticals, with particular reference to those factors applicable in India and noting the general importance of R+D. We then consider aspects of the Indian culture, at national and organisational levels, which distinguish it from competitor nations but which also potentially impact on the success of KM strategies. Finally we survey how KM is currently being undertaken in major Indian companies and especially compare pharmaceutical companies against other major organisations in relation to their knowledge management capabilities and strategic choices.

Knowledge Management and Industry

Knowledge management (KM) remains a central issue for large organisations. Having moved beyond being seen as a short-term fad, it is now widely recognised as critical to the success of knowledge-intensive industries, such as pharmaceuticals. Such industries, where the key organisational resource is knowledge, and which are often characterised by a focus on innovation and high research and development activity, are seen as taking on increased importance in the future economy (OECD, 1999). This has led to significant commercial and academic activity in information systems, in human resource management, accounting, economics and other disciplines. Surveys of CEO priorities, and numerous consultancy reports, dedicated journals, conferences and professional seminars indicate its continuing importance, as does the increased availability of vendor "solutions" and corporate appointments and internal KM initiatives. An indicative Google search uncovered (February, 2003) about 1,150,000 web pages. In this flurry of recent activity, definitions and understandings have been contested and, while work has separately focussed on IT, economic and human capital aspects, a more sophisticated understanding is emerging of its integrating potential. Earl (2001) has distinguished several schools that emphasise one or another of these various aspects and other frameworks and taxonomies have been proposed to integrate the extensive research underway.

KM, however, is not merely an academic exercise. Major companies have been quick to realise the importance of the assets implied by their data resources, the knowledge of their employees, and the communication of that knowledge in the work context. IT has allowed documents to be electronically preserved, emails to be archived, data to be warehoused, and computer activity to be logged, with management systems placed around those to search, discover patterns and organise for reuse or repurposing. These all, however, require *explicated* knowledge: the ability to form an intelligent query, to recognise a significant pattern, to relate ideas and to recognise a colleague's worth. In short, to make *use* of information in documents and databases is a human ability. And humans may not be able to express what they know, may not be willing to share it, and may not have had an opportunity to articulate information of relevance, such as a key connection between something of current organisational interest and something they have learned elsewhere. The concept of tacit knowledge, due originally to Polanyi (1958) and modified, elaborated and reinterpreted by later writers, has come to refer to that aspect in which unarticulated skills, intuitions and personal connections can be brought to bear in useful processes of knowing. According to Polanyi (1958), we know more than we are able to express in words. At the same time we rely on our awareness of what we cannot articulate. "While tacit knowledge can be possessed by itself, explicit knowledge must rely on being tacitly understood and applied. Hence all knowledge is either tacit or rooted in tacit knowledge. A wholly explicit knowledge is unthinkable" (Polanyi, 1969). Knowledge, therefore, can be formalized only in a limited way and any formal system will by necessity be incomplete. "The legitimate purpose of formalization lies in the reduction of the tacit coefficient to more limited and obvious informal operations, but it is nonsensical to aim at the total elimination of our personal participation" (Polanyi, 1958). However, many knowledge management initiatives rely on codification and formalization of knowledge and "tacit knowing is the fundamental power of the mind, which creates explicit knowledge, lends meaning to it and controls its uses" (Polanyi, 1969). Organisations dread losing employees with the ability to mobilise their knowledge in the organisation's service, hence the attempts to make it explicit and codified in transferable forms. The literature, unnecessary to rehearse further here, is replete with considerations of these issues, methods and "solutions" and with critiques of their philosophy. A clear distinction between tacit and explicit knowledge, which seems to underpin many knowledge management strategies does therefore not exist. Although the focus on explicit knowledge, particularly of technology-driven approaches to knowledge management, has significant implications for their success and usefulness.

Practically, there are many activities that have been conducted in an attempt to manage a particular organisation's knowledge, as we will see later. Many of these have been adopted piecemeal in a project context, in addressing a particular problem, or as pilot studies at the business-unit level. Maier and Remus (2002) propose contextualising KM activity centrally within a process-oriented strategy and enumerate eight sets of "strategies" identified from the literature. These include: (1) *mapping sources of internal expertise* (e.g., expert directories); (2) *establishing new knowledge roles* (e.g., create a new unit or position for knowledge-related tasks); (3) *creating a virtual work environment* (e.g., networked knowledge workers); (4) *supporting knowledge flows* (e.g., communication tools adapted for knowledge seekers and providers); (5) creating *innovation and new knowledge* (e.g., research and development focused on these). The other three strategic activity sets aim at managing customer information, intellectual assets, and integration with other business strategies.

Maier and Remus (2002) surveyed the top 500 German companies, as well as the 50 major banks and insurance companies in relation to their use of KM systems, and found a lack of process orientation in KM strategy. These authors also considered the numerous KM activities identified in the literature as confounding strategy, supporting activities and instruments. Reframing these activities within a process-oriented KM strategy, relating the activities to business processes, is seen by these authors as advantageous compared to other extant approaches. This is because of the value of an integrated approach, based on business processes.

Integration, focused around IT, has been understood by the Indian company Wipro, which recently achieved recognition for their leadership in knowledge management (Wipro, 2002). The international KM reality award recognises "implementation of knowledge management practices and processes by realizing measurable business benefits." The unified framework developed by Wipro cuts "across the boundaries of Culture, Content, Communities and Business Processes" and has resulted in a widely accessible knowledge base. "All of Wipro's initiatives like Six Sigma, PCMM, CMMi feed into the central knowledge management repository on a continuous basis" (Wipro, 2002).

Recent developments in information technology have inspired many Indian companies to imagine a new way for staff to share knowledge and insights. Instead of storing documents in personal files and sharing insights within a small circle of colleagues, they can store documents in a common information base and use electronic networks to share insights with their entire community. Most companies soon discover that leveraging knowledge is actually very hard and involves more community building than information technology (Gunnerson, Lindroth, Magnusson, Rasmusson and Snis, 2000). This is not because people are reluctant to use information technology, but due to the fact that they often need to share knowledge that is neither obvious, nor easy to document, and typically requires a human relationship to think about, understand and share (Swan, Newell and Robertson, 1999). However, with the growth in information technology capabilities, a clear operational distinction can be drawn between knowledge management as a technology and knowledge management as a strategy. The former can be captured, stored and transmitted as explicit knowledge in digital form (Marwick, 2001). The latter can only exist in an intelligent system (people) and uses information technology as a medium to create and share knowledge (Marwick, 2001). It is vital therefore to identify the interaction between knowledge and information technology and the appropriate balance between them.

The IT infrastructure in these approaches is seen as a key *mediating* component for explicit knowledge management. This is because information systems, enabling data or knowledge intensive processes operate in large, centralised or distributed organisations and typically require underpinning technologies specifically relevant to the nature of the knowledge work. IT-underpinned strategies have been implemented in several pharmaceutical companies with success.

Snis (2000) for example has described ways in which explicit knowledge in a Danish pharmaceutical company has been managed through, *inter alia*, IT support mechanisms such as intranet and "narrow-casting" of emails based on user profile matching. Such profiles identify processes and functions of specific concern to that group. Document management systems are also in use, with time-related status codes and access controls on operational documents, and this mechanism, with associated meta-information, allows relevant filtering of effective documents to applicable organisational groups or functional levels. User-owned and designed templates are also at work in functional areas allowing procedures and "better practices" to be shared. These are subject to internal quality controls before acceptance as a local way of working, and are framed by the legislative requirements of the external environment. Although the IT tools reported in her study certainly enabled effective knowledge management to occur, their success is surely dependent on the positive attitudes to knowledge management of those using them and Snis stresses that the IT should be seen in its mediating function. We return to this aspect of organisational culture later.

Knowledge Management and Healthcare

The consulting group KPMG describe various successful healthcare KM systems in their report, "The Knowledge Journey: Pathways to Growth" (KPMG, 2000). These include: Eli Lilly's globally spread intranet providing current information to the field sales force; NovaCare's system for providing regulatory and good practice knowledge as well as other information throughout the company; and Hoffman LaRoche's acceleration of new drug development through making information and knowledge available at every stage.

Eli Lilly, in particular, has led in the area of knowledge sharing by its strategic decision to emphasise alliances, e.g., with universities and biotechnology firms. They have developed tools which identified gaps in knowledge sharing and allowed effective remedial action to take place, in this case a discussion database that overcame geographical dispersion of partners (Futtrell et al., 2001). NovaCare's system is described in Quinn, Anderson and Finkelstein (1996), emphasizing its organisation around the frontline therapists' professional knowledge, in which detailed information on therapeutic care is recorded for use by a range of stakeholders. The (best practice) knowledge the company builds up over time is thus available to its professionals. Like Eli Lilly, Hoffman-La Roche's development of a new drug in conjunction with a range of strategic partners was another catalyst for a KM solution (Davenport and Prusak, 1997). In this case, collaboration tools and the development of a culture of sharing led to success (Vincente, 2002). Sharing knowledge is common to the above examples, and clearly addresses the human activities involved, with the technologies acting as effective supporting mechanisms.

Apart from the Roche example, Vincente (2002) recently summarised some other current KM initiatives of big pharmaceutical players and best practices identified by research. These included successful document management and collaboration at Amgen, and a portal and search solution to manage "overwhelming" unstructured information at AstraZeneca. He notes that the focus to date had been on document management and regulatory compliance, but portals and collaboration technologies are growing. As these latter technologies gain hold, the cultural factors affecting their usage will become significant. Indeed the field has for some time recognised the limits of equating KM with IT-based capture of existing knowledge, moving toward processes that *enable* new knowledge creation through tacit knowledge sharing, fostering communities and contexts in which this activity can thrive. These activities are more in the domain of human resource management, and processes of knowledge enabling are detailed in Von Krogh et al. (2000). Such a migration of focus will increasingly entail managerial initiatives addressing organisational cultures, not merely adopting IT "solutions." This will thus look to address the human processes of knowledge creation, and what can work culturally.

These examples show some of the current activities in organisations of relevance here, and resonate with the typical range of KM initiatives in knowledge intensive companies, including those that Skyrme (1997) identifies:

*   Creation of knowledge databases: best practices, expert directories, market intelligence, etc.;
*   Active process management: of knowledge gathering, classifying, storing, etc.;
*   Development of knowledge centres: focal points for knowledge skills and facilitating knowledge flow;
*   Introduction of collaborative technologies: intranets or groupware for rapid information access;
*   Knowledge webs: networks of experts who collaborate across and beyond an organisation's functional and geographic boundaries.

It is clear that while these can be enabled by IT, strategically integrating them with processes that will work within the culture are required (Davenport and Prusak, 1997). This entails assessment of those processes, the available technologies and the perceived benefits and threats related to a KM strategy.

THE PHARMACEUTICAL INDUSTRY

Pharmaceutical companies have an aspirational mission — introducing innovative products to serve the market as quickly as possible followed by enhancing their commercial potential. Four traditional core processes involved include: discovery, development, manufacturing and marketing, and these are closely interrelated. The creation and direction of knowledge, however, is now seen as the newest or fifth process by which a pharmaceutical company creates competitive advantage: it is this that is recognised as "knowledge management" in the Indian pharmaceutical sector.

The inaugural issue of the Pfizer journal (Pfizer, 1997) provided a useful assessment of the global pharmaceutical industry at the start of the new century. Challenges identified in its suite of articles include: market pressure to reduce costs, the R+D impact of biotechnology advances and mergers occurring among significant players, generic competition and "patent pirates," and changing societal demographics and expecta-tions.

These challenges translate into pressures to continue effective innovation, to streamline processes and to establish alliances (e.g., with biotechnology companies) to share findings as Pfizer, for example, has done (Pfizer, 1997, p. 19), and other major players likewise. All of these challenges are clearly critical knowledge-based activities. Innova-tion is recognised as a required continuing activity in the industry and to support this, growing larger, through mergers and alliances, has been a constant of pharma companies' strategies in recent times (Rasmussen, 2002). The value of scale has been stressed in a McKinsey study (Garg, Berggren and Holcombe, 2001) which notes that greater size "increases the number of bets a company can place on new technologies," as well as allowing faster completion of clinical trials, providing an advantage in launching blockbuster drugs, and increasing "its desirability as a licensing partner." Beyond a certain size, however, communities of practice begin to lose effectiveness and simply increasing size as a strategy is insufficient. Garg et al.'s analysis goes on to suggest that, with respect to new knowledge creation, a restructuring entailing smaller, federated specialist units is likely to be more productive and indicates that some major companies are already moving in this direction.

In addition to industry level challenges, the international and national legislative frameworks shape what is politically possible. For many countries, healthcare is a significant part of the national budget, and one that straddles public and private sector organisations. Although our focus here is primarily on pharmaceutical companies, it is to be noted that healthcare in general is a vastly larger concern, affecting these companies.

In India for example, a new national policy (the first in almost two decades) has been announced in which health sector expenditure is targeted to reach 6% of GDP by 2010 (PTI, 2002). The majority of this, however, is not centrally funded, with the policy aiming to decentralise services to district level and to achieve "gradual convergence of all health programmes under a single field administration" (Sharma, 2002). Currently India has a three-tier public health system, with central responsibility for major disease control (for example) and state governments funding the other two tiers. A convergence in which the responsibility devolves to the district level, and the central government's role becomes reduced to monitoring and funding of essential drug supplies, clearly implies knowledge management activity. Other aspects of the policy therefore indirectly address knowledge management issues, in which an integrated disease control network crossing the tiers of public healthcare can bring the goal of evidence-based policy-making closer. Interconnectivity, training and data integrity issues are indicated here (PTI, 2002), implicating both IT and human resource initiatives. There is a tight link between legislation for healthcare generally and pharma specifically. With respect to our focus on the pharmaceutical industry the policy notes the following two relevant points. Firstly, to avoid dependence on imports at least half of required vaccines or sera would be sourced from public sector institutions, and secondly, production and sale of irrational (understood here as not being science-driven) combinations of drugs would be prohibited (PTI, 2002).

It is not just national policies that impact on the pharmaceutical sector, however. Kuemmerle (1999) has shown that foreign firms invest in R&D sites abroad in order to augment their knowledge base or in order to exploit it. He states that foreign direct investment in Asia is expected to continue growth, with "more firms expected to carry out home-base-exploiting investments in China and India because of the future attractiveness of these countries' markets." The analysis by Atul (2002), however, qualifies this by noting specific relative advantages China has currently secured compared to India and shows how specific national policies have obtained these current advantages. Ganguli (1999) also expects a "sea-change in the pharmaceutical sector in India vis-a-vis business processes and intellectual property rights" due to changes in the patent laws occasioned by required compliance with the provisions of the Trade Related Intellectual Property Rights (TRIPS) following the GATT Uruguay. These particularly concern patent applications and marketing rights but also impact on research and development investments, and on foreign direct investment in R+D.

Policy settings will naturally impact on the strategic initiatives within the industry. With a market of about US$2.5 billion, the Indian pharmaceutical industry is the 12th largest in the world (Ramani, 2002) and other figures suggest a growth rate of 10% annually (Atul, 2002). The Indian pharmaceutical industry has traditionally thrived on rapidly copying Western drugs, often within four to five years of their first appearance in the global market The reverse engineering time includes a lag while likely market success is ascertained, but is much more rapid: both Zantac's and Viagra's marketers respectively met Indian competitors at the Indian and the global launches (Lanjouw and Cockburn, 2001).

Noting that India will implement the WTO-GATT agreement in 2005 (which will bar Indian firms from replicating innovations patented in Western countries), Ramani (2002) discusses approaches to research and development strategy and expenditure in this sector. In the Indian biopharmaceutical sector, this is linked not to firm size, but to research orientation, described in terms of the acquisition, disclosure, and internal creation of knowledge with market performance strongly correlated with a firm's (human) knowledge stocks. Examining a number of biotechnology firms on data from the mid-1990s, they found the counterintuitive result that patents, publications and academic collaborations all correlated negatively with R+D qualification intensity. The explanation provided recognizes the extent of tacit knowledge in biotechnology companies: literature is cited showing that because much of the knowledge created is tacit, residing in individuals or groups, it is hard to explicate, leading to a disincentive to patent. Although the imminent changes in the Indian patent law have led to a slight increase in patents recently (Desai and Agarwal, 2002), patent application processes and infrastructure were also reportedly inefficient at the time of writing, providing further disincentive. Publications and collaborations however do not have this latter problem, so managerial orientation is considered a more likely reason. Ramani (2002) concludes that since increased knowledge stocks impact positively with market performance of large firms, they might wish to reconsider whether increasing the knowledge disclosure parameters through publications and academic collaborations would increase longer term competitive advantage. Managing the intellectual property involved is thus likely to become vital.

It is the ability to create, generate or source knowledge that will provide sustainable advantage, but Kummerle (1999) has suggested that there are only a few outstanding academic clusters generating knowledge in the pharmaceutical industry and therefore, "foreign direct investment in R&D might be geographically more concentrated in only a few countries and regions than is the case in other industries." A WTO consultant (Prakash, 1998) interviewed the director of the Indian Drug Manufacturer's Association. His view was that the big foreign companies had never, and would not in future, conduct R+D outside their own countries, and there was little new internal investment and only a small overall amount in R+D. Without change there would be no indigenous innovation and the industry would be "stagnant." A study by Mansfield (1994) cited in Lanjouw (1999) confirms that the prevailing intellectual property laws in India were seen as so weak as to preclude it from being an acceptable location for basic R+D by multinationals, although there have been a small number of exceptions. The Indian government (2002) has recently announced its upgraded position on patents to comply with the Trade Related IPR agreements of its entry to WTO. The announcement also notes the related Doha declaration's (WTO, n.d.) stress on the affordability and availability of medicines for all. Pharma is not only big business: there are basic humanitarian issues in healthcare at issue. The debates and documents involved in relating IP rights to access to essential medicines are beyond the scope of this paper to review but one relevant source of further information is the Consumer Project on Technology website (http://www.cptech.org/).

Atul (2002) describes the comparative state of the pharmaceutical industries in China and India, and suggests China poses a threat to the Indian industry post 2005. He observes that foreign direct investment in the Chinese pharmaceutical industry is currently 18 times more than in India: a gap that is expected to increase "if India delays implementation of product patents and IPR laws." It is worth noting though that Chomsky (1994) has drawn parallels between the destruction of the French chemical industry when product patents were introduced and the likely impact of GATT on the Indian pharmaceutical industry. Lanjouw (1999) has considered this in some detail and suggested that there are signs that R+D will increase in India and that some companies will emerge as more innovative. But clearly in a sector that is having to change its model from reverse engineering of existing products towards indigenous innovation, the ability to create and share knowledge will be vital. This ability however, rests ultimately within the people making up an organisational and a national culture, and simply having enabling technologies is not sufficient to ensure success.

CULTURAL FACTORS IN RELATION TO KM STRATEGY AND IMPLEMENTATION

Knowledge sharing is essential for the effective implementation of knowledge management. The coupling between behaviour and technology is two-way: the introduction of technology may influence the way individuals work. People can and do adapt their way of working to take advantage of new tools as they become available, and this adaptation can produce new and more effective communication within teams. The history of information systems however is full of examples of user resistance to imposed developments that were "not invented here" or which did not fit the organisational culture or established way of working.

Staples and Jarvenpaa (2000), in a study of collaborative technology use in a Canadian and an Australian university, found that although task and technology factors were salient, indeed organisational culture factors did influence collaborative technology use for information sharing. Issues of trust and power are central here, and in an industry increasingly characterised by strategic partnering, the development of shared trust and a broad base of power is essential for generating a creative environment (Lendrum 1995). Although culture is learned, and ultimately plastic, both national culture and organisational culture have deeply held characteristics that may help or inhibit particular behaviours. Effective knowledge creation is critically dependent on willing workers within the organisation, and their propensity to share their knowledge. It is recognised that although local factors may override any particular predominant stereotype (Maruyama, 1994), such as a hierarchical and bureaucratic culture, entrenched national as well as organisational cultures are likely to play a significant role in determining this propensity.

Cultural factors at the national level, for example, have been shown to apply in a recent study of KM practice and understanding in Hong Kong (Poon Kam Kai Institute, 2000) whose summary of key findings notes the "paternalistic management style of Chinese companies" as being in evidence. Such factors translate into the typical practices of organisations in specific countries — Japan has had economic success in manufacturing through Kaizen (Imai, 1986), an ingrained philosophy to which it is culturally suited. But, when western manufacturers adopted integrated production "their divisions appear to lack the level of liaison and trust that exists between a Japanese manufacturer and its suppliers" (Imai, 1986). Again, the success of any particular organisational process must be attuned to what will work culturally.

The classic work-identifying dimensions by which national cultures are constructed and thereby differ is Hofstede (1980). A statistical analysis of two surveys was conducted in 1968 and 1972 totaling over 116 000 responses from employees of a large multinational firm (IBM was the empirical source). His book shows how his findings correlate to other extant studies and indicators. Considerable research has followed, including the introduction of a fifth dimension (short vs. long-term orientation), more countries and methodological critiques, which are addressed in a later book, revisiting the study and extending its implications (Hofstede, 1991; 1997). Although national culture and organisational culture are not "identical phenomena" (Hofstede, 1997), and the study of national differences has only been partly useful for understanding organisational cultures, organisational practices are shown to be culturally dependent. In the case of Indian companies, Hofstede (1997) suggests that the implicit model of organisation is the extended family, in which authority is concentrated along lines of seniority. In the original work, culture is characterised as "collective programming of the mind." Hofstede scored each of 40 countries on the following dimensions: power-distance, individualism, uncertainty-avoidance and masculinity. These dimensions are generally held to be stable, culturally entrenched and descriptively useful in illuminating cross-cultural differences. Two of these are particularly relevant here.

The first of these dimensions, *power-distance*, in organisational terms relates to the unequal distribution of power in a hierarchy, accounting for phenomena in which deference, sycophancy and servility are normal organisational behaviours. Hofstede's (1980) original definition is as follows:

"the power distance between a boss B and a subordinate S in a hierarchy is the difference between the extent to which B can determine the behaviour of S and the extent to which S can determine the behaviour of B."

India's score on this index is the fourth highest of all the countries, 77, where the mean is 51. This index has been theoretically related to trust and organisational innovation. It is worth noting that Hofstede (1980) reports other studies where a high score on this index correlates with relatively lower interpersonal trust. In other countries with high scores on power distance, low cooperativeness among employees and a relative lack of identification with cohesive work groups have also been shown. Such a climate would not be conducive to knowledge sharing. In contrast, Denmark has one of the lowest scores (18) on the power-distance dimension. The study reported earlier by Snis (2000) considered the issue of power, and found that in that (Danish) pharmaceutical organisation knowledge sharing was viewed as important and not seen as jeopardising an employee's position of expertise.

The second dimension in which cultures differ is uncertainty-avoidance, defined as "the extent to which members of a culture feel threatened by uncertain or unknown situations" and entails concepts such as the need for security and dependence upon experts and rules. On this index India scores 40, (seventh lowest overall) and well below the mean of 64. Some connotations of a lower value include more risk taking, acceptance of foreigners as managers, and a view that conflict in organisations is natural (Hofstede, 1980). It is also notable that those countries with lower values are held to be "more likely to stimulate basic innovations (but are) at a disadvantage in developing these to full-scale implementation" (Hofstede, 1997). The Australian Financial Review (Mills, 1994) published an assessment of Asian economies in which it viewed India as a "country of great creativity with a deep scientific and mathematical base" despite its commercial markets being "a haven of plagiarism and intellectual piracy." It also considered, however, that India was "a country of competing self-interest, and little concern for the common good." If the culture and incentive schemes are oriented towards knowledge hoarding, rather than sharing, innovation is likely to stall.

India's scores on Hofstede's other two dimensions are around the mean values and are not considered further here. The scores of particular organisations on the dimensions will also be moderated by local factors: Hofstede (1980) reports one study showing differences in structure and control systems between indigenous Indian and U.S. subsidiaries based in India. Although in the Indian pharma industry, the big players are mostly multinationals, Hofstede's original study was with IBM employees and the differences identified could thus be attributed to national factors. Since the employees in Indian pharma companies are predominantly Indian, whilst naturally remaining cautious in making attributions, the values learned in a particular culture can be expected to apply.

Puhlman and Gouy (1999) examined internal barriers to innovation in the international pharmaceutical industry, and noted that sharing knowledge is a major factor in successful companies, defined as those in the top 20% based on product introductions and sales. A lack of knowledge management leading to repeated mistakes was one of the five most common problems in innovation. Success was also seen to be enhanced by innovation in business systems, with information exchanged and disseminated faster, but also targeting the acquisition of new skills and information. Puhlman and Gouy's study showed that companies that use innovation tools and support knowledge management have considerably higher success rates, and note America's comparative advantages in process and strategy definition. They conclude with ten key self-assessment questions pertaining to innovation, addressing, *inter alia*, the gathering and systematic assessment of new ideas, the dissemination of knowledge, and the conduciveness of the company's culture.

SURVEY

Having covered the cultural issues that may impact on KM strategy success, we now look at some specific approaches to KM strategy in India through a 2002 survey of Indian Fortune 100 companies[1], which include leading indigenous companies in the pharma and healthcare sector. In particular the survey, which had 17 respondents, looked beyond a conception of KM as being purely IT-based and emphasised its relation to corporate strategy. However India, which has a recognised strength in IT, has often tended to equate KM activity with IT capabilities and solutions. The following summarises the key points gleaned from the survey.

To determine the technological infrastructure for implementing knowledge management within an organization, respondents were asked the following question:

Has your organization implemented or is it planning to implement the following technologies?

Figure 1 shows the responses.

Figure 1: Technologies Used for Knowledge Management

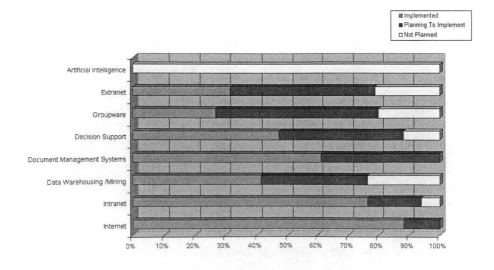

In the context of technology, respondents were looking at implementing both Internet and Intranet to develop a strong external and internal flow. In the context of the current scenario, developing a strong internal information backbone is of primary interest. This resulted in "document management systems" being the third most effective technology helping respondents in managing information. It is important to note though that technology in itself does not constitute a knowledge management programme; rather it facilitates one, especially in large, geographically dispersed organizations, typical of the participants in this survey. Another important aspect recognized was that, unlike such previous initiatives as Total Quality Management (TQM) and Business Process Re-engineering (BPR), the cost of implementation was not budgeted by the IT function, suggesting a whole business strategic perspective.

The state of knowledge management implementation was also addressed, and respondents were asked the following question:

When, if at all, do you intend to do any of the following, or has your organization done them already?

Figure 2 shows that facets of knowledge management practice such as implementing enterprise resource planning, creating a knowledge management strategy and benchmarking the current situation score more than establishing knowledge policies, incentives for knowledge working, creating a knowledge map or measuring intellectual capital. The majority of those interviewed were planning to use these measure to ensure success, but their preliminary focus was on having sound IT systems to facilitate knowledge within the organization. This confirms that less attention had been paid to the non-IT aspects.

The survey questions on strategy began by asking *Does your company have a Knowledge Management Strategy?* Seventy-five percent of respondents said that their organization had a knowledge management strategy in place, 19% stated there was no usage of any KM strategy, while 6% were completely unfamiliar with the term knowledge

Figure 2: Knowledge Management Processes

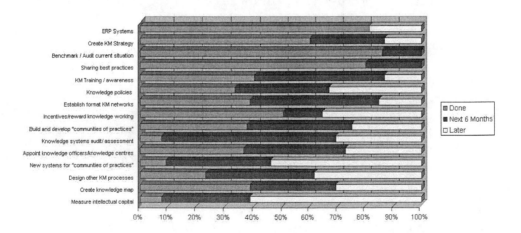

management. The above results demonstrate that most large organizations, including a major pharma, are not only informed about knowledge management but also are making efforts to successfully implement this strategy. However one company, which develops healthcare systems, had no internal KM strategy at the time of the survey despite an otherwise strong emphasis on information management solutions in the sector.

To examine the current position of knowledge management programmes within the 75% of organizations with a knowledge management strategy in place, a set of statements was presented and participants were asked: *How accurately does each statement reflect your organization?* Results revealed that 50% of companies have initiated knowledge in a nonuniform manner with pilot approaches in place. This is a fairly typical "entry-level" approach to KM. Only 12.5% of respondents said their organization had knowledge management as an integral part of their business process where the value of organizational knowledge is reported to their stakeholders.

Most participating organizations in the survey have, however, prioritised knowledge management initiatives on their business agenda. To identify the level at which these organizations have planned to initiate knowledge management activities, the respondents were asked the following question:

Which according to you is the most appropriate level in your organization to initiate knowledge management?

Reflecting an understanding of KM's organisational centrality, 50% of initiators of knowledge management are preparing to initiate knowledge management at all levels, and foresee implementing knowledge management organization-wide. This indicates that at least some drivers of the concept visualize knowledge management activities to spread across the organization. However, 12.5% of respondents plan to initiate knowledge management activities at the business unit or division-level and 37.5% identify the departmental level to be the most suitable, although no pharma companies were in these latter groups.

Another set of questions identified the general issues businesses foresee to encounter within the next five years, beginning with an importance rating on previously identified KM issues. The major issues selected as being important for pharmaceutical companies included *responsiveness*, in terms of time-to-market, *adaptability* and *quality* with, to a lesser extent in the case of pharma, *cost-productivity, alliance-networking* and *outsourcing* all seen as relatively important. However, this was generally true across all companies survey, not just pharma, though it is a bit surprising that alliances were not seen as more important than they were. In view of the 1997 (East Asian) recession, which caused a downturn in turnover in the majority of the companies, the biggest threat identified by the respondents was the ability to reduce the time to market to realize competitive advantage. Cost reduction and improved productivity follow this issue. Quality of the product was one of the major concerns but was not identified as an immediate threat to business sustainability.

Respondents were also asked to make a selection from the list of benefits on basis of short-term and long-term gains, through the following question:

Out of the following, what are the short-term and/or long-term benefits of implementing a knowledge management strategy?

Figure 3: Long-Term and Short-Benefits of Knowledge Management

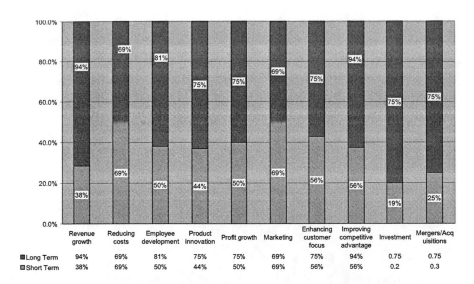

	Revenue growth	Reducing costs	Employee development	Product innovation	Profit growth	Marketing	Enhancing customer focus	Improving competitive advantage	Investment	Mergers/Acquisitions
■ Long Term	94%	69%	81%	75%	75%	69%	75%	94%	0.75	0.75
▨ Short Term	38%	69%	50%	44%	50%	69%	56%	56%	0.2	0.3

The responses indicated in *Figure 3* reveal that the potential benefits on a long-term basis would be in context of improving "revenue growth" and further enhancing competitive advantage. Another potential long-term benefit identified was "employee development" and "product innovation," which are very critical parameters in measuring the success of a knowledge management implementation.

Key short-term benefits expected by respondents would be "reducing costs," "improving marketing strategies," "enhancing customer focus" and "facilitating profit growth." The results indicate that knowledge management is not focused at enhancing a particular business process, but is implemented to achieve all-round benefits for the organization. It reflects more of a traditional conception of companies than a knowledge-centric view and innovation, acquisitions and investment are all seen as of more benefit in the relatively longer term, with less than half of respondents in each case seeing primarily a short-term value. For all categories one major pharma company saw all the benefits as long-term only, at odds with a range of companies in other sectors, the majority of whom also saw short-term benefits in a number of categories.

To measure the success of a knowledge management implementation, it is important also to ascertain the potential threats. Respondents who had a knowledge management strategy in place or were planning to implement a sound knowledge management strategy were thus asked to select the most likely threats from the list provided led by the question: *Of the following, what are the most likely threats towards achieving the benefits mentioned in the previous section?* The results are shown in *Figure 4*.

According to the respondents, as indicated in *Figure 4*, the integration of knowledge into everyday use in a normal work place and the lack of use or uptake due to insufficient communication were seen as the major threats. In addition, threats such as users not being able to perceive personal benefits and lack of participation from the senior management toward developing a sound knowledge management strategy were

Figure 4: Threats for Knowledge Management

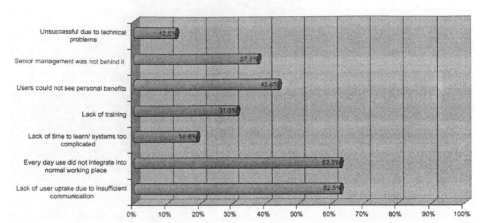

the prime areas of concern. The responses confirmed the fundamental flaw, i.e., viewing knowledge management only as a technology issue. We may assume from this that it is not the technology that is holding organizations back but a failure to initiate knowledge management into the organization's day-to-day operations and its culture. The communication issues identified as relevant barriers to KM comport with the low cooperativeness found in cultures with high power distance. Lack of senior support is also a substantial barrier for any culture formed along hierarchical authority lines.

CONCLUSIONS

In this concluding section we attempt to identify the current status and implications of knowledge management in organizations currently initiating knowledge management. Characteristics of national culture may at least in part be responsible for the anticipated and actual problems firms encounter in their knowledge management initiatives. They could also explain the focus on technology-driven approaches, as well as the failure to make knowledge management strategies an integral part of organizational life. Understanding of national and organizational culture and selecting a strategy that takes these factors into account seems a necessary prerequisite for successful knowledge management. In particular, barriers due to a prevalent cultural reluctance to share information mitigate against successful KM strategy implementations. Yet the nature of the industry environment in pharma requires effective knowledge sharing processes.

KM was primarily seen as having long-term, not short-term, benefits in pharma, yet the industry itself is having to change its model rapidly toward one based on innovation. In the survey data, in general however, there were few areas in which a particular sector (in particular pharmaceutical) was significantly divergent from norms in other sectors of Indian industry. The "knowledge management" projects within most of the respondents' organizations are just getting initiated and seem more heavily IT-oriented than HR and process-focused. It is vital to understand how indigenous organizations make an attempt to move beyond this concept and what measures they take to successfully initiate knowledge management. The big challenge, according to comments made by the senior executives who participated in this survey, will be to integrate the "pie in the sky" theories with actual use of "tools and technologies." A narrowly technical focus is likely to limit the potential for knowledge sharing unless coupled with effective human processes, and seeing knowledge as constructed through processes of social interaction among communities of practices means that issues of social networking, power and social inclusion/exclusion come to the forefront. In other cases information technology may actually undermine knowledge sharing and creation by reducing opportunities for informal contact or strengthening electronically the existing organizational walls, based on functional or geographical differentiation. Such issues may be at odds with the prevailing culture. However, although the pharma industry has several large multinational players located in India, our study is primarily concerned with the cultural capability of indigenous players to compete in knowledge intensive industries. Thus careful attention is needed to the potential impact of information technology on knowledge management for businesses in relation to existing social networks and communities within organizations.

REFERENCES

Atul, C. (2002). *Threat of China to Indian Pharmaceutical Industry*. Retrieved from the World Wide Web: http://www.indiainfoline.com/bisc/thre.html.

Davenport, T. & Prusak, L. (1997). *Working Knowledge: How Organizations Manage What They Know*. Harvard Business School Press.

Desai, P. & Sandhu, K. (2002). *Knowledge Management in India 2002*. Retrieved from the World Wide Web: http://www.knowledgepoint.com.au/knowledge_ management/index.htm.

Chomsky, N. (1994). *Noam Chomsky on India, GATT and Pharmaceutical Patents, and 3rd World*. Lumpen. Retrieved from the World Wide Web: http://www.cptech.org/pharm/noam.html.

Earl, M. (2001). Knowledge management strategies: Toward a taxonomy. *Journal of Management Information Systems, 18*(1), 215-33.

Futrell, D., Slugay, M. & Stephens, C. H. (2001). Becoming a premier partner: Measuring, managing and changing partnering capabilities at Eli Lilly and Company. *Journal of Commercial Biotechnology, 8*(1), 5-13.

Ganguli, P. (1999). Towards TRIPs compliance in India: The patents amendment Act 1999 and implications. *World Patent Information, 21*, 279-287.

Garg, R., Berggren, R. & Holcombe, M. (2001). The value of scale in pharma's future. *Vivo, 19*(8), 2-7. Retrieved from the World Wide Web: http://www.mckinsey.de/_downloads/kompetenz/healthcare/INVIVO_value_of_scale901.PDF.

Government of India. (2002). Press Information Bureau, Ministry of Law & Justice (press release), *India Upgrades Legal System For Patent Related Litigation*. Retrieved from the World Wide Web: http://pib.nic.in/archieve/lreleng/lyr2002/rdec2002/23122002/r231220021.html.

Gunnerson, M., Lindroth, T., Magnusson, M., Rasmusson, P. & Snis, U. (2000). *Less is more when IT comes to KM. Proceedings of IRIS 23*. Retrieved from the World Wide Web: http://iris23.htu.se/proceedings/PDF/110final.PDF.

Hofstede, G. (1980). *Culture's Consequences: International Differences in Work-Related Values*. Newbury Park, CA: Sage.

Hofstede, G. (1991/1997). *Cultures and Organizations: Software of the Mind*. London: McGraw-Hill.

Imai, M. (1986). *Kaizen*. New York: Random House.

KPMG. (2000). *The Knowledge Journey*. Retrieved from the World Wide Web: http://www.kpmgconsulting.co.uk/research/othermedia/wf2_kbase.pdf.

Kuemmerle, W. (1999). Foreign direct investment in industrial research in the pharmaceutical and electronics industries—results from a survey of multinational firms. *Research Policy*, 28, 179-193.

Lanjouw, J. O. (1999). The Introduction of Pharmaceutical Product Patents in India: Heartless Exploitation of the Poor and Suffering? NBER working paper No. 6366. Retrieved from the World Wide Web: http://www.oiprc.ox.ac.uk/JLWP0799.pdf.

Lanjouw, J. O. & Cockburn, I. M. (2001). New pills for poor people? Empirical evidence after GATT. *World Development*, 29(2), 265-289.

Lendrum, T. (1995). *The Strategic Partnering Handbook*. Australia: McGraw Hill.

Maier, R. & Remus, U. (2002). Defining process-oriented knowledge management strategies. *Knowledge and Process Management*, 9(2), 103-118.

Mansfield, E. (1994). *Intellectual Property Protection, Foreign Direct Investment and Technology Transfer*. IFC Discussion Paper, 19. The World Bank.

Maruyama, M. (1994). *Mindscapes and Management*. Dartmouth: Aldershot.

Marwick, A. D. (2001). Knowledge management technology. *IBM Systems Journal* 40(4), 814-830.

Mills, S. (ed.). (1994). *Asian Business Insight*. Fairfax: Australian Financial Review Library.

OECD. (1999). *The Knowledge-Based Economy: A Set of Facts and Figures*. Paris: OECD.

Pfizer. (1997). The pharmaceutical industry at the start of a new century. *The Pfizer Journal*, 1. Retrieved from the World Wide Web: http://www.thepfizerjournal.com/TPJ01.pdf.

Polanyi, M. (1958). *Personal Knowledge: Towards a Post-critical Philosophy*. London: Routledge and Kegan Paul.

Polanyi, M. (1969). *Knowing and Being*. London: Routledge & Kegan Paul.

Poon Kam Kai Institute. (2000). Pilot Survey on Knowledge Management in Hong Kong. Retrieved May 2000 from the World Wide Web: http://www.pkki.business.hku.hk/pilot.htm.

Prakash, S. (1998). *Trade and development case studies - country studies: India*. Retrieved from the World Wide Web: http://www.itd.org/issues/india5a.htm.

PTI. (2002). Two-year rural posting must for new docs according to new NHP clearing. *Express Healthcare Management*. Retrieved from the World Wide Web: http://www.expresshealthcaremgmt.com/20020515/hospinews1.shtml.

Puhlmann, M. & Gouy, M. (1999, June). Internal barriers to innovation: An international investigation. *Pharmaceutical Executive*, 19(6), 85-95.

Quinn, J. B., Anderson, P. & Finkelstein, S. (1996, March/April). Managing professional intellect. *HBR*, 71-80.

Ramani, S. V. (2002). Who is interested in biotech? R&D strategies, knowledge base and market sales of Indian biopharmaceutical firms. *Research Policy*, 31, 381-398.

Rao, M. (2002). *What do KM and Cricket Have in Common?* Retrieved from the World Wide Web: http://www.destinationkm.com/articles/default.asp?ArticleID=982.

Rasmussen, B. (2002). *Implications of the Business Strategies of Pharmaceutical Companies for Industry Developments in Australia.* Centre for Strategic Economic Studies, Working paper. Retrieved from the World Wide Web: http://www.cfses.com/pharma/documents/01-Business_Strategy.PDF.

Sharma, D. C. (2002, May). India's new health policy aims to increase public investments. *The Lancet,* 359, 1587.

Skyrme, D. (1997, September). Knowledge management: Oxymoron or dynamic duo. *Managing Information,* 4(7), 16-18. Retrieved from the World Wide Web: http://www.skyrme.com/pubs/kmoxy.htm.

Snis, U. (2000). Knowledge is Acknowledged? A Field Study about People, Processes, Documents and Technologies. *Proceedings of the 33rd Hawaii International Conference on System Sciences,* (vol. 3, p. 3023).

Staples, D. S. & Jarvenpaa, S. L. (2000). Using electronic media for information sharing activities: A replication and extension. *Proceedings of the 21st International Conference on Information Systems,* Brisbane, Australia (pp. 117-133).

Swan, J., Newell, S. & Robertson, M. (2000). Limits of IT-driven knowledge management initiatives for interactive innovation processes: Towards a community-based approach. *Proceedings of the 33rd Annual Hawaii International Conference on System Sciences*, Maui, January. IEEE Computer Society Press.

Vincente, S. (2002). Retrieved from the World Wide Web: http://www.novonordisk-it.com/resources/km+conference+nice+-+stefano+vincenti+v1.pdf.

Von Krogh, G., Ichijo, K. & Nonaka, I. (2000). *Enabling Knowledge Creation: How to Unlock the Mystery of Tacit Knowledge and Release the Power of Innovation.* Oxford University Press.

Wipro. (2002). *Wipro recognised for global leadership in corporate-wide knowledge management.* Retrieved from the World Wide Web: http://www.wipro.com/news room/newsitem2001/newstory219.htm.

WTO. (n.d.). *The Doha declaration explained.* Retrieved from the World Wide Web: http://www.wto.org/english/tratop_e/dda_e/dohaexplained_e.htm.

ENDNOTE

[1]   The questions (please contact authors for a copy of survey if required) were derived from a similar European study in 2000 by consulting group KPMG (http://www.kpmg.nl/das).

Chapter XIX

"Do No Harm":
Can Healthcare Live Up to It?

Nat Natarajan, Tennessee Technological University, USA

Amanda H. Hoffmeister, Cookeville Regional Medical Center, USA

ABSTRACT

The healthcare sector is a very important one in many countries and faces numerous quality and performance problems of great significance to all citizens who live there. Although there are many performance parallels between healthcare and other sectors, there are also numerous special issues and terminology, as well. Recent publications on medical errors have put the spotlight on the issue of safety in healthcare. There are opportunities for the healthcare sector to learn from other industries where many techniques and practices for preventing errors have already proved their worth. It is important and beneficial to encourage healthcare specialists to learn from other sectors the concepts, best practices, and tools for preventing errors and improving safety. This chapter addresses the key issues and challenges relating to the management and transfer of such knowledge and places them in the context of quality and knowledge management.

INTRODUCTION

Public spending on healthcare in Germany, France, Canada, UK, US, Australia, and Japan is at least 5% of their respective Gross Domestic Products (GDPs). In the US, UK, Australia, and Canada major health reforms have been proposed (*The Economist*,

2003). The total spending (public and private) in the healthcare sector in the US accounts for roughly 14% of its national income. In the US, the federal and state governments are the largest payers for healthcare services. The last decade has witnessed increasing attention to the healthcare-related issues such as widening coverage for access to healthcare, cost containment, quality of care, and regulation. These issues have been debated in legislative, academic, and professional forums. Issues concerning safety and quality have recently been in the public limelight. Recent publications have increased public awareness of safety or lack thereof in healthcare systems. They are the Institute of Medicine's (IOM) study titled *To Err is Human: Building A Safer Health System* (Institute of Medicine, 2000) and the follow-up report that was triggered by it, *Report of the Quality Interagency Coordination* (QuIC) *Task Force to the President* (Quality Interagency Coordination Task Force, 2000). The second report of the IOM, *Crossing the Quality Chasm: A New Health System for the 21st Century* (Institute of Medicine, 2001) goes beyond safety and identifies other areas where the need for improvement is urgent. Safety is viewed as one of the dimensions of healthcare performance. Effectiveness, patient-centeredness, timeliness, efficiency, and equity are the other dimensions. One of the ten recommended principles to guide the design of health systems is that safety should be system property (Institute of Medicine, 2001). The patient safety issue is not confined to the US. In the UK, a report published in June 2000 estimated 840,000 incidents and errors occur in the National Health Service (NHS) every year (BBC News, 2001).

QUALITY MANAGEMENT IN HEALTHCARE

The traditional approach to quality management in healthcare has relied on licensure, certification and accreditation, and the use of chart review methods. Over the years, a number of organizations have been involved in the development and deployment of these structural quality assurance mechanisms. Most notable are the Joint Commission on Accreditation of Healthcare Organizations (JCAHO), Commission on Professional and Hospital Activities (CPHA), Regional Medical Programs (RMPs), Experimental Medical Care Review Organizations (EMCROs), Professional Standards Review Organizations (PSROs), and Peer Review Organizations (PROs). In one sense, these organizations form the backbone of the regulatory structure of the healthcare industry. Thus, the traditional quality management was externally driven. The positive aspect of this system is that it provides safeguards to the public in terms of standards of healthcare and minimal competence of the healthcare professionals and ensures at least minimal participation of those professionals in quality management activities (Williamson, 1991). Its shortcomings are that it uses the negative incentive of punishment in the cases of non-compliance, and the underlying premise seems to be that sanctions are needed to ensure quality. It does not promote learning. It also involves a lot of paperwork, absorbing time and effort while achieving only modest improvements.

In the last 15 years or so, there have been many instances where the healthcare organizations have used the principles that underlie the industrial quality control model (Chesanow, 1997). These are the principles of total quality management (TQM) and continuous quality improvements (CQI) that have been successfully implemented in the manufacturing sector.

Briefly, these principles can be summarized as follows (Berwick, Godfrey & Roessner, 1990a): (1) productive work is accomplished through processes; (2) sound customer-supplier relationships are absolutely necessary for sound quality management; (3) the main source of quality defects is problems in the process; (4) poor quality is costly; (5) understanding the variability of processes is a key to improving quality; (6) the modern approach to quality is thoroughly grounded in scientific and statistical thinking; (7) total employee involvement is critical; (8) quality management employs three basic interrelated activities: quality planning, quality control, and quality improvement.

There have been many case studies of applications of CQI in healthcare (Carey & Lloyd, 1995). However, the concepts and tools of CQI did not always find acceptance among healthcare administrators and providers. Skepticism such as: "How do we define and measure quality, which is a more subtle concept in healthcare?", "Isn't quality mainly a matter of the physician making the correct decision?", "Where is the uniform product in medical care when every patient is different?" were expressed.

It is difficult to generalize about the effects of TQM in healthcare from isolated examples. Fortunately, the National Demonstration Project (NDP) on Quality Improvement in Healthcare provides a collection of experimental projects whose purpose was to study if the TQM model will work in the healthcare setting (Berwick, Godfrey & Roessner, 1990a). The NDP brought together 21 experts in quality management to work with a leadership team in 21 healthcare organizations represented by health maintenance organizations (HMOs), hospitals, and group practices in the US. The experts (who were from major US companies, consulting firms, and universities) were to offer their expertise in transferring quality management concepts and tools to these organizations that were willing to try them out. The participating organizations were to report on the results eight months later. Even though not all of the 21 teams completed the projects and reported back, the experiences of all of them contributed to the following important lessons learned (Berwick, Godfrey & Roessner, 1990b): (1) quality improvement tools can work in healthcare; (2) cross-functional teams are valuable in improving healthcare processes; (3) data useful for quality improvement abound in healthcare; (4) costs of poor quality are high, and savings are within reach; (5) involving doctors is difficult; (6) training needs arise early; (7) non-clinical processes draw early attention; (8) healthcare organizations may need a broader definition of quality; (9) in healthcare, as in other industries, the fate of quality improvement is first of all in the hands of leaders.

Despite these important insights that were gleaned from these projects, as acknowledged by the initiators of the project, there were two major gaps that were associated with these projects (Berwick, Godfrey & Roessner, 1990b). First, only a few project teams addressed core clinical processes such as physician decision-making, diagnostic strategies, and medical treatments. This seems to be in agreement with other research findings on the application of TQM in healthcare (Shortell, Levin, O'Brien & Hughes, 1995). Most teams worked on business and service support processes such as appointment waiting times, Medicare billing, patient discharge processes, and the hiring and training of nurses. Here the problems were similar to the quality problems in other industries. Interestingly enough, not even one of the teams measured success in terms of improved health status of the patient! Another gap was that the projects did not try to change the organizational cultures. Clearly, both these gaps have to be addressed in any effort to reduce or eliminate medical errors.

ERRORS IN HEALTHCARE

It is instructive to consider some findings about the occurrence and the impact of errors in healthcare. These stylized facts bring home in a compelling way the significance and the enormity of the tasks that lie ahead in the prevention of these errors. According to the IOM report (Institute of Medicine, 2000):

- Preventable adverse events (see the following below) are a leading cause of death in the United States. When extrapolated to the more than 33.6 million admissions to US hospitals in 1997, the results of two studies (involving large samples of hospital admissions, one in New York and the other in Colorado and Utah) imply that at least 44,000 and perhaps as many as 98,000 Americans die in hospitals each year as a result of medical errors. Deaths due to preventable adverse events exceed the deaths attributable to motor vehicle accidents (43,458), breast cancer (42,297) or AIDS (15,516).
- The rate of healthcare errors is far higher than the error rate in other industries. In one study of intensive care units (ICU), the correct action was taken 99.0% of the time, translating to 1.7 errors per day. One out of five of these errors was serious and/or potentially fatal. If performance levels even substantially better than those found in the ICU (for example, 99.9%, a 10-fold reduction in errors) were applied to the airline and banking industries, it would still equate to two dangerous landings per day at O'Hare International Airport and 32,000 checks deducted from the wrong account per hour (Leape, 1994)! In these industries, such error rates would not be tolerated.
- Errors occur not only in hospitals but in other healthcare settings, such as physicians' offices, nursing homes, pharmacies, urgent-care centers, and care delivered in the home. Unfortunately, very little data exist on the extent of the problem outside of hospitals. The IOM report indicated, however, that many errors are likely to occur outside the hospital. For example, in a recent investigation of pharmacists, the Massachusetts State Board of Registration in Pharmacy estimated that 2.4 million prescriptions are filled improperly each year in the state (Agency for Healthcare Research and Quality, 2003b).

Errors in healthcare do not lend themselves to commonly agreed-upon definition and classification. This poses a challenge in the design and implementation of measures to prevent them. For instance, according to IOM, an **error** is defined as the failure of a planned action to be completed as intended or the use of a wrong plan to achieve an aim. However, QuIC (Quality Interagency Coordination Task Force, 2000), in order to address all the relevant issues, has expanded the IOM definition as follows: An **error** is defined as the failure of a planned action to be completed as intended or the use of a wrong plan to achieve an aim. Errors can include problems in practice, products, procedures, and systems.

Medical error is defined through adverse events. An **adverse event** is an injury caused by medical management rather than the underlying condition of the patient. An

258 Natarajan and Hoffmeister

adverse event attributable to error is a **"preventable adverse event."** **Negligent adverse events** represent a subset of preventable adverse events that satisfy legal criteria used in determining negligence, i.e., whether the care provided failed to meet the standard of care reasonably expected of an average physician qualified to take care of the patient in question (Institute of Medicine, 2000).

Medical error is an adverse event or near miss that is preventable with the current state of medical knowledge. Note that consideration of errors is broadened beyond preventable adverse events that lead to actual patient harm to include "near misses," sometimes known as "close calls." A **"near miss"** is an event or situation that could have resulted in an accident, injury, or illness, but did not, either by chance or through timely intervention. The broader definition of error allows learning from close calls as well as from incidents leading to actual harm (Quality Interagency Coordination Task Force, 2000). Such learning has proved to be very valuable in other industries, such as aviation and nuclear power. It is also worth noting that not all adverse errors are preventable. **Unpreventable adverse event** is defined as an adverse event resulting from a complication that cannot be prevented given the current state of knowledge.

The implication of these definitions and classifications is that a single approach to error reduction and prevention is not fruitful. Different types of errors call for different approaches.

Error Prevention in Other Industries

Error prevention strategies in other industries have been part of an overall strategy for process improvement. The important features of these strategies can be summarized as follows:

1. *They have emphasized the control of the variation in the process.* Sets of tools that help to monitor, identify, and eliminate the root causes of process variations were utilized. How the responses of management can reduce or amplify the variation in the process was understood by considering the common and special causes of variation. The important lesson was that only management could and must do something about common causes of variation. Control charts were used to monitor process stability and signal the presence of special causes of variation. It must be pointed out that in Complex Adaptive Systems (CAS) like healthcare one has to carefully distinguish between meaningful variation resulting from innovation and variation which leads to waste (Institute of Medicine, Appendix B, 2001).

2. *Processes were simplified; standards were developed, documented, and adhered to.* One of the principles of lean manufacturing is to simplify the process and make it transparent to the workers (Womack, Jones & Roos, 1990). Simple and visual signals like *kanban* cards and a system of lights are used in the pull system of Just-in-Time (Schonberger, 1986). Errors can be easily detected and prevented in a visual factory. Standardization of work methods — which implies reduction of variation — is considered an important aspect of *kaizen* or continuous improvement. Once a process is improved using tools like the Plan Do Check/Study Act (PDC/SA) cycle, it is documented for future use. Standardization encompassed all aspects of the process. For instance, a system like the 5S encompassed housekeeping and promoted safety in the work place (Shaw & Gillard, 1996). Food production and service is an industry where safety is of paramount importance. As part of its efforts

to enhance the safety of food supply system in the US, the Food and Drug Administration (FDA) has mandated Hazard Analysis and Critical Control Point (HACCP) systems as a prevention standard. HACCP systems represent a systematic approach to the identification and control of the biological, chemical, and physical hazards that are reasonably likely to occur in a particular food in a particular production process.

3.   *Inexpensive but effective solutions were used to design errors out.* Poka-yoke or error proofing is a powerful, simple, and often inexpensive technique for eliminating mistakes from occurring in the first place or to provide early warning that a mistake is about to occur. The basic ideas behind mistake-proofing were first developed and applied by Shigeo Shingo under the rubric of Zero Quality Control (Shingo, 1986). Shingo felt that defects have to be prevented by preventing the mistakes that cause them. And this has to be designed into the elements of the process, i.e., into the equipment, procedures, the operating environment, and training of the employees. Of late, the principles of mistake-proofing have also been applied to service processes. An application in healthcare is the use of indented trays in surgical procedures to prevent surgeons from leaving any particular instruments inside the patient!

It is important to note that, in services, often the customer is an active participant in the service creation and delivery processes. Customer mistakes can occur at the stages of: (1) preparing for the service encounter; (2) during the encounter; and (3) post-encounter resolution (Chase & Stewart, 1995). This has important implication for application in healthcare — mistake-proofing efforts must be directed not only at the equipment and employees of the providers but customers of healthcare as well. For example, if you are a patient in a hospital, consider asking all healthcare workers who have direct contact with you whether they have washed their hands (Agency for Healthcare Research and Quality, 2003a). There is great potential for the application of mistake-proofing in healthcare.

4.   *Automation, information, and simulation technologies were used to reduce and prevent defects.* It is well known that computer-based automation in manufacturing has led to increased process consistency enabling much tighter tolerances to be met. For instance, robots can weld and paint more uniformly than humans. Information technology has been used in service industries to improve quality and customer service, e.g., by Ritz Carlton hotel chain (Bounds, 1996). Simulation and modeling has also proved to be very valuable in providing insights about the functioning of processes. Flight simulators are routinely used in aviation for training and education. Healthcare organizations can learn from the military as well. The healthcare profession can use computer simulation and military-based teamwork training as a means of training. Human factors engineering and ergonomics is incorporated into the design of processes and systems in industries such as nuclear power. By designing jobs, machines and operations that take into account human limitations, human errors can be prevented or reduced (Rooney, Heuvel & Lorenzo, 2002).

5.   *Trained and empowered employees implemented error prevention methods. They often worked in a multi-disciplinary team structure.* There was a cultural shift. Process improvement was no longer the responsibility of management alone. Employees were now responsible for not only doing the job but also improving it.

The leadership in the organization provided the support. Employees were encouraged to report on errors and devise solutions. In some of the companies that implemented Just-in-Time (JIT), the workers were given the authority to stop the line to prevent defects from being passed down stream. Once the line was stopped, problem-solving teams were formed on the spot to address the problem (Suzaki, 1987). The aviation reporting system, which the IOM and others have suggested as a model that healthcare should emulate, depends on the collection of as much information as possible about close calls as well as errors that actually resulted in harm. In the aviation industry, the identity of those who report and those who are involved in the incident are protected. This encourages people to report errors and makes the information available quickly.

6.   *Organizations have benchmarked their processes to identify and close performance gaps in critical processes.* The best-in-class processes — which were not necessarily in the same industry — were benchmarked. For instance, the activities of pit crews during pit stops in the motor racing circuit have been studied to benchmark worker changes on assembly lines (Walleck, O'Halloran & Leader, 1991). Granite Rock, a building materials supplier, has benchmarked its concrete mix delivery process with Domino's pizza delivery process (Bounds, 1996)!

7.   *Process improvement strategies focused on multiple dimensions of process performance.* The Six Sigma approach that was pioneered by Motorola in the 1980s and now being utilized by many manufacturing and service companies aims at *simultaneous* reduction of defect rates, cost, and cycle time in the process (Bounds, 1996). Six Sigma has been applied to manufacturing and non-manufacturing (service and business) processes (Chassin, 1998). Linking costs to quality and cycle times is a relatively new concept in healthcare (Castañeda-Méndez, 1996).

What is Different About Healthcare?

There are some characteristics of the healthcare industry that distinguish it from other industries. Although the managerial processes in the healthcare industry are similar to those of other industries, the prevalent norms, culture, practices, and the regulatory framework can promote or hinder efforts to improve safety. These characteristics also influence the extent to which the best practices for error prevention in other industries are relevant and transferable to the healthcare sector.

1.   Healthcare systems are very complex systems in terms of its constituent elements (e.g., patients, physicians and other healthcare professionals, purchasers of healthcare, payers, insurers, regulators, accrediting and licensing bodies, healthcare administrators, and professional groups), the web of relationships between them, and the knowledge, skills, and technologies that are utilized (Institute of Medicine, 2000). These groups have their own definition of errors and quality in healthcare. The interests of some of these groups are also in conflict.

2.   It is difficult in healthcare systems to establish precise linkages between the inputs and the resulting outcomes (Garvin, 1990). Therefore, it is not always possible to study and model the delivery of clinical care as a "process" as it is done in manufacturing. The outcomes in terms of patients' physiological and psychological states lag — sometimes in years — the treatments they receive. The outcomes

are also dependent on the cooperation and the compliance of patients themselves. In this sense, healthcare systems are quite different from other industries such as airlines, nuclear power, and food supply where safety is a critical issue. Hence, it becomes quite difficult to implement the principle that quality gurus like Dr. Deming have emphasized — quality can be improved only by improving the process. Lack of process knowledge could also be one of the factors that lead to litigation being viewed as the only recourse in the case of adverse outcomes. In fact, many legal cases in healthcare involve scrutiny of the underlying clinical processes in the courtroom.

3.   In healthcare, there is an information asymmetry between the care provider and the patient. The professional judgment of the caregiver determines the nature of the clinical care that is provided. Thus, the patient often cannot judge the quality or the safety of clinical care that he or she is receiving. In this respect, healthcare may not be very different from other professional services (e.g., accounting, legal, education) where such asymmetry exists and professional judgment influences the outcomes. Nevertheless, it underscores the difficulties in developing and monitoring quality and safety standards for clinical practices. This makes the healthcare market one in which the consumers do not have the requisite information about quality, safety, and utility to make informed choices. Thus consumers cannot adequately exert their power in the market place — as it happens in other industries — to bring about changes in healthcare providers.

4.   In many healthcare institutions, there are dual lines of authority — one involving the medical staff and the other the administrative staff. This complicates decision-making concerning design and implementation of safety improvement projects. In other industries, the managerial core has control over the technical core.

5.   Healthcare organizations are concerned about litigation in the context of tracking and reporting medical errors. This inhibits the relevant information from being shared within and between healthcare organizations. Legal constraints on access to and sharing of information relating to patients also prevent the dissemination of the information, which could be useful in preventing errors.

6.   In other industries like the automotive, large customers routinely exert pressure on their suppliers for continuous improvements in quality and costs. This is just beginning to happen in healthcare as large group purchasers want the healthcare organizations to improve their performance, but this has not become standard industry practice so far.

7.   Mechanisms and institutions for research and dissemination of research on safety in healthcare are still in a developmental stage (Institute of Medicine, 2000; Quality Interagency Coordination Task Force, 2000). The difficulties are compounded by the fact that advances in clinical knowledge, medications, and technologies in healthcare are taking place very rapidly.

8.   There are powerful subcultures in healthcare organizations based on occupation and specialization, e.g., physicians, nurses, and pharmacists. Their interests and functional orientations do not facilitate a systems approach to the promotion of safety (Zabada, Rivers & Munchus, 1998).

Prospects for Improving Safety in Healthcare

In the 1990s, many healthcare facilities and health plans placed an increasing emphasis on improving healthcare quality. Since 1999, it has become a requirement for managed care plans that contract directly with Medicare (Scott, 1998). However, these programs have not sufficiently addressed the problem of medical errors.

There are a number of factors that reduce the effectiveness of existing programs to prevent medical errors (Institute of Medicine, 2000). Performance measurement and improvement programs within healthcare organizations do not directly address the problem of medical errors. Programs that have been specifically developed to prevent medical errors often operate in isolation. Efforts by external organizations to monitor errors also face limitations. For example, JCAHO has experienced significant difficulty in securing hospitals' participation in its "sentinel events" reporting system because of concerns about legal vulnerabilities or punitive actions. A number of different programs exist to detect adverse health events, although no one system is designed to detect the full scope of medical errors. Systems designed to hold organizations or individuals accountable for bad outcomes are commonly limited by underreporting of adverse events.

Clearly, the quality improvement programs within healthcare organizations could be enhanced or adapted to address errors. However, there are serious obstacles such as: (1) a lack of awareness that a problem exists; (2) a traditional medical culture of individual responsibility and blame; (3) the lack of protection from legal discovery and liability. This causes errors to be concealed; (4) the primitive state of medical information systems, which hampers efficient and timely information collection and analysis; (5) inadequate allocation of resources for quality improvement and error prevention throughout the healthcare system. No insurer pays hospitals for safety initiatives, no matter how beneficial they are. And in most hospitals, revenues are declining as private and government insurers try to cut reimbursements; (6) inadequate knowledge about the frequency, causes, and impact of errors, as well as effective methods for error prevention; (7) a lack of understanding of systems-based approaches to error reduction (such as those used in aviation safety or manufacturing); (8) there are even greater barriers to error reduction in non-hospital settings, where the general absence of organized surveillance systems and lack of adequate personnel hinder local data collection, feedback, and improvement.

The IOM report and the action agenda developed by QuIC will go a long way in addressing these barriers. The QuIC report identified the actions that have already been taken and will be taken to reduce medical errors. They included, among others, plans of Department of Defense (DoD) to implement a new reporting system in its 500 hospitals and clinics serving approximately 8 million patients. This confidential reporting system will be modeled on the system in operation at the Department of Veterans Affairs and will be used to provide healthcare professionals and facilities with the information necessary to protect patient safety. DoD providers will inform affected patients or their families when serious medical errors occur.

The Food and Drug Administration (FDA) will develop new standards to help prevent medical errors caused by proprietary drug names that sound similar or packaging that looks similar, making it easy for healthcare providers to confuse medications. The agency will also develop new labeling standards that highlight common drug-drug interactions and dosage errors related to medications.

The Department of Veterans Affairs is considered as one of the nation's leaders in patient safety, having instituted patient safety programs in all of its healthcare facilities serving 3.8 million patients nationwide. The Veterans Administration (VA) healthcare system will form an innovative alliance with NASA to develop a medical error reporting system similar to the system NASA has operated successfully for the Federal Aviation Administration (FAA) since 1975. Aviation errors are reported by pilots, air-traffic controllers, mechanics, and all others involved in air transportation, to the Aviation Safety Reporting System (ASRS).

In 2001, the Department of Defense (DoD), investing $64 million, began the implementation of a new computerized medical record, including an automated order entry system for pharmaceuticals, that makes all relevant clinical information on a patient available when and where it is needed. It will be phased in at all DoD facilities over three years.

The QuIC member agencies, including DoD, Veterans Administration (VA), and the Agency for Healthcare Research and Quality (AHRQ), began a collaborative project with the QuIC Task Force and the Institute for Healthcare Improvement (IHI) to reduce errors in "high hazard areas," such as emergency rooms, operating rooms, intensive care units, and labor and delivery units.

Information Technology

The federal government has played a pivotal role in the application of information technology to healthcare. It has some of the earliest research on computerized patient records, studies evaluating the impact of computer reminder systems on laboratory testing errors, and research on the effect of computers on drug ordering. VA and DoD are recognized national leaders in the implementation of electronic medical records and decision-support tools.

QuIC can have an impact through its participants' activities in the area of electronic records and order entry. Most healthcare providers currently work with handwritten patient notes, which are often difficult to read, not readily available, incomplete, and prone to alteration, destruction, and loss. Structured, electronic order entry systems that require complete data entry remove ambiguities that arise from incomplete information or illegible writing. Real-time decision support is a powerful technological tool for error proofing. Decision-support systems can intercept errors, such as interactions between incompatible medications and the prescription of drugs to which the patient's electronic medical record notes an allergy. Bar-coding of medications and use of robotics in dispensing medications can ensure that the appropriate medication is provided to the right patient at the right time.

Information technology can also play a very important role in preventing errors in the delivery of clinical care itself. Electronic medical records and interactive decision-support tools have the potential to allow healthcare providers timely knowledge of a patient's health history and improve clinical care. Often physicians are overwhelmed with the changes in the knowledge base and find it hard to keep up with the literature — now they can turn to information technology for help. New England Medical Center has done work in the areas of Decision Support Systems (DSS) and Expert Systems (ES) that help physicians in making accurate diagnosis in emergencies and in selecting the best course of treatments for individuals and groups. Choices are developed by ES in the form of decision trees which incorporate individual risk preferences and special medical conditions (Grossman, 1994).

STEPS IN THE RIGHT DIRECTION

- One hospital in the Department of Veterans Affairs uses hand-held, wireless computer technology and bar-coding, which has cut overall hospital medication error rates by 70% (Agency for Healthcare Research and Quality, 2003b). This system is to be implemented in all VA hospitals. VA has an exemplary patient safety program, and the DoD is developing one that is modeled after that of VA.

- The specialty of anesthesia has reduced its error rate by nearly seven-fold, from 25 to 50 per million to 5.4 per million, by using standardized guidelines, protocols and simple mistake-proofing devices, redesigning and standardizing equipment (Agency for Healthcare Research and Quality, 2003b).

- In the UK, a missed diagnosis that almost resulted in the death of a three-year-old spurred her parents to set up a charity to develop a computer system to prevent such mistakes. The online system, called ISABEL, is free to all doctors. The rapid system uses pattern recognition software to search for information in pediatric textbooks, once it is given the symptoms. It even builds in other doctors' experiences of making mistakes (News Telegraph, 2002).

- The VA/Stanford simulation center for crisis management in healthcare at Palo Alto, California, uses a simulator that can execute all the physiological functions and mimic many complex and realistic clinical crisis scenarios. Instructors can alter these scenarios. By simulating an actual patient during surgery as much as possible, doctors can get quick feedback on if they injected the wrong drug, made incorrect interpretations and other errors. In the future, such simulators are likely to be part of medical education (Institute for Healthcare Improvement, 2000).

- SSM Healthcare became the first winner of the Baldrige award in the healthcare sector (National Institute of Standards and Technology, 2003). Sister Mary Jean Ryan, the CEO of SSM for last 17 years, said she once failed to report her own error in medicating a patient, so SSM has created a "blame-free" zone for reporting not only errors but near-misses. "Half the reported incidents lead directly to system improvements," she said (Broder, 2002).

- General Motors (GM), which has 1.25 million people in its health plans, is the largest private purchaser of healthcare in the US. It is working with partners in the healthcare industry to teach them principles of lean organization such as standardized work; workplace organization and visual controls; error proofing; employee process control; planned maintenance; and reduction of variation (Shapiro, 2000). Some hospitals have tried to be proactive in adapting such best practices from manufacturing by implementing patient-focused care teams analogous to manufacturing cells (Taylor, 1994).

- "The Medical Center of Ocean County has embraced an approach that has put the facility in Brick, New Jersey, on the cutting edge of medication system developments" (Darves, 2002). The new system involves using pharmacy technicians both on nursing units and in the emergency department and implementing Just-in-Time (JIT) delivery of medications to replace the traditional 24-hour cart system. Patient safety has improved, time savings have accrued, and nurse and patient satisfaction has increased.

- In an important development in the dissemination of comparative data, the federal centers of Medicare and Medicaid have developed a massive database, including in it every one of the 17,000 Medicare and Medicaid-certified nursing homes in every state in the US. This data is now available online (Medicare, 2003) and also on a toll-free telephone number, 1-800-MEDICARE (Medicare, 2003). For the first time, objective comparisons on several quality measures and inspection results can be made. It also provides individual nursing homes a database to benchmark, learn, and improve quality of care.

Other than the initiatives spawned by the above-mentioned federal agencies and taskforces, a number of other non-governmental programs have also been launched. For instance, the Leapfrog group was formed by the Business Roundtable in 2000. Leapfrog is a coalition of more than 135 public and private healthcare organizations and a voluntary program which has as part of its mission "... to help save lives and reduce preventable medical mistakes by mobilizing employer purchasing power to initiate breakthrough improvements in the safety of healthcare and by giving consumers information to make more informed hospital choices" (Leapfrog Group, 2003). It has focused on three patient safety practices that it believes have the potential to save lives by reducing preventable medical mistakes in hospitals. They are: Computer Physician Order Entry, Evidence-Based Hospital Referral, and Intensive Care Unit Physician Staffing. The group gathers data from hospitals on their status with regard to these practices and makes the information available to the consumers and communities.

The American Society for Quality (ASQ) is partnering with the National Patient Safety Foundation (NPSF) to offer solutions for reducing errors and increasing patient safety. Successful applications of methods such as Six Sigma will be shared in the events organized by them. ASQ is also influencing public policy in this area. It has presented a paper to the congressional health policy staff advocating the wider adoption of proven quality methods in an effort to reduce medication errors (American Society for Quality, 2002).

In the UK, where the National Health Service (NHS) is the major provider of healthcare, the National Public Safety Agency (NPSA) has been created. It is a special health authority created in July 2001 to coordinate the efforts of the entire country to report, and more importantly to learn from, adverse events occurring in NHS-funded care. The NPSA will collect and analyze incident and other patient safety information and provide timely and relevant feedback to healthcare organizations, clinicians, and other healthcare professionals, and patients (National Patient Safety Association, 2003).

While these success stories and developments contribute to the application of knowledge management systems to improve patient safety, a word of caution may be in order. The success stories may indicate what has worked in specific instances, but given the nature of the industry not too much is going to be heard about failures. The knowledge about what does not work may be lacking.

In one sense, the task of transferring best practices is made easier in the case of healthcare. In the 1980s, when the manufacturing sector in the US faced a crisis with respect to product quality and competitiveness, not many role models and forums for sharing best practices were available. The Baldrige Award was set up to address that gap. But today, there is no shortage of knowledge or the mechanisms to disseminate that knowledge. The Baldrige framework has been extended to the healthcare sector. Award winners such as SSM Healthcare can serve as role models. There are many other state and local quality award programs that provide avenues for sharing best practices. Within healthcare itself, organizations like the National Coalition for Healthcare, Institute for Healthcare Improvement, Leapfrog Group, and The National Patient Safety Foundation disseminate the best practices.

These forums and mechanisms are indeed necessary, but they are not sufficient to ensure the actual transfer of these best practices. For instance, it has been noted that the National Safety Partnership publicized a list of 16 proven and accepted best practices in medication safety. Many of them have been known for years but most are not used in a majority of hospitals. The case of the healthcare industry in Japan also reinforces this point. Despite having a manufacturing industry known for its world class quality management system, the healthcare system in Japan did not undergo a similar quality revolution (Wocher, 1997). The reasons for this are rooted in the institutional characteristics of the Japanese healthcare sector. According to Wocher, the Japanese healthcare sector lags far behind US in terms of efficiency, overall management, and the application TQM and CQI ideas (Wocher, 1997).

All this leads one to conclude that there has to be a "felt need" for industry-wide, effective prevention of errors, and improving patient safety. At the level of an individual healthcare organization, this "felt need" will be generated by a mixture of factors. They are: (1) the organizational leadership that is willing and able to overcome the internal obstacles; (2) economic incentives from the market place that affect the bottom-line; (3) external compulsions by the consumers, purchasers, payers, accreditors, and regulators; and (4) the leadership role and the role models of the federal agencies. Earlier discussion of the above issues suggests that, of late, there are encouraging signs that some traction for improving patient safety has been created by these factors. And that portends well for patient safety and knowledge management for patient safety as well.

REFERENCES

Agency for Healthcare Research and Quality. (2003a). *20 tips to help prevent medical errors*. Patient Fact Sheet. AHRQ Publication No. 00-PO38. Rockville, MD: Agency for Healthcare Research and Quality. Retrieved from the World Wide Web: http://www.ahrq.gov/consumer/20tips.htm.

Agency for Healthcare Research and Quality. (2003b). *Medical errors: The scope of the problem*. Fact sheet, AHRQ Publication No. 00-P037. Rockville, MD. Retrieved from the World Wide Web: http://www.ahrq.gov/qual/errback.htm.

American Society for Quality. (2002, September). ASQ lends a hand at reducing healthcare errors. *Quality Progress, 35*(9), 29.

BBC News. (2001, April). NHS aims to improve patient safety. *Health*. Retrieved from the World Wide Web: http://news.bbc.co.uk/l/hi/health/1281329.stm.

Berwick, D. M., Godfrey, A. B. & Roessner, J. (1990a). Symptoms of stress in healthcare systems. *Curing Healthcare: New Strategies for Quality Improvement* (pp. 1-17). San Francisco, CA: Jossey-Bass.

Berwick, D. M., Godfrey, A. B. & Roessner, J. (1990b). Ten key lessons for quality improvement. *Curing Healthcare: New Strategies for Quality Improvement* (pp. 144-157). San Francisco, CA: Jossey-Bass.

Bounds, G. M. (ed.) (1996). *Cases in Quality.* Homewood, IL: Richard D. Irwin.

Broder, D. S. (2002, April). A beacon for better healthcare. *The Washington Post.*

Carey, R. G. & Lloyd, R. C. (1995). *Measuring Quality Improvement in Healthcare: A Guide to Process Control Applications.* New York: Quality Resources.

Castañeda-Méndez, K. (1996). *Value-based Cost Management for Healthcare: Linking Costs to Quality and Delivery.* New York: Quality Resources.

Chase, R. B. & Stewart, D. M. (1995). *Mistake-proofing: Designing Errors out.* Portland, OR: Productivity Press.

Chassin, M. (1998). Is healthcare ready for Six Sigma quality? *Milbank Quarterly,* 76(4), 565-1.

Chesanow, N. (1997, August). Making doctors' lives easier — and patients happier. *Medical Economics,* 1, 118.

Darves, B. (2002, December). Just-in-time drug delivery pays off. *The Newsletter of Quality Issues in Healthcare.* Retrieved from the World Wide Web: www.qualityindicator.com.

The Economist. (2003, March). Regime change for doctors. *The Economist Global Agenda.* Retrieved from the World Wide Web: http://www.economist.com/agenda/displayStory.cfm?story_id=1626257.

Food and Drug Administration. (2001). Retrieved from the World Wide Web: http://www.fda.gov/ola/2001/foodsafety1010.html.

Garvin, D. A. (1990). Afterword: Reflections on the future. In *Curing Healthcare: New Strategies for Quality Improvement*, (pp. 159-165). San Francisco, CA: Jossey-Bass.

Grossman, J. H. (1994). Plugged-in medicine. *Technology Review,* 97(1), 22-29.

Hoerl, R. W. (1998, June). Six Sigma and the future of the quality profession. *Quality Progress,* 1(6), 35-42.

Institute for Healthcare Improvement. (2000, February). Reducing medical errors and improving patient safety: Success stories from the front lines of medicine. *Accelerating Change Today.* Retrieved from the World Wide Web: www.ihi.org.

Institute of Medicine. (2000). *To Err is Human: Building a Safer Healthcare System.* L. Kohn, J. Corrigan & M. Donaldson (eds.). Washington, DC: National Academy Press. The on-line versions of the report can be found at the website of National Academy Press. Retrieved from the World Wide Web: www.nap.edu.

Institute of Medicine. (2001). *Crossing the quality chasm: A new health system for the 21st century.* Washington, DC: National Academy Press. The on-line version of the reports can be found at the website of National Academy Press. Retrieved from the World Wide Web: www.nap.edu.

Leape, L. L. (1994). Error in medicine. *Journal of the American Medical Association,* 272, 1851-57.

Leapfrog Group. (2003). Retrieved from the World Wide Web: http://www.leapfrog group.org/about.htm.

Medicare. (2003). Retrieved from the World Wide Web: www.medicare.gov.

National Institute of Standards and Technology. (2003). Baldrige National Quality Program. *SSM Healthcare.* Retrieved from the World Wide Web: www. quality.nist.gov.

National Patient Safety Association. (2003) Retrieved from the World Wide Web: http://www.npsa.nhs.uk.

News Telegraph. (2002, June). *Parents who did something positive.* Retrieved from the World Wide Web: www.news.telegraph.co.uk.

Quality Interagency Coordination Task Force (QuIC) Report to the President. (2000, February). Doing what counts for patient safety: federal actions to reduce medical errors and their impact. *Retrieved from the World Wide Web:* http://www.quic.gov/ report/.

Rooney, J. J., Heuvel, L. V., & Lorenzo, D. K. (2002, September). Reduce human error. *Quality Progress,* 35(9), 27-36.

Schonberger, R. (1986). *World Class Manufacturing: Lessons of Simplicity Applied.* New York: Free Press.

Scott, J. S. (1998, October). Questing for quality: QISMC-ly cutting the QAPI. *Healthcare Financial Management,* 52(10), 32.

Shapiro, J. P. (2000, July). Taking the mistakes out of medicine. *U. S. News & World Report,* 129(i3), 50.

Shaw, A. & Gillard, J. (1996). Partnering the Honda way. In G. Bounds (Ed.), *Cases in Quality,* (pp. 26-56). Homewood, IL: Richard D. Irwin.

Shingo, S. (1986). *Zero Quality Control: Source Inspections and the Poka-Yoke System.* Portland, OR: Productivity Press.

Shortell, S., Levin, D., O'Brien, J. & Hughes, E. (1995). Assessing the evidence on CQI: Is the glass half empty or half full? *Journal of the Foundation of the American College of Healthcare Executives,* 40, 4-24.

Suzaki, K. (1987). *The New Manufacturing Challenge: Technique for Continuous Improvement.* New York: Free Press.

Taylor, S. (1994, January). The medical center takes proactive approach to healthcare reform. *Industrial Engineering,* 26(1), 20-23.

Walleck, S., O'Halloran, D. & Leader, C. (1991). Benchmarking world-class performance. *McKinsey Quarterly,* 1, 7.

Williamson, J. W. (1991). Medical quality management system in perspectives. Chapter 2 in J. B. Crouch (Ed.), *Healthcare Quality Management for the 21st Century.* The American College of Physician Executives, Tampa, FL: American College of Medical Quality.

Wocher, J. C. (1997). TQM/CQI efforts in Japanese hospitals—why not? In V. A. Kazandijian (Ed.), *Effectiveness of CQI in Healthcare: Stories from a Global Perspective,* (pp. 49-108). Milwaukee, WI: Quality Press.

Womack, J. P., Jones, D. & Roos, D. (1990). *The Machine that Changed the World.* New York: R. A. Rawson.

Zabada, C., Rivers, P. A. & Munchus, G. (February 1998). Obstacles to the application of total quality management in healthcare organizations. *Total Quality Management,* 9(1), 57-59.

Section IV

Managing Knowledge
as an Asset in
Healthcare Organizations

Chapter XX

Temporary Communication Infrastructures for Dynamic KM in the Complex and Innovative Environment of Palliative Care

Graydon Davison, University of Western Sydney, Australia

ABSTRACT

Research in Australia on the management of innovative practices in multidisciplinary palliative care teams reveals the central role of knowledge as an enabler of holistic care in an environment where sometimes little, apart from the result of the end of life process, is operationally predictable. While palliative care organisations provide, and regulators require, opportunities for formal exchange, recording and review of patient-based information and patient care processes; the members of care teams require and construct more frequent opportunities for the exchange of information and the generation and application of knowledge. Multidisciplinary patient care teams are resourced to and capable of constructing real-time temporary communication infrastructures between the team's different disciplinary representatives, between teams as necessary and between teams and the organisation, for individual patient situations. This chapter describes the organisational capabilities and levers necessary for providing an environment within which these infrastructures can be created and the individual behaviours and team tools that are used in the process, based on a wide ranging literature review and the results of research interviews.

PALLIATIVE CARE

Palliative care is an environment where multi-profession teams work collegeately with patients who are dying and with the patient-based carers who support them so that the primary issue becomes and remains patient comfort (Meyers, 1997). Palliative care is delivered by multidisciplinary teams (McDonald and Krauser, 1996) that comprise a number of disciplines including nursing, medicine, pharmacology, physiotherapy, occupational therapy, social work, spiritual care, grief counseling and administration. In this environment people are the centre, not diseases, and care results from the understanding of the causes of distress (Barbato, 1999). Successful provision of palliative care is dependent upon understanding the causes of distress, whether the cause is physical, emotional or spiritual or whether it is known or unknown (McDonald and Krauser, 1996; Witt Sherman, 1999). The patient's end-of-life state and central role in efforts to manage that state makes the patient a participatory member of the palliative care team who maintains a level of autonomy and control in relation to the other team members (McDonald and Krauser, 1996; McGrath, 1998). The arrival of a patient at an end-of-life experience requiring palliative care brings the certainty that life will end, generally within a relatively short period of time. This single fact aside, uncertainty is the basis of the end-of-life experience. In addition to this, each patient is experiencing the end-of-life on two distinct levels, the conscious and the unconscious, and the depth of the experience at each level varies from patient to patient (Kearney, 1992). Palliative care is an uncertain, dynamic environment with a certain conclusion. Prior to arriving at that certain conclusion, it is the uncertainty that directs all attempts to provide care. For the professions involved, this creates a working environment requiring ongoing work-based learning, governed by an uncertain direction of care that must follow a trajectory of need, of which the patient is the major informant (Henkelman and Dalinis, 1998). The palliative care environment is one of multi-causal uncertainty. This is addressed with individualized care for patients and their personally based support systems, using cross-functional, collaborative, multidisciplinary teams that include the patient and patient-based carers.

CAPABILITIES ENABLING KM IN THE MULTIDISCIPLINARY TEAM

A number of capabilities are necessary for palliative care organisations: managing knowledge; managing information; multidisciplinary operations; collaborative operations; managing technology; and managing change and its effects (Davison and Hyland, 2003). Research in Australia has confirmed the necessity of these capabilities from interviews with palliative care managers. Of this list, the first two are obviously and directly relevant to this chapter. However, given the predominant role in palliative care of knowledge and information creation across boundaries and using a large range of sources and targets, it is proposed that multidisciplinary and collaborative operations also have relevance to this chapter.

The manifold nature of palliative care demands multidisciplinary operations as a capability (McDonald and Krauser, 1996; Myers, 1997). The usefulness of multidisciplinary operations in palliative care is the opportunity that this provides for teams to mobilise and learn from each other's skills and experiences in patient care in any of the palliative environments; home care, inpatient, outpatient or hospice (Witt Sherman, 1999). McDonald and Krauser (1996) note the need within effective palliative care to remove traditional territorial thinking and interests and to raise new partnerships in the carer networks.

Collaboration across professional groups in healthcare is capable of increasing levels of satisfaction in carers, requires common purpose, is built on trust arising from the honest communication of information, and requires the alignment of the values of the collaborators to occur successfully (Liedtka et al., 1998). The operationalization of multidisciplinary collaboration in healthcare is dependent on the recognition of alternative perspectives on the part of the collaborators, combined with the use of communication styles that facilitate collaboration (Van Ess Coeling and Cukr, 2000). Witt Sherman (1999) writes that physicians, nurses and members of other disciplines need to work collaboratively to deliver holistic care over time, to assist patients and families to come to terms with the issues of death and dying and to move beyond the management of symptoms. Collaboration is also necessary in the creation of knowledge and the provision of information within a context such as palliative care.

Knowledge management includes knowledge generation, capture, exploitation and dissemination. Managing and cultivating knowledge is a method of building, changing, displaying and evidencing organisational competence (Brown and Duguid, 1998). Knowledge can be described as information that has been contextually processed and enriched via analysis and interpretation and information as data that have been organised and interpreted (Duffy, 2000). This view is supported by Davenport et al. (1998), who describe knowledge as a contextual combination of experience, interpretation and reflection. Palliative care is delivered by multidisciplinary teams that include any person relevant and available to the patient's needs (McDonald and Krauser, 1996), including family and friends of the patient (Lewis et al., 1997; Rose, 1997). In palliative care, the carer network that uses knowledge in this environment is widespread, multi-leveled, and dynamic. Each member of each patient's dynamic carer network will join the network with an existing level of knowledge and experience, an ability to learn and communicate and differing requirements for knowledge. Managing knowledge across and through the carer network includes the opportunistic capture and exploitation of knowledge from sources other than the carer network. Dynamic carer networks are rich in terms of the number and type of individuals involved. This richness is evidenced in the diversity of experience, information, intellect, biases, skills and training that are brought to the inter and intra-network use and generation of knowledge (Brown and Duguid, 1998). Palliative care networks are knowledge-based networks.

Information is viewed in this chapter as distinctly different to knowledge. Certainly knowledge and information are linked, with Abell (2000) describing information as a precursor and the foundation of knowledge. Knowledge can be recorded, archived and distributed and one of the primary formats or vehicles for the transport and distribution of knowledge is information (Berman, Brown and Woodland, 1999). In smaller, singularly focused healthcare organisations the usefulness and importance of information is related to informing the reorganization of services, policies and structures to better suit patients and to remotely manage patients (Alemi, 2000). The nature of palliative care drives a need to manage information from disparate sources within and between disciplines and dynamic carer networks and related networks in the broader healthcare community and the general community. According to Brown and Duguid (1991), information exchanged through story telling is used in work situations with complex social networks as a mechanism for groups to apply accumulated learning to changing situations. The richness of the knowledge available and necessary across and within the dynamic carer networks of palliative care requires a sophisticated, multi-role use and management of information. The role of information in palliative care is threefold and each role is of equal priority: (1) it is essential to the effective operation of carers, administrators and decision makers (Austin et al., 2000); (2) it is, as already noted by Abell (2000), a foundation of knowledge; and it is also (3) a vehicle for the transport of knowledge (Berman, Brown and Woodland, 1999).

LEVERS FOR THE KM ENVIRONMENT

Important to the operation of knowledge management processes at the team level is the use of a number of levers that have "substantial influence on the attitudes and practices of individuals and groups with regard to improvement and learning" and "facilitate characteristic behaviour and activity" (Gieskes, 2001). An interesting characteristic of palliative care operations is that the heads of disciplines, as well as being managers, are also practicing members of the multidisciplinary teams.

Multidisciplinary palliative care teams contain a functional and demographic diversity that is established by the context. A primary component of these diversities, mentioned by a number of authors (Reese and Sontag, 2001; Coopman, 2001; Duncker, 2001), is knowledge. Cohen and Levinthal (1990) note that the diversity of the knowledge held by individuals within groups, provided communication is sufficient, enables the creation of novel linkages and relationships, which these authors call innovation. Sethi et al. (2001) state that this creation of novel linkages and relationships is a fundamental reason for creating a cross-functional team. Multidisciplinary teams are collaborative by requirement (Jassawalla and Sashittal, 1999; Reese and Sontag, 2001; Sethi et al., 2001). With specific regard to palliative care practice, Coopman (2001) describes multidisciplinary healthcare teams as self-managing, needing to share information among members and giving particular priority to the participation of members.

Sethi et al. (2001), describing factors affecting the ability of cross-functional product development teams to innovate as required, note that one of the keys to the successful operation of these types of teams, at the project level, is balance. According to these authors, an appropriate balance must be struck on a number of fronts, all affecting the ability of the team to innovate. Among these are: (1) functional diversity, (2) social cohesion, and (3) superordinate identity. Functional diversity is described as referring to "the number of functional areas represented on the team whose members are fully involved in the project" (Sethi et al., 2001). An increase in functional diversity creates an increase in views and opinions, although there is a warning about information overload and failure to resolve differences that can accompany high levels of diversity. Eagleson et al. (2000) suggest that, at least in management teams, the level of diversity is a function of the context of the team's operation. Other authors regard functional diversity, when combined with demographic diversity, as requisite for the success of multidisciplinary team operations (Reese and Sontag, 2001; Coopman, 2001) and management team operations (Simons et al., 1999; Eisenhardt et al., 1997; Schoenecker et al., 1995).

Social cohesion "refers to the strength of interpersonal ties among team members" (Sethi et al., 2001, p.75). It is necessary for the team to generate a level of social cohesion for the basic functioning of the team. According to Bernthal and Insko (1993), social cohesion is based in the value team members place on social relationships within the team, while task cohesion is based in the value team members place on demonstrating task competence as a member of an effective team. Coopman (2001) makes the point that high levels of task cohesion are positively correlated with high team effectiveness. Bernthal and Insko (1993, p.81) write among their conclusions that, "These findings imply that the likelihood of groupthink tendencies was lowest when social-emotional cohesion was low and task-oriented cohesion was high." It would seem that balance is an issue in cohesion within multidisciplinary teams. However, it seems that the balance is perhaps not one between too little and too much social cohesion, as suggested by Sethi et al. (2001), but one between task cohesion and social cohesion.

Superordinate identity "refers to the extent to which members identify with the team (rather than merely with their functional areas) and perceive a stake in the success of the team" (Sethi et al., 2001, p.75). It is important to strike a balance between a team member's functional identity and an identity with the cross-functional team. The value of a cross-functional team is the access to diverse information, knowledge and opinions located in the functional area and provided through team members. However, if a cross-functional team member retains a heavily functional identity, then "integration is difficult to achieve in cross-functional settings because people from different functional areas hold biases and stereotypes toward one another" (Sethi et al., 2001, p.75). The corollary to this is when a cross-functional team member identifies strongly with the cross-functional team that it shuts down or severely limits access to the knowledge, information and opinions available from the member's functional area. Balance is required in the establishment and maintenance of an individual's identity within various teams.

A characteristic of palliative care multidisciplinary teams is that they operate interdependently with the disciplines that resource them. This is an interesting relationship because it enables the disciplines to supply externally accessed information and knowledge directly to team operations. It also enables the team members to supply locally derived information and knowledge through the disciplines to specific external environments. Tasi (2001) writes that knowledge transfer within organisations is a socially based function where units are interdependent. In this networked environment, the links between organisational units are fundamental to learning by and within units. Also important to learning, according to Tasi (2001), is a unit's position within the network and the ability of the unit to absorb the necessary information and knowledge. In palliative care the multidisciplinary patient care team is at the operational centre of the organisation. This location is likely to enhance the practices of units because of the access to information and knowledge from contributing units and, at the same time, allow contributors early, often immediate, access to new operational knowledge.

As for the ability to absorb information and knowledge, Tasi (2000) describes this as absorptive capacity. Tasi notes that it is an organisational unit's ability to "assimilate and replicate new knowledge gained from external sources" (p.998) and adds that the definition also covers the unit's ability to apply the knowledge opportunistically. Cohen and Levinthal (1990), writing specifically on absorptive capacity and its relationship with learning and innovation, note that access to outside knowledge is critical to the innovation process at any level. These authors describe absorptive capacity as a collection of abilities central to an organisation's innovative efforts. These abilities include, "the ability to evaluate and utilize outside knowledge," "the ability to recognize the value of new information, assimilate it, and apply it" and "knowledge of who knows what, who can help with what problem, or who can exploit new information" (Cohen and Levinthal, 1990, p.128, p.133). Crucial to the application of these abilities is prior knowledge of related fields. Interestingly, these authors include shared language as a basic skill related to prior knowledge and a fundamental requisite of absorptive capacity. Another interesting point made by Cohen and Levinthal (1990) is that prior related knowledge can include knowing how to learn and learning how to learn.

In summary, it appears that a small number of levers is necessary for influencing and maintaining the knowledge management environment for the multidisciplinary teams. The first, collaboration, is used to integrate resources, access knowledge, access information and manage communications. Next, balance, in terms of access to knowledge and information and the ability to use them, team and discipline identities, team diversity and team cohesion. Then absorptive capacity, for the ability to recognise the value of and utilise knowledge and information available outside the team, to know where to look for this knowledge and information and the ability and knowledge to learn.

KNOWLEDGE AND INFORMATION MANAGEMENT BEHAVIOURS

The management of knowledge and information in palliative care is based on two sets of behaviours, each of which utilises its own set of tools. Sometimes these overlap. Patients, patient-based carers and palliative care professionals seek to establish and exchange knowledge and information in an attempt to ensure the creation of understanding that enables the monitoring of change (Lewis et al., 1997; Kearney, 1992). The foundation of this process is to know the patient and the patient-based carers, described as being core and pivotal to the successful provision of palliative care by Luker et al. (2000). Individual patients bring individual care contexts into the palliative network. This means that each patient must be known individually. Within this environment relationships based on trust and integrity are constructed between the palliative care professionals and the patient and patient-based carers to facilitate the provision of care at all levels (McDonald and Krauser, 1996; Keaney, 1999; Krishnasamy, 1999). The vulnerability of patients, patient-based carers and professionals is a persistent issue (Rose, 1995; Henkelman and Dalinis, 1998; Krishnasamy, 1999) because of the interdependent nature of their relationships. Directly related to vulnerability is trust (Lewicki et al., 1998), which is an essential precursor to the generation and exchange of information and knowledge and to the development of learning (Nonaka and Konno, 1998).

In palliative care the imminent end of life can not be given a specific timeframe for each patient because the timing cannot be known. This uncertainty brings a temporal pressure to the environment that results in a population of temporary groups and temporary systems, characterised by Meyerson et al. (1996, p.167) as containing groups that, "have a finite life span, form around a shared and relatively clear goal or purpose, and their success depends on a tight and coordinated coupling of activity." These are groups where "there isn't time to engage in the usual forms of confidence-building activities that contribute to the development and maintenance of trust in more traditional, enduring forms of organisation." Importantly, according to Meyerson et al. (1996, p.170), in temporary systems, "Swift judgements about trustworthiness can't be avoided, because they enable people to act quickly in the face of uncertainty."

According to Schein (1993), the issue of time in relationship building in cross-cultural environments can be, to a large extent, overcome by the ability of some professionals to offer a stable social unit based on the use of organizational artifacts. This stable social unit is generally located within an organisational culture of some sort and, therefore, facilitates a newcomer's enculturation. The facilitation is important because it situates the newcomer within a social system, authenticating and giving meaning to the activities, concepts and learning that will follow (Brown et al., 1989). Palliative care professionals can use artifacts such as the credibility provided by the organisation's reputation, their own experience and the organisation's experience in situations anticipated by the patient and the close relationships developed in small, tightly focused teams. Trust is important because it reduces feelings of uncertainty and vulnerability (Meyerson et al., 1996; Lewicki et al., 1998). Thus, the generation and exchange of knowledge and information between patient, patient-based carers and professional carers can be facilitated and the monitoring and management of change is enabled by the establishment of trust. Situating in a cultural context that reflects social cohesiveness is important because the context will influence the learning that takes place within it. The palliative organisation is therefore offered the opportunity to shape the necessary learning for the patient, with an emphasis on interdependence. The value of the relationship between the situation within a cultural context and learning that is directly related to the context is in the immediate relevance of knowledge generated from participation and collaboration. The knowledge and the act of its creation are both owned by the collaborators, as noted by Brown et al. (1989) and Henning (1998).

In complex environments a method of achieving a shared understanding is articulated in Senge's (1990) concept of openness. Openness is an organisational characteristic where, "both the norm of speaking openly and honestly about important issues *and* the capacity to continually challenge one's own thinking" (Senge, 1990, p.274) is a positive contributor to the generation of shared views. Senge's (1990) theme is the generation of trust to facilitate the sharing of mental models in order to reach shared understandings based on the need to achieve common interests and to optimally leverage the knowledge and information contained in relationships at the local level. In palliative care the drivers for the effort to produce an open environment are the reduction of the levels of uncertainty accompanying each patient and establishment of a trustworthy environment for the development and use of knowledge and information. None of these can be achieved without the generation of shared understandings at the team and individual levels. According to Senge (1990, p.10), an important tool for the development and maintenance of openness is dialogue, described as, "the capacity of members of a team to suspend assumptions and enter into a genuine 'thinking together.'"

The need to know the patient quickly, establish social stability and trust and do so in a climate that acknowledges the patient's impending death requires a mode of learning that can address underlying value-based causes of concern and distress. Such a method is described by Argyris (1989) as double-loop learning. Double-loop learning encourages "cooperative, inquiry-oriented, high trust and high risk-taking dynamics" (Argyris, 1989) in groups. High risk-taking refers to the personal social risk attached to an individual's willingness to expose underlying values, causes of perceptions and behaviours. Typical behaviours encountered in this type of learning system include, "sharing power with anyone who has competence and who is relevant to deciding or implementing the action" (Argyris, 1989). This encompasses descriptions of the requirements of the palliative environment by a number of authors (McDonald and Krauser, 1996; Krishnasamy, 1999; McGrath, 1998; Luker et al., 2000). Shared information that is useful and valid in terms of the participants can be generated using dialogue (Senge, 1990; Schein, 1993; Brown and Duguid, 1991). Dialogue is also described as a component of psychosocial care supplied by nurses in hospice care (Rassmussan and Sandman, 1998) and as a fundamental device for learning about and knowing patients (Perry, 2000).

The behaviours evidenced in front of the patient that support knowledge management are: (1) The use of artifacts such as role credibility of professional carers and organisational reputation and experience to enable rapid creation of trust and enculturation of the patient and patient-based carers appears to facilitate inclusion in, and maintenance of, a socially stable structure and culture. This, in turn, enables (2) the establishment and maintenance of an ability to generate meaning from the palliative experience and to address values-based issues. The inclusive, supportive exchange of knowledge and information across all boundaries enables (3) the monitoring and management of change and the provision of care suited the patient's situation at any given time. This leads to (4) understanding the patient's situation as the basis for care.

For the palliative professionals, palliative care means teamwork (McDonald and Krauser, 1996). Professional members of palliative care teams are often members of several teams simultaneously, but not necessarily permanent members of the same teams. Teams and team members in palliative care utilise what Nabeoka (1995) describes as a concurrent transfer strategy, where a new care project transfers knowledge, information and technologies from older projects or from a base of collective palliative experience while other care projects are still in train. This requires continuous interactions and communications between teams and, in return, increases the efficiency of the design of care for patients. The ties between teams, because of the overlapping memberships, are strong. This means at least a two-way interaction that can assimilate non-codified knowledge that is created because the nature of the teams' relationships and interactions invite and enable testing, mistakes and instruction, particularly with complex knowledge (Hansen, 1999). The generation of shared meaning, particularly in complex issues, can increase the effect of integrative behaviours, validating them as useful social processes that bind group members with a common language, assumptions and beliefs (Beech and McCalman, 1997).

Language is an important issue in the operation of multidisciplinary teams. Reese and Sontag (2001) note the importance, in hospice teams, of the creation of a commonly understood language used to communicate moral and ethical issues and meanings. When disciplines collaborate to enable the operation of a multidisciplinary team that must communicate successfully within itself and with other teams, the team needs a language common to team members (Duncker, 2001). Add to this the fact that patients and patient-based carers become members of patient care teams (McGrath, 1998) and the importance of an ability to generate and use common languages is brought into sharp relief. Language is a fundamental enabler of communication and, therefore, of knowledge and information generation, transfer and management.

The tool that Brown and Duguid (1991) propose as central to the generation of work-based knowledge in evolving circumstances is story telling, or narrative. Reflecting this view, Schein (1993) notes the value of experience in reaching shared understanding in groups, reaching decisions based on that understanding and implementing actions as they were meant to be implemented by the group.

The nature of the work of the palliative care professional is highly collaborative and requires that team members are capable of persistently overcoming the common obstacles to collaboration such as confusion over autonomy and responsibility, territoriality and indecision about trust (Liedtka et al., 1998). Others, including Lewicki et al. (1998), describe trust as a foundation for collaboration, relationship driven and occurring within a social context. Schweikhart and Smith-Daniels (1996) note trust as a key issue in organisational views on autonomy and decision-making in healthcare delivery.

The issue of ambivalence is also important in collaborative environments because it provides an obstacle to collaboration. Ambivalence is described by Lewicki et al. (1998) as occurring in individuals in relationships "when positive and negative attitudes toward a single target coexist." The continual mixing and changing of team memberships creates inevitable situations where people who have, for some reason or another, negative attitudes toward one another or one to another are repeatedly required to work together. In working together, however, these individuals are positioned so that, in an effort to achieve organisational, professional and ethical goals, positive attitudes must surface at some level.

The behavioural focus of the palliative care professionals when dealing with each other appears to be one of acknowledging and accommodating the heterogeneity of professional teams as a basis for learning, sense-making, information and knowledge exchange and the planning and provision of care, via a number of behaviours: (1) working in teams provides multidisciplinary input to care; (2) collaboration in the generation of knowledge and information via inter-project and situational learning enables utilisation of contextually sensitive knowledge and information within and between patient care teams; and (3) ambivalence is managed to reduce the obstacles to care that can occur in multidisciplinary, collaborative teams.

TOOLS FOR TEMPORARY COMMUNICATIONS INFRASTRUCTURES

When multidisciplinary team members interact with patients and patient-based carers the following tools appear to be used: (1) Trust, used to remove socially-based uncertainties that could prevent the generation and exchange of knowledge and information and the generation of meaning (Lewicki et al., 1998; Meyerson et al., 1996); (2) Openness, used to provide a discourse related to the situation and the honest communications necessary (Senge, 1990). Within this, (3) dialogue is used to exchange knowledge, information and meaning and to understand the values and attitudes related to those things (Schein, 1993; Brown and Duguid, 1991; Rassmussan and Sandman, 1998; Perry, 2000). (4) Double-loop learning provides a method by which underlying values and causes can be surfaced and contextualized (Argyris, 1989). (5) The sharing of power (Argyris, 1989) provides a way to maintain the patient's centrality, facilitating the generation of knowledge and information about the patient's situation. This tool also facilitates collaborative operations between the patient and the organisation.

When multidisciplinary team members interact between themselves away from patients and patient-based carers another, slightly different set of tools has been identified: (1) Narrative, primarily used between professionals when exchanging knowledge and information about patients, situations and results of care efforts, between teams and individuals while away from formal organisational communication opportunities (Brown and Duguid, 1991); (2) Dialogue, primarily used between professionals when exchanging knowledge and information about patients, situations and results of care efforts, between teams and individuals while utilizing formal organisational communication opportunities (McGrath, 1998); and (3) Trust and distrust, both tools in the management of ambivalence (Lewicki et al., 1998) between team members.

Applying the Tools and Using the Infrastructures

Results of research interviews in palliative care organisations in Australia are used here to describe the use of tools by multidisciplinary teams to establish temporary communications infrastructures. Trust is an issue that is raised by team members throughout the interviews, referring to understanding the patient's situation, delivering care and working together in teams. With regard to understanding the patient's situation, there is a need to understand as quickly as is necessary, indicated by the situation itself. An inpatient team noted that, "we need to have a couple of days to work on trust," while an outpatient team reported that, "it depends on how sick the patient is. If we get a late referral, we need to develop that trust fairly quickly if you can see that there's a lot of issues to resolve. If they're relatively stable when you get the referral you've got a bit more time." Being able to demonstrate artifacts such as skill and knowledge that are immediately beneficial to the patient or patient-based carers is another way of building early trust. From an inpatient team, "I think people bring their own life experiences and how they trust or don't trust, and I use some of my skills as a social worker to try and make them feel safe. If they feel safe I think trust can develop." From an outpatient team, "If you've been able to sort out medications that they've been taking wrongly, or give them a reason for why they're taking them, that builds up trust faster."

With regard to openness, teams note that they encourage an honest view of the situation on the part of the patient and patient-based carers. Sometimes patients request that families are not informed of the true situation and sometimes the reverse occurs. The response to these types of requests, from members of one team was that, "people handle it (the end of life situation) in different ways and you have to be respectful of people's coping strategies. You can't force your boundaries and terminologies on people. We're very much listening to the patient and the family to hear what their values are, and their ways of coping." This was immediately followed by, "It's a cultural thing, too, and if they are in a culture where they don't want the mother or father to know that they're dying, we do respect that most definitely. But we will always say to the families that if the patient asks are they going to die then we will answer them truthfully. We would do it with all due respect to the family, but we would do it."

Team members note that it is important for patients and patient-based carers to feel included: "The patients need to know who they're basically dealing with," and "They have to feel that they can ask questions." This becomes even more important when attempting to deal with deep seated issues in relationships and families so that care can be better framed or that issues can be brought to the surface and dealt with as part of the end of life experience. An inpatient team noted, "Sometimes when you look in the notes you see some horrific, some very difficult issues, and you can understand why some things might not work, why some approaches might not work. And once you understand, then it makes it easier to cope with." This level of understanding opens the way for the use of dialogue.

As for double-loop learning, there is an acknowledgment that the patient is an expert. An inpatient team noted, "We're looking for them to tell us what their needs are because often we can, with the nursing assessment or the medical assessment, and like all the other assessments where you have, I guess, a list of things that we feel would be beneficial for the patient, but if the patient sort of doesn't see that the same way, then we can be working at cross purposes." This was followed by, "It's really the situation from their perspective rather than from our perspective and our solutions put on to them."

The use of narrative was noted when discussing the issue of holistic care as a driver of the need to gather and exchange a broad range of information about patients and patient-based carers. A team member noted, "constantly, formally and informally, probably definitely more informally than formally, you can see everyone's having these little conversations all over the place, bouncing ideas. Trying to decide if there are any more ideas. So that you are not doing it on your own, but its a team." An outpatient team member reported, "There's constant talking. I think there's a big effort made, like when you've seen a patient, to, you know, fill in all the other people involved when you get back. Even if its quick, for a couple of minutes." And another said, "We all talk amongst ourselves. I mean, we'll sit down and talk about the troubles that a patient might be having at home. Is there something that can be done? Would this benefit the patient? Do you think that if you saw them this would help? So that's how we all talk together about these sorts of things." Members of individual disciplines observe aspects or requirements of care outside of their disciplines when dealing with patients and patient-based carers. One team member talked about observing "issues that might relate to another professional so that I could give that person an idea that they were needed. They have particular specialist skills and knowledge. We all have the overview." There is a conscious willingness to share information and knowledge (Davison and Sloan, 2002).

The interviews report that ambivalence is an issue to be managed formally and informally because of its ability to detract from the performance of the teams. There is a conscious acknowledgment that multidisciplinary teams bring with them the possibility of discipline-based or paradigm-based conflicts. Asked about how they managed problems within the team, both types of teams gave similar responses. These are typified by an outpatient team member who said, "I mean, at least at first you'd try and talk to the person and get their reason and their side of the story. If you were talking about patient care and you felt something should be happening and they felt the opposite, then maybe if you got their clinical reason you'd understand where they're coming from." A team leader notes, "From my perspective, there have been things that have happened between team members, differences of opinion and things. And often when it fails it's because there hasn't been absolute communication because of time limits." The teams interviewed highlighted the roles of communication and respect between team members in the establishment and maintenance of trust, "respecting each person's discipline, respecting the boundaries and your own discipline, too."

It appears that the need for temporary communications infrastructures and the use of the tools indicated in the literature do exist in practice.

Before progressing, however, it would be useful to come to an understanding of the difference between multidisciplinary palliative care teams and other healthcare delivery teams, in the view of palliative care team members. The great bulk of palliative care team members interviewed had arrived at palliative care after a generally long period of time spent elsewhere in healthcare delivery organisations. Team members were asked at interviews what the difference was between working in a multidisciplinary palliative care team and a multidisciplinary team in other healthcare situations that they had experienced. Replies were commonly based around three fundamental differences: (1) Levels of stress were relatively lower for team members in palliative care than in, for example, a hospital. Team members suggested that this was a result of being in a care environment where the pressure for a cure was removed, although the stresses of dealing only with the dying still had to be managed. (2) Frequency of communication was higher and the communication networks were more sophisticated in palliative care than in other healthcare delivery situations. A number of reasons were offered for this situation. It was suggested that this situation resulted from more disciplines being involved, often simultaneously, with individual patients than would be the case in other places. It was also suggested that this situation could result from the uncertain timing of changes in a patient's situation and from the involvement of patient-based carers, for example, families, in the palliative care process. (3) The high level of support for members found within the palliative care team. This, it was suggested, resulted from the palliative care ethos of holistic care and the understanding that this required collaborative team-based care delivery. An interesting point was made by some team members who stated that working within a palliative care team after working in other parts of healthcare was a learned skill because of the high frequency of communication over relatively large networks.

LESSONS LEARNED

The creation of situation-specific temporary communication infrastructures does not happen by chance. Even a talented team that instinctively recognises the need and attempts to create these types of infrastructures will not generate a sustainable effort without the support of the organisation. The organisations discussed in this chapter work to ensure that a combination of organisational capabilities and facilitating levers is in place to support behaviours within the teams that can utilise sets of tools capable of bridging discipline-based, organisational and social boundaries as the situation demands. This must occur so that the situation can inform and be informed. Understanding the patient's situation is the basis for care.

The organisational effort with regard to these infrastructures is anthropocentric rather than technocentric. Perhaps this arises from an understanding that knowledge creation is a human activity, as suggested by Davenport and Volpel (2001). These authors suggest another concept that appears applicable here and that is the concept of a personalized approach to knowledge transfer, where direct contact between, in this case team members, is the preferred method of transfer rather than interaction with a codified knowledge repository. This seems evident in the interview responses reported above, where team members referred to the value of frequent face-to-face communications. Davenport and Volpel (2001) also describe the difference between tacit knowledge, held, according to these authors, embedded in individuals and explicit knowledge, easily codified for use between people.

Nonaka and Konno (1998) describe a knowledge creation approach that seems somewhat similar to the approach taken in palliative care, the SECI approach. The SECI Model contains four steps: socialization, externalization, combination and internalization. According to Nonaka and Konno (1998) socialization "involves the sharing of tacit knowledge between individuals" and in practical terms, "involves capturing knowledge through physical proximity." Socialization also involves transferring knowledge. Externalization "requires the expression of tacit knowledge and its translation into comprehensible forms that can be understood by others." Externalization involves converting tacit knowledge to explicit knowledge. Combination "involves the conversion of explicit knowledge into more complex sets of explicit knowledge." This involves systematizing the knowledge. Internalization "of newly created knowledge is the conversion of explicit knowledge into the organisation's tacit knowledge." This step is involved in a process of learning by doing, by accessing organisationally held tacit knowledge available through membership of the team.

Each step of this model is reflected in the palliative care team environment. Socialization occurs as a result of working in collaborative teams on complex issues in dynamic situations. Palliative care organisations provide the environment for this to occur and the teams provide the tools. Externalization can be said to occur as a part of the generation of common languages between the disciplines when creating and exchanging information and knowledge about changing patient situations. Combination occurs when available communication networks, such as those provided by the disciplines or those provided by informal meetings of carers, are put to use to generate and transfer knowledge. Internalization is produced when the team retains the explicit knowledge generated collectively, but held by each member.

It seems, also, that a primary reason for this organisational awareness of the need for temporary infrastructures is the fact that, in the main, management also works in the operational multidisciplinary teams. This provides management with firsthand knowledge and experience of the requirements and uses of the tools and the infrastructures at the level where the organisation meets its reason for being. The theme found to be common between authors such as Davenport and Volpel (2001) and Nonaka and Konno (1998) and the organisations described in this chapter is that people are knowledge managers. The formal provision and resourcing of organisational capabilities and levers to influence the knowledge environment at its most basic level is just the beginning of adequately resourcing knowledge management in organisations. The organisations described here are at the fringe of social consciousness and of the public sector bureaucracies that regulate and fund them. They are small, with a particular ethos and without commercial targets. Yet they recognise the central role of knowledge and the necessity to resource its management and use on an organisational basis but at a human level.

It becomes apparent that without a willingness to understand and resource the knowledge management process on a human scale resourcing on any other scale is suboptimised.

REFERENCES

Abell, A. (2000). Skills for knowledge environments. *Information Management Journal*, 34(3), 33-41.

Alemi, F. (2000). Management matters: Technology succeeds when management innovates. *Frontiers of Health Services Management*, 17(1), 17-30.

Argyris, C. (1989). *Reasoning, Learning, and Action*. San Francisco, CA: Jossey-Bass.

Austin, J. C., Hornberger, K. D., Shmerling, J. E. & Elliot, M. W. (2000). Managing information resources: A study of ten healthcare organizations. *Journal of Healthcare Management*, 45(4), 229-239.

Barbato, M. (1999, May). Palliative care in the 21st century - Sink or swim, *Newsletter of the New South Wales Society of Palliative Medicine*.

Beech, N. & McCalman, J. (1997). Sex, lies and videotropes: Narrative and commitment in high technology teams. *Journal of Applied Management Studies*, 6(1), 77-92.

Berman Brown, R. & Woodland, M. J. (1999). Managing knowledge wisely: A case study in organisational behaviour. *Journal of Applied Management Studies*, 8(2), 175-198.

Bernthal, P. R. & Insko, C. A. (1993). Cohesiveness without groupthink. *Group and Organization Management*, 18(1), 66-87.

Brown, J. S. & Duguid, P. (1991). Organizational learning and communities of practice: Toward a unified view of working, learning, and innovation. *Organization Science*, 2(1), 40-57.

Brown, J. S. & Duguid, P. (1998). Organizing knowledge. *California Management Review*, 40(3), 90-111.

Brown, J. S., Collins, A. & Duguid, P. (1989). Situated Cognition and the Culture of Learning. *Educational Researcher*, 18(1), 32-42.

Cohen, W. M. (1990). Absorptive capacity: A new perspective on learning and innovation. *Administrative Science Quarterly*, 35, 128-152.

Coopman, S. J. (2001). Democracy, performance, and outcomes in multidisciplinary health care teams. *The Journal of Business Communication*, 38(3), 261-284.

Davenport, T. H. & Volpel, S. V. (2001). The rise of knowledge towards attention management. *Journal of Knowledge Management*, 5(3), 212-221.

Davenport, T. H, De Long, D. W. & Beers, M. C. (1998). Successful knowledge management projects. *Sloan Management Review*, 39(2), 43-57.

Davison, G., & Hyland, P. (2003). Pallative care: An environment that promotes continuous improvement. In E. Geisler, K. Krabbendam & R. Schuring (Eds.), *Technology, Healthcare, and Management in the Hospital of the Future*, pp. 103-123, Westport, CT: Praeger Publishers.

Duffy, J. (2000). Knowledge management: What every information professional should know. *Information Management Journal*, 34(3), 10-16.

Duncker, E. (2001). Symbolic communication in multidisciplinary cooperations. *Science, Technology and Human Values*, 26(3) 349-386.

Eagleson, G., Waldersee, R. & Simmons, R. (2000). Leadership behaviour similarity as a basis of selection into a management team. *The British Journal of Psychology*, 39(2), 301-308.

Eisenhardt, K. M., Kahwajy, J. L. & Bourgeois, L. J., III. (1997). Conflict and strategic choice: How top management teams disagree. *California Management Review*, 39(2), 42-62.

Gieskes, J. F. B. (2001). Learning in product innovation processes: Managerial action on improving learning behaviour. *Doctoral Thesis*, University of Twente, Print Partners Ipskamp.

Hansen, M. T. (1999). The search-transfer problem: The role of weak ties in sharing knowledge across organization subunits. *Administrative Science Quarterly*, 44(1), 82-111.

Henkelman, W. J. & Dalinis, P. M. (1998). A protocol for palliative care measures - part 2. *Nursing Management*, 29(2), 36C 36G.

Henning, P. J. (1998). Ways of learning: An ethnographic study of the work and situated learning of a group of refrigeration service technicians. *Journal of Contemporary Ethnography*, 27(1), 85-136.

Jassawalla, A. R. & Sashittal, H. C. (1999). Building collaborative cross-functional new product teams. *Academy of Management Executive*, 13(3), 50-63.

Kearney, M. (1992). Palliative Medicine - just another speciality? *Palliative Medicine*, 6, 39-46.

Krishnasamy, M. (1999). Nursing, morality, and emotions: Phase I and phase II clinical trials and patients with cancer. *Cancer Nursing*, 22(4), 251-259.

Lewicki, R. J., McAllister, D. J. & Bies, R. J. (1998). Trust and distrust: New relationships and realities. *The Academy of Management Review*, 23(3), 438-458.

Lewis, M., Pearson, V., Corcoran-Perry, S. & Narayan, S. (1997). Decision making by elderly patients with cancer and their caregivers. *Cancer Nursing*, 20(6), 389-397.

Liedtka, J. M., Whitten, E. & Jones, J. S. (1998). Enhancing care delivery through cross-disciplinary collaboration: A case study. *Journal of Healthcare Management*, 43(2), 185-205.

Luker, K. A., Austin, L., Caress, A. & Hallett, C. E. (2000). The importance of 'knowing the patient'; community nurses' constructions of quality in providing palliative care. *Journal of Advanced Nursing*, 31(4), 775-782.

McDonald, K. & Krauser, J. (1996). Toward the provision of effective palliative care in Ontario. In E. Latimer (Ed.), *Excerpts from OMA Colloquium on Care of the Dying Patient*.

McGrath, P. (1998). A spiritual response to the challenge of routinization: A dialogue of discourses in a Buddhist-initiated hospice. *Qualitative Health Research*, 8(6), 801-812.

Meyers, J. C. (1997). The pharmacist's role in palliative care and chronic pain management. *Drug Topics*, 141(1), 98-107.

Meyerson, D., Weick, K. E. & Kramer, R. M. (1996). Swift Trust and Temporary Groups. In R. M. Kramer & T. R. Tyler (Eds.), *Trust in Organizations: Frontiers of Theory and Research* (pp. 166-195). London: Sage.

Nabeoka, K. (1995). Inter-project learning in new product development. *Academy of Management Journal (Best Papers Proceedings)*, 432-436.

Nonaka, I. & Konno, N. (1998). The concept of 'ba': Building a foundation for knowledge creation. *California Management Review*, 40(3), 40-54.

Perry, M. A. (2000). Reflections on intuition and expertise. *Journal of Clinical Nursing*, 9(1), 137-145.

Rasmussen, B. H. & Sandman, P. O. (n.d.). How patients spend their time in a hospice and in an oncological unit. *Journal of Advanced Nursing,* 28(4), 818-828.

Reese, D. J. & Sontag, M. A. (2001). Successful interprofessional collaboration on the hospice team. *Health and Social Work,* 26(3), 167-175.

Rose, K. (1995). Palliative care: The nurse's role. *Nursing Standard,* 10(11), 38-44.

Rose, K. (1997). How informal carers cope with terminal cancer. *Nursing Standard,* 11(30), 39-42.

Schein, E. H. (1993). On dialogue, culture, and organizational learning. *Organizational Dynamics,* 22(2), 40-51.

Schoenecker, T. S., Daellenbach, U. S. & McCarthy, A. M. (1995). Factors affecting a firm's commitment to innovation. *Academy of Management Journal,* Special Volume/Best Papers Proceedings, 52-56.

Schweikhart, S. B. & Smith-Daniels, V. (1996). Reengineering the work of caregivers: Role definition, team structures, and organisational redesign. *Hospital & Health Services Management,* 41(1), 19-35.

Senge, P. M. (1990). *The Fifth Discipline — The Art and Practice of the Learning Organisation.* New York: Doubleday Currency.

Sethi, R., Smith, D. C. & Park, C. W. (2001). Cross-functional product development teams, creativity, and the innovativeness of new consumer products. *Journal of Marketing Research,* 38(1), 73-85.

Simons, T., Pelled, L. H. & Smith, K. A. (1999). Making use of difference: Diversity, debate, and decision comprehensiveness in top management teams. *Academy of Management Journal,* 42(6), 662-673.

Tasi, W. (2001). Knowledge transfer in intraorganizational networks: Effects of network position and absorptive capacity on business unit innovation and performance. *Academy of Management Journal,* 44(5), 996-1004.

Van Ess Coeling, H., & Cukr, P. L. (2000). Communication styles that promote perceptions of collaboration, quality, and nurse satisfaction. *Journal of Nursing Care Quality,* 14(2), 63-74.

Witt Sherman, D. (1999). Training advanced practice palliative care nurses. *Generations,* 23(1), 97-90.

Chapter XXI

Managing Healthcare Organizations through the Knowledge Productivity Measurement

Jae-Hyeon Ahn, KAIST, Korea

Suk-Gwon Chang, Hanyang University, Korea

ABSTRACT

Understanding the contribution of knowledge to business performance is important for efficient resource allocations. It is very true for healthcare organizations. For the best utilization of scare medical expertise in the successful medical service delivery process, knowledge management will play a more important role in the future. In this paper, a performance-oriented knowledge management methodology or KP^3 methodology was applied to the medical domain. Through actual data from the six OB/GYN specialty hospitals in Korea, the contribution of knowledge to performance was assessed. Specifically, the productivities of knowledge entities were calculated using DEA (Data Envelopment Analysis) approach to give some important managerial insights for knowledge management activities.

INTRODUCTION

For the economic growth of the country and the success of individual corporations, knowledge plays an increasingly important role (Cole, 1998). Knowledge is considered as an explicit third factor for the creation of value besides the traditional input factors;

capital and labor. Additionally, knowledge can be an important source of sustainable competitive advantage because of its difficulty to create and imitate (Peteraf, 1993; Prahalad & Hamel, 1990; Teece, 1998; Winter, 1987). Naturally it has to be nurtured and well-managed (Lubit, 2001; Maria & Marti, 2001; Ndlela & du Toit, 2001).

It is equally true for the healthcare organizations. Typical healthcare organizations can be considered as "data-rich" because they generate massive amount of data, such as electronic medical records, clinical trial data, hospital records, administrative reports, benchmarking findings and so on (Abidi, 2001). To be useful, the data needs to be mined as a usable form of knowledge, classified, shared, and disseminated among the related stakeholders such as patients, medical professionals, and government agencies. However, the data is rarely mined and then used for strategic decision-support resources (Adidi, 2001). Therefore, there are lots of opportunities for the knowledge management approach to improve the productivity of healthcare organizations.

Recently, we proposed a performance-oriented knowledge management approach or KP^3 methodology (Ahn & Chang, 2004). The methodology assesses how much knowledge contributes to actual business performance. Using business performance data, which is the result of applying knowledge to business operations, the methodology enables us to assess the contribution of each knowledge entity to business performance. Knowledge contribution to the business performance was estimated using the Data Envelopment Analysis (DEA) approach in comparison with knowledge entities for better business performance.

To satisfy the need for the efficient management of healthcare organizations, it is necessary to understand the contribution of medical knowledge to the performance of the organizations. In this chapter, the KP^3 methodology is applied and validated in the medical domain to achieve the goal. To validate the methodology, data were collected from seven hospitals and the performance measures, such as revenue and annual number of patients cared for per each medical personnel were estimated.

The assessment of knowledge contribution to performance provides an important understanding of the productivities of healthcare organizations and knowledge entities. Specifically, the assessment would highlight very useful information for evaluating and compensating medical knowledge workers, and for allocating and developing human capital. Therefore, through this approach, medical professionals and managers in healthcare organizations could address the knowledge management issues such as knowledge productivity measurement, developing human capital, and employee evaluation and compensation, systematically.

The rest of the chapter is organized as follows: In the next section, the background of the methodology is explained. The components and relationships among them are then explained. This is followed by a section where linkage matrices are estimated using the data from the six OB/GYN specialty hospitals and knowledge productivity concept is discussed. The chapter then concludes with an agenda for further research.

BACKGROUND

To survive in today's competitive, regulated, and litigious medical market place, it is no longer enough for a doctor to have impeccable diagnostic abilities and bedside manner. Doctors need to have business savvy and organizational skills (Dordick, 2001).

It implies that required knowledge for a doctor to survive in the changed environment has changed.

Representing these changes, the Accreditation Council for Graduate Medical Education (ACGME) initiated a program in the late 1990s to assess physicians' competence to reform residency training programs (Lee, 2002; Swing, 2002). Based on their study, the ACGME and the American Board of Medical Specialties (ABMS) adopted six competencies: (1) *patient care*, (2) *medical knowledge*, (3) *practice-based learning and improvement*, (4) *interpersonal and communication skills*, (5) *professionalism*, and (6) *systems-based practice*. The detailed explanation for each competency is available in the Appendix. In addition to these, the American Board of Ophthalmology (ABO) has proposed to add another one, surgical competency (Lee, 2002). The surgical competency can be measured by several ways such as the American Board of Surgery In-Training Examination (ABSITE) and the global rating scale of operative performance (Scott et al., 2000). The global rating could be measured by items such as respect for tissue, time and motion, instrument handling, knowledge of instruments, flow of operation, use of assistants, knowledge of specific procedure and overall performance. Because the competency measures are proposed and used by the organizations of authority such as ACGME, ABMS, and ABO, they could be used as the component of knowledge or knowledge entities in the knowledge management framework.

In the following, the KP³ methodology is reviewed from the medical knowledge management perspective. In the KP³ methodology, *K* means *k*nowledge and *P³* means *p*roduct, *p*rocess, and *p*erformance. In the medical domain, product can be interpreted as the medical services that are delivered to the patients. Process is the steps and supporting activities that enable the efficient delivery of medical services. Performance is the result of the medical service.

The KP³ methodology enables us to assess the contribution of knowledge entities to business performance. If we consider medical service from the perspective of business, business performance is the performance of the medical service. The methodology establishes logical links between knowledge and business performance through product and process concepts, and suggests various areas for improving business performance. A number of linkage matrices were introduced for that purpose. With the help of those linkage matrices, the contribution of knowledge to business performance can be assessed. Because the direct link between knowledge and business performance and its assessment are difficult from the perspective of practical implementation, a *two-step* approach was proposed by employing *Product* and *Process* as intermediaries.

One of the major building blocks of the KP³ methodology is knowledge. In fact, knowledge is viewed from many different perspectives. Polanyi (1966) suggested two types of knowledge: tacit knowledge and explicit knowledge, and Nonaka (1994) used them in the theory of organizational knowledge creation. Collins (1997) related knowledge types to their accessibility: symbol-type knowledge, embodied knowledge, embrained knowledge, and encultured knowledge. There are other views on knowledge types, which include Spek and Spijkervet (1997), Quinn et al. (1996), etc. In the framework of the KP³ methodology, knowledge helps to achieve business performance through product and process. It's our view that product and process serve as key intermediaries when we relate knowledge to performance, and accordingly the associated knowledge should be managed separately by *product knowledge* and *process knowledge*.

To assess business performance, financial performance and organizational performance were used in this paper. Incidentally, several research findings in the area of human resource management show that human resources increase the financial and organizational performance and serve as the source for sustained competitive advantage (Becker & Gerhart, 1996; Huselid, 1995; Lado & Wilson, 1994). In a study which assesses the impact of human resource management practices on the business performance, Harel and Tzafrir (1999) used similar performance measures: organizational performance and market performance in relation to the company's competitors. The assessment of the contribution of knowledge and the measurement of the impact of human resource management practices share common characteristics. They both involve the assessment of the contribution of human capital. Therefore, financial and organizational performance could be used to measure the contribution of knowledge to business performance.

THE KP³ METHODOLOGY

Figure 1 shows the overview of the KP³ methodology. The basic building blocks of the KP³ methodology consist of four components: Knowledge, Process, Product, and Performance. Knowledge is further classified into two types: Product-related knowledge and Process-related knowledge.

The arrows in *Figure 1* with solid lines represent the fact that the four components are linked together through four linkage matrices: *the Knowledge-Product matrix, the Product-Performance matrix, the Knowledge-Process matrix, and the Process-Performance matrix.* The purpose of the linkage matrices is to link knowledge to business performance through product and process. Specifically, product knowledge is linked to product by the Knowledge-Product matrix and further linked to financial performance by the Product-Performance matrix. On the other hand, process knowledge is linked to process by the Knowledge-Process matrix and further linked to organizational performance by the Process-Performance matrix. Process and organizational performance are indirectly linked to product and financial performance respectively, and the linkages are represented as dotted lines.

It is important that the four components in the KP³ methodology are linked logically. The logical linkage would enable the monitoring of the status of financial and organizational performance, and it would take necessary actions to improve them through knowledge management activities. The solid line in *Figure 1* represents presumably direct relationships that can be formally stated with logical or mathematical expressions. It means that the contributions of knowledge are possibly quantified and monitored so that we influence them to improve business performance. The dotted line represents indirect relationships that exist but cannot be expressed explicitly. It means that it is hard to measure organizational contribution in monetary terms and their influence is rather indirect.

Components of the KP³ Methodologies

In the next section, four components of the KP³ methodology (Knowledge, Process, Product, and Performance) and four linkage matrices (*the Product-Performance matrix, the Process-Performance matrix, the Knowledge-Product matrix, and the Knowledge-Process matrix*) are explained in more detail.

Figure 1: Overview of the KP³ Methodology

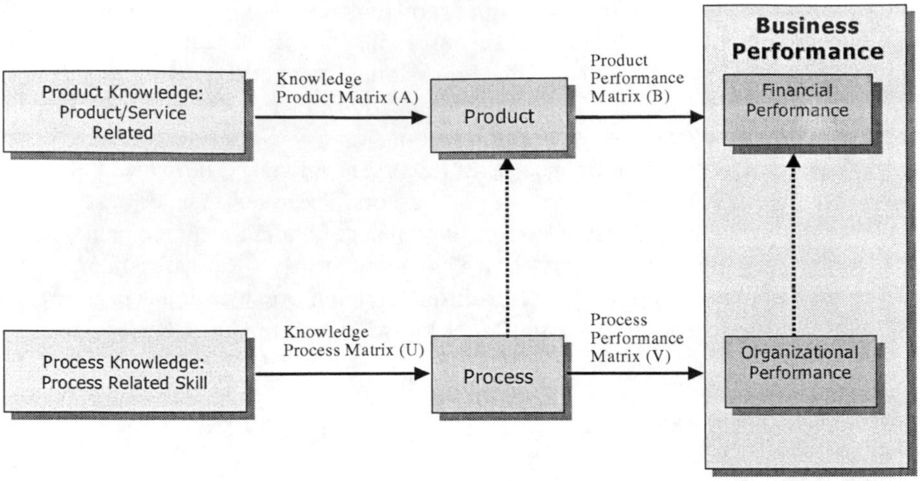

Knowledge

According to Nonaka and Konno (1998), knowledge created in a knowledge platform emerges in individuals, working groups, project teams, informal circles, temporary meetings, e-mail groups, and at the front-line contact with the customer. Two typical forms of knowledge are created and shared among organizational members. Explicit knowledge is a type of knowledge which can be formed and expressed as data, scientific formulae, specifications, manuals and the like, while tacit knowledge is another type which is highly personal and hard to formalize like subjective insights, intuitions and hunches.

In the framework of the KP³ methodology, knowledge helps to achieve business performance through product and process. Therefore, knowledge is classified as product-related knowledge or product knowledge and process-related knowledge or process knowledge.

Product knowledge is knowledge directly related to the company's specific product. Based on the studies by Hall (1992), Day (1994), and Hitt et al. (2000), we identify in this paper three key product knowledge entities: (1) *technology related*, (2) *operations related*, and (3) *market related*. Technology-related product knowledge includes manufacturing know-how and understanding of technical functions for a specific product like semiconductor, medicine, software, contents, and so on. Operations-related product knowledge is related with the value chain activities for a specific product. According to Hall (1992), it is considered the most important area of employee know-how. Finally, market-related product knowledge is product-specific know-how or understanding in relation to the behavior of the suppliers, competitors, and customers.

Process knowledge is the knowledge associated with the activities performed in each stage of a value chain from inbound logistics to customer care. Compared to product knowledge, which is directly related to the provision of products or services, process knowledge is a kind of glue that brings the organizational knowledge assets together and

Table 1: Medical Knowledge Entities in the KP³ Methodology

Knowledge in KP³ methodology		Medical context
Product Knowledge	Technology-related knowledge	Medical knowledge
	Operations-related knowledge	Surgical competence
	Market-related knowledge	System-based practice
Process Knowledge	Leadership capability	Professionalism
	Problem solving capability	Patient care
	Communication capability	Interpersonal and communication skills
	Learning capability	Practice-based learning and improvement

enables the achievement of better financial and organizational performance (Day, 1994). A number of studies deal with various types of human capability or tacit process knowledge in our terms. They include problem solving, problem finding, prediction, social interaction (Leonard & Sensiper, 1998), leadership expertise, social judgment skills (Connelly et al., 2000), learning capabilities (Lynn, 1998), and political skill (Ferris, Perrewe, Anthony & Gilmore, 2000). Based on the previous studies, we identify four key process knowledge entities: (1) leadership capability, (2) problem-solving capability, (3) communication capability, and (4) learning capability.

The seven knowledge entities in the KP³ methodology are defined to be generic in the business context. However, it turns out that they can be used in the medical area without major modification. In the medical context, competencies adopted by ACGME and ABO can be matched quite well with three product knowledge and four process knowledge identified in the KP³ methodology. Based on the description of ACGME competencies (see Appendix), they can be classified as shown in *Table 1*.

Product

Products are the output of value chain activities. If the company or organization in discussion were a service company, product would mean service in that context. In the medical context, the product is the medical services delivered to the patients.

Process

The process of delivering a product or service can be divided into a number of linked activities, each of which adds value for customers (Porter, 1985). The value chain is a framework for analyzing the contribution of each activity to the business performance. Various activities that make up the value chain are important individually, but they are perhaps even more important in combination. Overall value for the customer is created not by individual value chain activities, but by groups of activities that come together to form what are known as core processes (Miller & Dess, 1996). Miller and Dess consider three processes: (1) product development process, (2) demand management process, and (3) order fulfillment process as core processes. Based on their studies, we identify these as core processes.

Because the core processes are a set of critically important activities that produce products and eventually determine the performance of a company, they need to be well managed. Process knowledge would make the core process the most efficient and productive contributor to both the financial and organizational performance.

In the medical context, process is the steps and supporting activities that enable the efficient delivery of medical services. Typically, a patient goes through an admission process once the patient arrives at the hospital. Then, a doctor performs a differential diagnosis with an interview, physical examination, and necessary medical tests. Then, a doctor takes an action to treat a disease based on the conclusion from the differential diagnosis. Finally, a patient would be discharged from the hospital after having the necessary medical services. Those sub-processes can be grouped as medical service process.

Performance

Performance or business performance is both financial and organizational. Financial performance is directly influenced by how the product or service performs in the market. Depending on the characteristics of the product and service, different metrics can be used. The typical monetary metrics for measuring financial performance are revenue, EVA (Economic Value Added), profit, etc. Especially, financial performance is considered quite essential considering the fact that real financial improvement has to be demonstrated before knowledge management activities are adopted and diffused into the regular business activities.

Meanwhile, organizational performance is usually defined with non-monetary metrics, thus relatively difficult to measure. Though it could be measured indirectly using some "intermediate" measures like the number of new ideas, the number of new products, and job satisfaction level, the contribution of knowledge management activities to the organizational performance is hard to be translated into tangible benefits. Organizational performance is as important as financial performance because the organizational quality would indirectly influence financial performance serving as a moderating factor.

In the medical context, metrics for financial and organizational performances can be chosen similarly depending on the knowledge management purposes.

Linkage Matrices

To represent the relationships of knowledge to business performance over product and process, four linkage matrices are employed to link four components of the KP^3 methodology. They are *the Knowledge-Product matrix, the Product-Performance matrix, the Knowledge-Process matrix,* and *the Process-Performance matrix*. They are represented by matrix A, B, U, and V, respectively as shown in *Figure 1*. Knowledge-Product matrix links product knowledge to product. Product-Performance matrix links product to financial performance. Knowledge-Process matrix links process knowledge to process. Process-Performance matrix links process to organizational performance.

Conceptually each matrix has its own meaning. For example, the element a_{ij} in the Knowledge-Product matrix A represents the input level of product knowledge i in association with product j. The element b_{jk} in the *Product-Performance matrix* B represents financial performance of a product j in terms of financial performance metric k. Once we define matrix A and B, then we can define Product Knowledge-Financial

Performance matrix (matrix C). The Product Knowledge-Financial Performance matrix or matrix C represents the contribution of product knowledge i to financial performance metric k. It can be calculated by multiplying the elements of matrix A and B and by summarizing them over products.

In the similar manner, U, V, and W matrices can be estimated. For example, the element u_{ij} in the Knowledge-Process matrix U represents the input level of process knowledge i in association with process j. The element v_{jk} in the *Process-Performance matrix V* represents organizational performance of a process j in terms of organizational performance metric k. Once we define matrix U and V, then we can define Process Knowledge-Organizational Performance matrix (matrix W) which represents the contribution of process knowledge i to organizational performance metric k. For a more detailed description, refer to the work by Ahn and Chang (2004).

A CASE EXAMPLE

In the previous section, the KP³ methodology is reviewed from the medical perspective. The methodology itself makes sense. However, it is difficult to verify its real-world applicability because of insufficient empirical data availability at this early stage of development. Given this limited data availability, this section demonstrates the applicability of the methodology to the OB/GYN specialty hospitals in Korea.

Data Collection

Data were collected from six representative OB/GYN specialty hospitals in Korea, ranging in size from 31 to more than 1,500 beds. In order to exclude the effect of structural differences among different medical disciplines, only OB/GYN hospitals were investigated. Though the size of the hospitals differs, all of them are basically OB/GYN specialty hospitals. *Table 2* summarizes the high level data.

Table 2 shows four input factors for the six OB/GYN specialty hospitals and two performance metrics, number of bed-days and total annual revenue. The number of bed-days can be considered an interim performance metric toward total annual revenue which is the ultimate financial performance metric. This is clear from the fact that total annual revenue tends to grow as the number of bed-days becomes larger. But a larger number of bed days does not necessarily lead to larger total annual revenue. In fact, revenue per bed-day ranges from $0.09K for Hospital 6 to $0.53K for Hospital 3, denying the positive relationship. Therefore, the number of bed-days seems to be related to the organizational performance, while total annual revenue is related to financial performance.

As for the input factors, four proxy measures were collected. The fixed asset measures the capital input and the number of employees measures the labor input. These two input factors are very important because they form the hospitals' production function along with the knowledge input of medical professionals.

The remaining two input factors are the most important ones in our analysis. They measure the knowledge input. Although we suggested seven exhaustive knowledge entities in the previous section, we used two types of knowledge: Product knowledge and Process knowledge at the aggregate level. The two knowledge types aggregate the seven knowledge entities agreed in the medical society. The product knowledge aggregates medical knowledge, surgical competence, and system-based practice, while the process knowledge aggregates professionalism, patient care, interpersonal and communication skills and finally practice-based learning and improvement.

In order to estimate the knowledge level of each hospital, an evaluation committee of three was organized with the OB/GYN specialty doctors who have enough information about the investigated hospitals. They were provided with reference data such as home page information, brochures, government documents, and analysis reports of hospital consulting company. Then, each member of the committee was asked to evaluate each hospital's knowledge level from 0 to 1 in view of our knowledge categorization. The knowledge input level of each hospital was then estimated by calculating the simple arithmetic mean of each member's assessment. The total knowledge input was then estimated by multiplying the knowledge level by the number of specialty doctors for each hospital.

Traditional Productivity Analysis

OB/GYN specialty hospitals may be more knowledge-intensive, while others may be capital or labor-intensive. Depending on the characteristics of the hospitals, it can be conjectured that productivity of knowledge or the contribution of knowledge to the performance of the hospital can be affected.

In order to capture the overall view of the characteristics of the hospitals, some productivity indices were calculated as shown in *Table 3*. Additionally, *Figure 2* shows the amount of fixed asset per employee and number of specialists per employee with respect to the revenue per employee.

In general, revenue per employee is a good metric for business performance. The metric can be improved as the hospital is equipped with better facilities or becomes more capital-intensive. The degree of capital-intensiveness can be captured by the amount of fixed asset per employee. The metric can be also improved as the hospital keep personnel with better medical expertise or becomes knowledge-intensive. The degree of knowledge intensiveness can be captured by the number of specialists per employee. From *Figure 2*, it can be observed that the relationship between revenue per employee and fixed asset per employee shows positive relationship at p-value 0.11.

According to the analysis shown in *Table 2*, Hospitals 3 has the highest revenue per employee, amount of fixed asset per employee, and number of specialists per employee among all the other hospitals. Therefore, it can be conjectured that Hospital

Table 2: Input Factors and Performance Data for Each Investigated Hospital

Hospital ID	1	2	3	4	5	6
Fixed asset (in $K)	1,043	3,334	29,555	9,968	544	17,003
No. of employees	82	100	740	487	34	1867
No. of specialty doctors	7	10	93	33	3	135
Product knowledge	4	6	74	24	2	68
Process knowledge	5	6	86	27	2	115
Number of bed-days	17,925	14,361	89,599	71,699	2,890	474,562
Total annual revenue (in $K)	1,705	2,280	47,383	18,307	569	94,516

Table 3: Some Performance and Operation Indices for the Hospitals

Hospital ID Indices	1	2	3	4	5	6
Revenue per employee (in $K)	20.80	22.80	64.03	37.59	16.74	50.62
Amount of fixed asset per employee (in $100K)	0.15	0.40	0.48	0.25	0.19	0.33
No. of specialists per employee	0.09	0.10	0.13	0.07	0.09	0.07

Figure 2: Relationships Between Productivity Indices

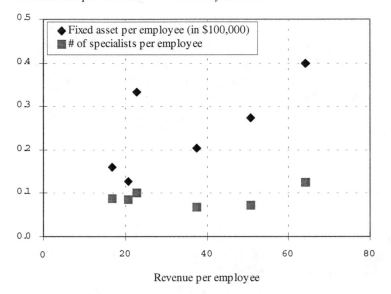

Revenue per employee

3 is very efficient in itself and at the same time it is both capital-intensive and knowledge-intensive. It implies that Hospital 3 may be equipped with high value-adding facilities like 3D ultra-sonogram, CT, MRI as well as well-trained medical experts.

On the other hand, Hospital 2 has relatively low revenue per employee but with relatively high amount of fixed asset per employee and number of specialists per employee. That is, Hospital 2 is not efficient in terms of revenue per employee even though it is relatively capital-intensive and knowledge-intensive. The problem is that the Hospital 2 may have been managed relatively poorly even though it has the potential to be efficient because of its capital-intensiveness and knowledge-intensiveness. However, traditional productivity analysis cannot easily find out the real cause of the problem.

Therefore, productivity of knowledge or the contribution of knowledge to the performance of the hospital can be properly measured once we understand that the current hospital is operated efficiently or not comparing with other hospitals. In the following, we will demonstrate how the DEA (Data Envelopment Analysis) approach finds out the hypothetically efficient hospital and will show the way to estimate knowledge productivity of a hospital by comparing it with the hypothetically efficient hospital.

Knowledge Productivity Analysis by DEA

Data Envelopment Analysis (DEA) is a quite useful tool to find the most productive input composition and their linkage to business performances. It is an application of linear programming that has been used to measure the relative efficiency of operating units with the same goals and objectives (Ahn & Chang, 2004).

In the section titled "The KP³ Methodology," the methodology was explained in terms of A, B, C, U, V, and W matrices. However, for the purpose of simplicity, we will represent the linkage matrices only with A, B and C treating product and process knowledge together. Furthermore, this example deals with one product (OB/GNY specialty service) and one process (one overall process for total medical service) case. If relevant data for the multiple products and multiple processes are collected, similar analysis can be done.

As an example, let's consider Hospital 2 again. The problem of finding the most productive input composition for Hospital 2 is formulated as:

Min e_2

subject to

$$1043w_1 + 3334w_2 + 29555w_3 + 9968w_4 + 544w_5 + 17003w_6 - 3334e_2 \leq 0$$
$$82w_1 + 100w_2 + 740w_3 + 487w_4 + 34w_5 + 1867w_6 - 100e_2 \leq 0$$
$$4w_1 + 6w_2 + 74w_3 + 24w_4 + 2w_5 + 68w_6 - 6e_2 \leq 0$$
$$5w_1 + 6w_2 + 86w_3 + 27w_4 + 2w_5 + 115w_6 - 6e_2 \leq 0$$
$$1705w_1 + 2280w_2 + 47383w_3 + 18307w_4 + 569w_5 + 94516w_6 - 2280 \leq 0$$
$$17925w_1 + 14361w_2 + 89599w_3 + 71699w_4 + 2890w_5 + 474562w_6 - 14361 \leq 0$$
$$w_1 + w_2 + w_3 + w_4 + w_5 + w_6 = 1$$
$$w_1, w_2, w_3, w_4, w_5, w_6, e_2 \geq 0$$

where w_i is the weight applied to inputs and outputs for Hospital i, $i = 1, ..., 6$, and e_2 (efficiency index for Hospital 2) is the fraction of Hospital 2's input required by the composite hospital. For the detailed explanation for DEA applications, refer to Ahn and Chang (2004).

If we solve the above problem, we can obtain the optimal solution, $w_1^* = 0.3087$, $w_2^* = 0$, $w_3^* = 0$, $w_4^* = 0$, $w_5^* = 0.067681$, $w_6^* = 0.0145$, and $e_2^* = 0.7604$. The value $e_2^* = 0.7604$ implies that the Hospital 2 is only 76% efficient as compared to the hypothetically most efficient composite hospital which is the combination of Hospitals 1, 5, and 6 with the corresponding weights, w_1^*, w_5^* and w_6^*. Theoretically, the composite hospital can produce the same revenue and the total number of bed-days with at most 76% of the resources Hospital 2 has used. The input for the composite hospital is calculated by taking the weighted average of six hospitals' input levels with weights w_1^*, w_2^*, ..., w_6^*.

Table 4: Comparison Between Hospital 2 and Its Ideal Composite Hospital

Hospital Input level	Current input for Hospital 2	Input for composite hospital
Fixed asset (in $1,000)	3334	936.4
Number of employees	100	75.4
Product knowledge	6	3.6
Process knowledge	6	4.6

Based on the above result, we can estimate matrices **A**, **B** and **C** associated with the most efficient composite hospital for Hospital 2. The **C** (actual) is estimated by allocating the actual performances with the weights from the most efficient combination of input factors.

In performing knowledge management activities, knowledge productivity for each knowledge entity provides valuable information. From the above DEA output, we can estimate the relative productivity of each input factor by dividing each element in **B** (actual) by the corresponding the element on **B** in *Figure 3*. *Table 5* shows that one unit of labor (number of employees) and the process knowledge input contribute more to the performance than that of the product knowledge, and that the fixed asset contributes the least.

Figure 3: Estimated Matrices A, B, and C — Actual vs. Ideal

A(actual)	B(actual)		C(actual)	
3334	0.628	3.995	2093	13185
100	1.685	10.612	168	1061
6	1.331	8.368	8	50
6	1.700	10.707	10	64

A	B	=	C	
936.4	2.236	14.081	2093	13185
75.4			168	1061
3.6			8	50
4.6			10	64

Table 5: Relative Productivity of Input Factors for Hospital 2

Performance Metric Input	Annual revenue	No. of bed-days
Fixed asset	0.281	0.281
No. of employees	0.754	0.754
Product knowledge	0.596	0.596
Process Knowledge	0.760	0.760

Table 6: Optimal Solutions Obtained from DEA

Hospital ID	w_1^*	w_2^*	w_3^*	w_4^*	w_5^*	w_6^*	e_i^*
1	1.0000	0.0000	0.0000	0.0000	0.0000	0.0000	1.0000
2	0.3087	0.0000	0.0000	0.0000	0.6768	0.0145	0.7604
3	0.0000	0.0000	1.0000	0.0000	0.0000	0.0000	1.0000
4	0.0000	0.0000	0.0000	0.0000	0.8112	0.1888	0.8643
5	0.0000	0.0000	0.0000	0.0000	1.0000	0.0000	1.0000
6	0.0000	0.0000	0.0000	0.0000	0.0000	1.0000	1.0000

Not only for Hospital 2, but we can apply the DEA to the other five hospitals and solve them to find the associated most productive composite hospitals. *Table 6* summarizes the optimal solution for each hospital.

Table 6 shows that Hospital 2 and 4 have their ideal composite hospital. This means that Hospital 2 and 4 can definitely improve their performance by changing input composition. On the other hand, Hospitals 1, 3, 5, and 6 have their own distinct portfolios of input factors, which are not dominated by any composite hospitals. However, this does not necessarily mean that Hospital 1, 3, 5, 6 are more productive than Hospital 2 or 4.

Discussions

From the conventional view of the productivity discussed in *Table 3* and *Figure 2*, a clear understanding about the contribution of various input factors to business performance is hardly obtained. This is clearly reflected in *Table 3* by the fact that the apparently capital-intensive and knowledge-intensive hospital (Hospital 2) is poor in revenue per employee. Furthermore, it is not clear which input factors are scarce resources for the purpose of enhancing the overall business performance.

Contrary to the conventional productivity analysis, the DEA procedure in the KP[3] methodology provides a clear view on the productivity or marginal contribution of knowledge and other input factors. Additionally, it provides us valuable information on the scarce or binding resources when resources are allocated for better performance.

For the comparative analysis, the relative productivity of the input factors for Hospital 4 was calculated, and shown in Table 7. Based on the relative productivities shown in *Tables 5* and *7*, it can be found that the most contributing and binding input factor is the process knowledge for both Hospital 2 and Hospital 4. This result demonstrates the need to nurture process knowledge with the highest priority for better performance. This is a valuable insight derived from the DEA approach in the framework of KP[3] methodology which is not available from the traditional productivity analysis.

In addition, Hospital 2 has more potential to improve than Hospital 4 considering the efficiency indices $e_2^* = 0.7604$ and $e_4^* = 0.8643$. From *Table 5*, we can observe that Hospital 2 is operated poorly, especially spending relatively much of its capital in vain on fixed assets. This can be also observed from the *Figure 2* that the data point of the

Table 7: Relative Productivity of Input Factors for Hospital 4

Performance Metric Input	Annual revenue	No. of bed-days
Fixed asset	0.366	0.286
No. of employees	0.780	0.609
Product knowledge	0.603	0.470
Process Knowledge	0.864	0.674

amount of fixed asset per employee for Hospital 2 is an outlier without following the general linear trend.

CONCLUSIONS

In the competitive, regulated, and litigious medical market place, more diverse knowledge is needed as well as the conventional ability such as good diagnostics and patient care. To be successful in the new environment, medical knowledge needs to be mined, stored, shared, and disseminated efficiently. Therefore, knowledge management becomes a very important principle that medical society has to adopt.

Recently, a general knowledge management methodology called KP[3] methodology was proposed with the principle that knowledge needs to be managed by focusing on its contribution to business performance. In this paper, the KP[3] methodology was applied to the medical domain.

Using the real data from six OB/GYN specialty hospitals in Korea, the applicability of the methodology was demonstrated in the medical domain. While applying KP[3] methodology, Data Envelopment Analysis (DEA) was very useful to find out the knowledge productivity of a hospital in comparison with the ideal composite hospital. From the analysis, it was found which hospital is more efficient than others and where to allocate resources to increase the business performance efficiently. We believe that healthcare organizations can be managed better and will benefit from this approach.

However, there are many theoretical and practical issues to be addressed for the applications of KP[3] methodology in the medical domain. First, better performance measures need to be developed for the wide acceptance of the knowledge management practice in the medical domain. For example, patient satisfaction would be a very good area to explore. Second, scales for the assessment of knowledge levels need to be developed. This would be even better if the scales are developed with the involvement of diverse medical professionals and their consensus.

REFERENCES

Abidi, S. S. R. (2000). Knowledge management in healthcare: Towards "knowledge-driven" decision-support services. *International Journal of Medical Informatics*, 63, 5-18.

Ahn, J. H. & Chang, S. G. (2004). Assessing the contribution of knowledge to business performance: The KP[3] ethodology. *Decision Support Systems*, 36(4), 403-416.

Becker, B. & Gerhart, B. (1996). The impact of human resource management on organizational performance: Progress and prospects. *Academy of Management Journal*, 39, 779-801.

Cole, R. E. (ed.) (1998). Introduction. *California Management Review*, 40(3), 15-21.

Collins, H. H. (1997). Machines and the structure of knowledge. In R. Ruggles (Ed.), *Knowledge Management*. Tolls: Butterworth-Heinemann.

Connelly et al. (2000). Exploring the relationship of leadership skill and knowledge to leader performance. *Leadership Quarterly*, 11(1), 65-86.

Day, G. S. (1994). The capabilities of market-driven organizations. *Journal of Marketing*, 58(4), 37-52.

Dordick, V. (2001). Medical knowledge alone can't keep a physician in business. *Capital District Business Review*, 27(51), 10B.

Ferris, G. R., Perrewe, P. L., Anthony, W. P. & Gilmore, D. C. (2000). Political skill at work. *Organizational Dynamics*, 28(4), 25-37.

Hall, R. (1992). The strategic analysis of intangible resources. *Strategic Management Journal*, 13, 135-144.

Harel, G. H. & Tzafrir, S. S. (1999). The effect of human resource management practices on the perceptions of organizational and market performances of the firm. *Human Resource Management*, 38(3), 185-200.

Hitt, M. A., Ireland, R. D. & Lee, H. (2000). Technological learning, knowledge management, firm growth and performance: An introductory essay. *Journal of Engineering Technology Management*, 17, 231-246.

Huselid, A. M. (1995). The impact of human resource management practices on turnover, productivity, and corporate financial performance. *Academy of Management Journal*, 38, 635-672.

Lado, A. A. & Wilson, C. M. (1994). Human resource systems and sustained competitive advantage: A competency-based perspective. *Academy of Management Review*, 19, 699-727.

Lee, A. G. (2002). Examining the examiner: New assessments will evaluate physician competence. *Ophthalmology Times*, 27(20), 4-6.

Leonard, D. & Sensiper, S. (1998). The role of tacit knowledge in group innovation. *California Management Review*, 40(3), 112-132.

Lubit, R. (2001). Tacit knowledge and knowledge management: The keys to sustainable competitive advantage. *Organizational Dynamics*, 29(4), 164-178.

Lynn, G. S. (1998). New product team learning: Developing and profiting from your knowledge capital. *California Management Review*, 40(4), 74-93.

Maria, J. & Marti, V. (2001). ICBS - Intellectual capital benchmarking system. *Journal of Intellectual Capital*, 2(2), 148-164.

Miller, A. & Dess, G. (1996). *Strategic Management* (second ed.). New York: McGraw-Hill.

Ndlela, L. T. & du Toit, A. S. A. (2001). Establishing a knowledge management programme for competitive advantage in an enterprise. *International Journal of Innovation Management*, 21(2), 151-165.

Nonaka, I. (1994). A dynamic theory of organizational knowledge creation. *Organization Science*, 5(1), 14-37.

Nonaka, I. & Konno, N. (1998). The concept of "Ba": Building a foundation for knowledge creation. *California Management Review*, 40(3), 40-54.

Peteraf, M. A. (1993). The cornerstone of competitive advantage: A resource-based view. *Strategic Management Journal,* 14, 179-191.

Polanyi, M. (1958). *Personal Knowledge.* Chicago, IL: University of Chicago Press.

Porter, M. (1985). *Competitive Advantage: Creating and Sustaining Superior Performance.* New York: Free Press.

Prahalad, C. K. & Hamel, G. (1990). The core competence of the corporation. *Harvard Business Review,* 68(3), 79-91.

Quinn, J. B., Anderson, P. & Finkelstein, S. (1996). Managing professional intellect: Making the most out of the best. *Harvard Business Review,* 74(2), 71-80.

Scott et al. (2000). Evaluating surgical competency with the American Board of Surgery in-training examination, skill testing, and intraoperative assessment. *Surgery,* 128(40), 613-622.

Spek, R. Van der & Spijkervet, A. (1997). Knowledge management: Dealing intelligently with knowledge. In Liebowitz and Wilcox (Eds.), *Knowledge Management and its Integrative Elements.* CRC Press.

Swing, S. R. (2002). Assessing the ACGME general competencies: General considerations and assessment methods. *Academic Emergency Medicine,* 9(11), 1278.

Teece, D. J. (1998). Capturing value from knowledge assets: The new economy, markets for know-how, and intangible assets. *California Management Review,* 40(3), 55-79.

Winter, S. (1987). *Knowledge and competence as strategic assets, in the Competitive Challenge.* D. Teece (ed.). New York: Harper and Row.

ENDNOTE

[1] We would like to thank Korea Health Industry Development Institute (KHIDI) for their support in collecting hospital data.

APPENDIX

Summary of the Six ACGME Competencies

1. *Patient Care*
*   Provide patient care that is compassionate, appropriate, and effective for the treatment of health problems and promotion of health.
*   Communicate effectively and demonstrate caring and respectful behaviors when interacting with patients and families.
*   Gather essential and accurate information about patients.
*   Make informed decisions about diagnostic and therapeutic interventions based on patient information and preferences, up-to-date scientific evidence, and clinical judgment.
*   Develop and carry out patient management plans.
*   Counsel and educate patients and their families.
*   Use information technology to support patient care decisions and patient education.
*   Perform competently all medical and invasive procedures considered essential for the area of practice.
*   Provide healthcare services aimed at preventing health problems or maintaining health.
*   Work with healthcare professionals, including those from other disciplines, to provide patient-focused care.

2. *Medical Knowledge*
*   Demonstrate knowledge about established and evolving biomedical, clinical, and cognate (e.g., epidemiological and social-behavioral) sciences and the application of this knowledge to patient care.
*   Demonstrate an investigatory and analytic thinking approach to clinical situations.
*   Know and apply the basic and clinically supportive sciences that are appropriate to their discipline.

3. *Practice-Based Learning and Improvement*
*   Investigate and evaluate patient care practices, appraise and assimilate scientific evidence, and improve patient care practices.
*   Analyze practice experience and perform practice-based improvement activities using systematic methodology.
*   Locate, appraise, and assimilate evidence from scientific studies related to patients' health problems.
*   Obtain and use information about your own population of patients and the larger population from which your patients are drawn.
*   Apply knowledge of study designs and statistical methods to the appraisal of clinical studies and other information on diagnostic and therapeutic effectiveness.
*   Use information technology to manage information, access online medical information, and support your own education.
*   Facilitate the learning of students and other healthcare professionals.

4. *Interpersonal and Communication Skills*
- Demonstrate interpersonal and communication skills that result in effective information exchange and teamwork with patients, their families, and professional associates.
- Investigate and evaluate your patient care practices, appraise and assimilate scientific evidence, and improve patient care practices.
- Create and sustain a therapeutic and ethically sound relationship with patients.
- Use effective listening skills and elicit and provide information using effective nonverbal, explanatory, questioning, and writing skills.
- Work effectively with others as a member or leader of a healthcare team or other professional group

5. *Professionalism*
- Demonstrate a commitment to carrying out professional responsibilities, adherence to ethical principles, and sensitivity to a diverse patient population.
- Demonstrate respect, compassion, and integrity; a responsiveness to the needs of patients and society that supercedes self-interest; accountability to patients, society, and the profession; and a commitment to excellence and ongoing professional development.
- Demonstrate a commitment to ethical principles pertaining to provision or withholding of clinical care, confidentiality of patient information, informed consent, and business practices.
- Demonstrate sensitivity and responsiveness to patients' culture, age, gender, and disabilities.

6. *Systems-Based Practice*
- Demonstrate an awareness of and responsiveness to the larger context and system of healthcare and the ability to call on system resources effectively to provide care that is of optimal value.
- Understand how patient care and other professional practices affect other healthcare professionals, the healthcare organization, and the larger society and how these elements of the system affect your own practice.
- Know how types of medical practice and delivery systems differ from one another, including methods of controlling healthcare costs and allocating resources.
- Practice cost-effective healthcare and resource allocation that does not compromise quality of care.
- Advocate for quality patient care and assist patients in dealing with system complexities.

Chapter XXII

Knowledge Strategic Management in the Hospital Industry

Ana Karina Marimon da Cunha, University of Vale do Rio dos Sinos, Brazil

Ely Laureano Paiva, University of Vale do Rio dos Sinos, Brazil

ABSTRACT

This work examines the role of knowledge in the strategic process in the hospital industry. The research method consists of multiple case studies with eight hospitals located in Brazil. We analyzed the relationship among information, knowledge and capability creation. The cases shown that knowledge dissemination is a current management practice. Nevertheless, just one case presented a clear idea of the strategic role of knowledge management. Based on this evidence, we propose a three-step theoretical model related to the strategic management of knowledge. Most of the cases analyzed are in the first stage of the proposed model. On the other hand, the hospital in the third stage presented the following characteristics: a clear strategic focus related to knowledge access, dissemination and application, a mix of formal and informal practices related to knowledge creation, and a propitious internal environment in order to develop its capabilities.

INTRODUCTION

Considering the complexity of hospital organizations, they have to keep up with ongoing advancements in technology, improvements in service throughout their facilities, new generations of medical equipment and continuous development of their competences.

Hospital organizations employ a high number of qualified professionals, offering highly specialized services. Thus, a hospital has a large demand for coordination of its activities. Its management systems have to be constantly developing, with a permanent need to seek and disseminate new knowledge.

Therefore, this study aims at presenting relevant aspects within the current competitive environment when investigating strategic knowledge management in hospitals. Organizational knowledge is one of its core aspects. In addition to that, there is also the concern of integrating this study in a context of its management: internal competencies, the use of internal and external information, and cross-functional activities. We describe SIPAGEH (Standardized Measurement Systems for Hospital Management) in detail as the main source of information for the hospitals studied.

Based on these assumptions, strategic knowledge management in hospitals is analyzed from a decision standpoint, which seeks creating and developing the organization's internal competences. That analysis encompasses the information used, the way the process is carried out, and the hospital's competitive environment.

This chapter is organized as follows: the theoretical framework regarding strategic knowledge, the method adopted by the study, the analysis of the relationship between information, knowledge and competence creation, and finally, conclusions.

THEORETICAL FRAMEWORK
Organizational Knowledge and the Current Context

Drucker (1999) maintains that in the new economy of knowledge, this knowledge is not only one more resource alongside traditional production factors — labor, capital and land — but, in effect, the only significant resource nowadays. The author argues that knowledge is becoming the main resource and is what makes the new society so unique. Drucker (1999) and Toffler (1994) share Quinn's (1980) view that the economy and production power of a modern company is based on its intellectual and service capabilities rather than its fixed assets such as land, facilities and equipments. In the hospital organization, this scenario is no different. In this context, understanding that knowledge is a differential factor that needs to be disseminated and internalized by the multi-professional team is still a present challenge. Creation of new knowledge is not only a question of learning from others or acquiring external knowledge. Knowledge must also be internally built, often demanding an intensive interaction between organization members.

Learning and shared skills must be internalized in order to generate knowledge – that is, modified, enriched and translated so as to adjust to the company's identity.

As organizational knowledge, we understand the capability of a company to generate and disseminate knowledge in the organization, incorporating it into products, services and systems (Nonaka, 1995). According to Davenport and Prusak (1998), knowledge is derived from information just as information is derived from data. Considering that knowledge is close to action, the employees' know-how feeds the organization's functioning. Knowledge underlying the company's routines and practices is transformed into valuable products and services, resulting in the main asset of organizations.

Knowledge, being imperfectly imitable and transferable, might lead to sustainable competitive advantage. The main source of competitive advantage is what a company knows collectively, the effectiveness with which it uses such knowledge, and the readiness with which it acquires and uses new knowledge (Grant, 1996).

To Nevis et al. (1995), knowledge is wider than information, since it aggregates meaning and interpretation. These characteristics give to knowledge a high degree of intangibility, since it includes cognition and skills that individuals use to solve problems (Probst et al., 2000).

Based on the literature, it is possible to state that knowledge is a set of elements possessed by people through their experiences and skills, originated from stored, organized and known data and information.

Knowledge Creation

The organization cannot create knowledge by itself. Knowledge creation needs an individual's efforts and interactions among groups (discussions, experience sharing and observation). Conflict and disagreement, among others, are dynamic interactions that help the transformation of individual knowledge in organizational knowledge.

According to Nonaka (1995), knowledge takes place at three levels: individual, group, and organization. Knowledge can also be classified in two ways: tacit and explicit. Tacit knowledge, hard to articulate in formal language, is arguably the most important type of knowledge. It is personal knowledge incorporated into individual experience and involves intangible factors such as: personal beliefs, perspectives, and value systems. Explicit knowledge is formalized, written, recorded (for instance, routine documents and task manuals). That type of knowledge is more easily accessed and transferred between individuals and organizations.

Knowledge Management and Competency Development

Knowledge management is a systematic, articulated and intentional process, based on generation, codification, dissemination and appropriation of knowledge in order to reach organizational excellence (Landini & Damiani, 2001). Therefore, knowledge management intends to establish ways of acquiring, keeping, recycling and using it as a tool for new knowledge creation. At the same time, knowledge management seeks to eliminate existing knowledge when it becomes obsolete (Lipparini et al., 2000).

Nevis et al. (1995) define three steps for the process of organizational learning:

a. *knowledge acquisition:* skill development or creation, insights and relationships;
b. *knowledge dissemination (exposure):* dissemination of what is being learned; and,
c. *knowledge application:* integration of knowledge and its wide accessibility; it can be generalized to other situations, thus creating the company's competencies.

According to the authors, most studies on this subject stress knowledge acquisition and dissemination. Few of them focus on the application step, where knowledge is largely made available as opposed to its individual or group-specific concentration. To the authors, knowledge assimilation and application embedded in these processes are the "organizational memory."

The three steps point out the importance of cross-functional activities. Such orientation allows organizational knowledge to reach higher levels by integrating existing knowledge. Within a healthcare organization, that means joint actions among different areas, such as managerial and medical areas.

The integration of all three steps poses a strategic challenge to organizations. Therefore, the steps described lead to creating the organization's competencies, generating competitive differentials. Hamel and Prahalad's (1990) classical definition of competence states that *"... corporate-wide technologies and production skills ... that empower individual businesses to adapt quickly to changing opportunities."* This definition reinforces the idea that competencies allow prospecting new businesses, improving existing business opportunities and making the company unique within the competitive market.

Considering the definition above, Leonard-Barton (1992) claims that the role of management is to prospect and to invest in the development of new competencies in such a way that they do not turn into "core rigidity." Such innovation-inhibiting rigidity is a result of the difficulty and the resistance that both people and companies have to change. This is especially present when behavior and managerial actions that need to be changed are the same that leveraged the business' success. Therefore, core competences should have a dynamic nature in order to prevent them from becoming a core rigidity.

The creation of the company's competencies through cross-functionality (i.e., joint action by different managerial functions) can be analyzed from the knowledge integration viewpoint (Grant, 1996). Knowledge integration will be the means for the company to widen its organizational knowledge and to create/reinforce its competencies. Hamel and Prahalad (1990) also see core competencies as based on coordinated cross-functional efforts.

We claim that the strategic process is both interactive and dynamic. It does not happen according to a sequence of pre-established events, as structured and "hierarchized" strategic planning has proposed (Zahra & Das, 1993). In this way, organizational knowledge provides the necessary conditions for the organizations to permanently analyze their internal and the external environments, which are the starting-points of the strategic process. Therefore, decision processes based on continuous environment evaluation can either reinforce existing competencies or create new ones, according to the competitive environment's dynamics. Following these assumptions, our theoretical model presents organizational knowledge as a key resource for the strategic process, built from information and resulting in the organization's competencies. Cross-functional actions related to the dissemination of knowledge generate a learning environment. Finally, organizational competencies may create a competitive advantage (*Figure 1*).

The Hospital as an Organization

The hospital, according to Mirshawka (1994), is an integral part of a medical and social organization. Its function is to provide the population with total medical assistance — curative and preventive — 24-hours-a-day, 365-days-a-year, educational and human resource training, and research center capabilities.

Gonçalves (1983) adds that technological advancements and the emergence of scientific medicine at the turn of the 20th Century revolutionized hospitals' role and

Figure 1: Key Components of Knowledge Management

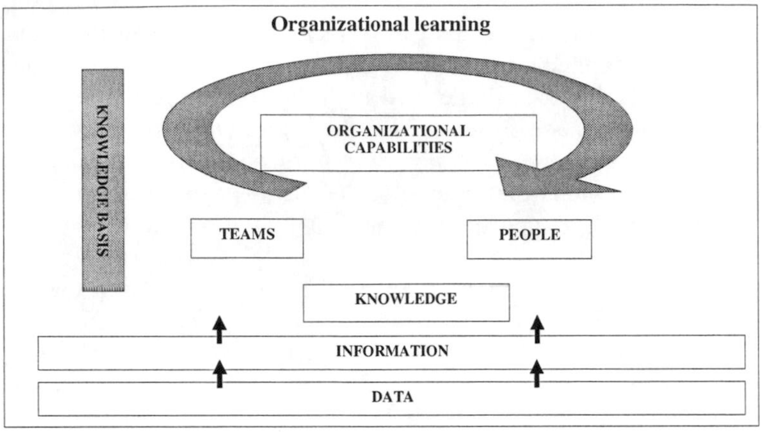

Source: Adapted from Probst et al. (2000) and Paiva et al. (1998)

functions. At that point, the hospital ceased to be a place where the poor and sick were taken to die and turned into the most important institution for the treatment of illnesses.

Today hospitals have changed their characteristics, goals, management, processes of delivering care and even the instruments they work with to provide that care. That fact generates an increasing need for coordination and planning in order to better serve the patient, considering their whole complexity.

Therefore, the characteristics of the processes in healthcare organizations are complexity, heterogeneity and fragmentation. Complexity is the result of the diversity in professions, practitioners, users, technologies used, social and interpersonal relations, work organization forms and work environments. Heterogeneity is related to the diversity of the different work processes that coexist within health institutions. These processes often have their own organization and function, which may not be properly articulated with other work processes. Fragmentation includes several dimensions. One is technical fragmentation, characterized by the increasing presence of specialized professionals. Another is social fragmentation, which sets stiff hierarchical and subordinate relations, configuring social division of labor among the various professional categories (Quintana, Roschke & Ribeiro, 1994).

Hospitals need to be able to face growing and those specific challenges that are due to their complexity, as mentioned by several authors such as Campos and Campos (1982), Ribeiro (1993) and Mirshawka (1994). Their increasing search for quality and effectiveness in the services they provide has also provided challenges for their managers. Carapinheiro (1998) adds to the aspects mentioned earlier, the power relations established within hospitals. According to the author, several studies carried out in different countries and distinct types of hospitals show that such institutions are organized according to multiple authority systems and multiple forms of professional power. Those organizational structures excluded a single reference to a well-defined set of objectives or the reference to a singular approach to management.

The literature on strategy in healthcare organizations is often related to strategic planning. We mention Bruton et al. (1995), Drain and Godkin (1996), Zuckerman (1998), and Popovich and Popovich (2000). Nevertheless, new views of the strategic process are also identifiable in the literature such as:

*   strategy as a process (Begun & Heatwole, 1999);
*   customer-driven strategic process (Lafferty, 2003; Scott, 2001);
*   balanced scorecard (Inamdar et al., 2002);
*   organizational learning (LeBransseur et al., 2002).

SIPAGEH: A Performance Information System

We claim that hospital management involves activities with a high degree of complexity, heterogeneity, and fragmentation. These three characteristics result from the diversity of professionals, customers and technologies applied. This context explains the wide range of processes in hospitals. Therefore, hospitals face increasing challenges when they are seeking effectiveness and service quality. In order to respond to these issues, a group of hospitals developed SIPAGEH with support of the *Universidade do Vale do Rio dos Sinos* (UNISINOS University — state of Rio Grande do Sul, Brazil), oriented by other performance measurement systems for hospitals such as APACHE II (George Washington University), QI Project of Maryland and PROAHSA (state of São Paulo, Brazil).

SIPAGEH is a first step to build a proposal for knowledge management in its founding group, considering that data and information are the main components for knowledge creation (Davenport & Pruzak, 1998).

This group of hospitals established and started to work on a set of managerial measurements, in order to meet the requirements from PNQ (Brazilian National Quality Awards) and PGQP (State Quality and Productivity Program): Brazilian equivalents to the Malcolm Balbridge Awards. The hospitals from this group compare performances, standardize information, and exchange experiences.

SIPAGEH started its operation in July 1999, in nine hospitals with ten measurements. After the first meetings, the original group identified the need for systematic information exchange. The system is based on the idea that a hospital's performance can be best evaluated if its information is compared to the information from similar hospitals. All systems mentioned above, such as Apache II and PROHASA, stress information and comparisons through service measurements (Cunha & Sordi, 2001). SIPAGEH's measurements are: private and public customer-satisfaction rates; turnover; absence rates; training hours per employee; frequency of work accidents; average stay — general, obstetric and pediatric; monthly rate of caesarian sections; mortality rate — general, obstetric and pediatric; infection rate — blood stream infection related to central venous catheter and hospital infection in clean surgeries; bed occupation rate; and liquid margin (see Appendix). SIPAGEH distinguishes itself from other existing systems for including managerial information and providing hospitals with market strategic information. Therefore, SIPAGEH is a structured, managerial hospital information system, regularly updated, which supports the managerial development in this group of hospitals.

CASE STUDIES

This study analyzed eight hospitals, seeking to identify distinct knowledge management stages. We based our analysis on the theoretical model for knowledge management and strategy according to *Figure 1* (Paiva et al., 1998; Prosbt et al., 2000). The hospitals studied have different sizes (from 260 to 1,775 beds), with a total of 4,170 beds. They have also different characteristics:

- public (three) or private (five),
- university owned (four),
- general focus on treatments (seven) or highly specialized (one).

The hospitals present the following characteristics:

Hospital	Characteristics	Beds
A	Public	260
B	Public	1587
C	Public	722
D	Private	224
E	Private	272
F	Private	1175
G	Private	309
H	Private	171

We analyzed the following aspects:
- the strategic process (Quinn, 1980);
- the steps of knowledge management — acquisition, dissemination and application (Nonaka, 1995; Nevis et al., 1995); and
- competency creation (Leonard-Barton, 1994; Hamel & Prahalad, 1990).

Analysis of the Types of Management

The strategic process was identified within two orientations (*Figure 2*), according to Mintzberg et al.'s (1998) definition:
- *Type 1:* Strategic planning limited to its content in this type. Multidisciplinary group meets periodically and establishes the institutions' guidelines for a certain period of time. Once those guidelines are defined, they are communicated to employees. The strategic process follows the traditional orientation from formal strategic planning. Hospitals A, D, E, F, G, and H qualify as Type 1.
- *Type 2:* There is a more dynamic strategic process in this case. Teams get involved in institutional guidelines and strategy setting. However, planning teams are open and all associates are invited to participate. There is ongoing work with no predictable end. Goals are periodically reviewed and analyzed, allowing their permanent adjustment to changes in the healthcare scenario. Hospitals B and C qualify as Type 2 and both are public teaching hospitals. They reached this stage when they identified that the strategic process would only be applicable when it was no longer a management's proposal. According to interviewees, in this case hospitals disregard their current conditions and work with an idealized context.

Figure 2 : Types of Strategic Processes Existing in the Hospitals Studied

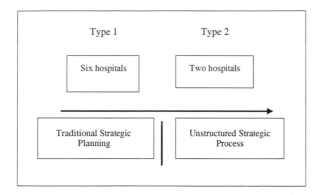

Knowledge Management Stages Identified

Among the cases studied, most hospitals stress internal knowledge dissemination. Knowledge acquisition has a focus that is notably internal to the organization. The most frequently cited forms of knowledge dissemination were: meetings, work and project development by multidisciplinary teams, internal seminars, lectures and courses. Strategic-focus acquisition was identified just in one case. Among the cases studied, only one hospital was identified in a more advanced stage of knowledge management. All others are in early stages.

Stages related to knowledge management present the following characteristics:

- *Stage 1:* In this stage, knowledge is not seen as a strategic resource.

  Acquisition is carried out from individual efforts, with no previous orientation by the institution. Dissemination is the main focus in knowledge management. The hospital's actions related to knowledge dissemination follow no structured forms. At the same time, knowledge application is not controlled. There is not a formal managerial control over the competencies created and results obtained from acquired and disseminated knowledge.

  Hospitals A, B, C, D, F and G are in this stage. They present similar actions regarding knowledge dissemination, considering that this is the only identifiable action related to knowledge management.

  For instance, even though hospital G's administrative manager mentions the importance of evaluating employees through their knowledge, that hospital is still in an early stage in all remaining items. It does not present a clear policy concerning knowledge management. This hospital keeps information limited to specific working groups. In this case, information from SIPAGEH is concentrated in the person who manages the system in the hospital. Similarly, that hospital has no strategic orientation in the search for knowledge and it only keeps existing competencies.

- *Stage 2:* In this stage, knowledge starts to appear in the hospital's strategic plans as a guiding element. Therefore, knowledge is acknowledged as a strategic resource of the organization.

  However, knowledge acquisition still depends upon individual efforts with weak orientation by the institution. Once again, the organization is more committed to knowledge dissemination. In this stage, hospitals start presenting structured forms for knowledge dissemination. Such policies allow associates to publicize acquired knowledge, especially externally. Internally, dissemination takes place in some clear ways, with a managerial discourse stressing the awareness about the importance of knowledge exchange and dissemination among areas and associates. Finally, knowledge application is not strongly controlled yet. Nevertheless, organizations create first formal controls related to measurement systems in this stage. The first efforts for capability identification and evaluation were also found. Hospital H is included in this stage, being the only one to present knowledge dissemination as a strategic principle. This stage was considered as an initial proposal for knowledge management, even though with clear gaps still to be bridged in the future.

This hospital has developed formalized ways in order to disseminate knowledge through meetings, workshops, and seminars, allowing associates to exchange information. These activities are included in the human resources plans. The gaps found are related to the informal ways for knowledge exchange in the internal environment and groups are not encouraged to develop their own practices. Managers establish the ways that knowledge is disseminated internally.

- *Stage 3:* In this stage, the hospital clearly acknowledges knowledge as a strategic resource, aggregating value to the services provided by the institution. Since its acquisition, there is a clear orientation by the institution pointing at the importance of new knowledge within the hospital's competitive environment. Knowledge dissemination is guided by the acknowledgment of the importance of exchange. The hospital previously establishes some forms of dissemination but allows other forms to be internally created by groups. Results from knowledge application are monitored by measurement systems in structured (such as SIPAGEH) or unstructured ways (informal systems).

Hospital E is in this stage, with the best practice in knowledge management. That hospital carried out the identification of strategically important knowledge and seeks such knowledge. It has clearly identified new service-provision needs in the market, seeking permanently to create new competencies.

Hospital E has identified new external knowledge through benchmarking, research, and studies of Brazilian and international cases of success. Its managers are able to identify existing competencies, using formal or informal processes. International accreditation is a result of their continuous research for strategic knowledge. Presently, hospital E is only the third hospital in Brazil with this type of accreditation.

Therefore, strategic knowledge management in hospital E includes knowledge acquisition, dissemination, and application (*Figure 3*).

Table 1 summarizes the main characteristics of the three stages for knowledge strategic management found in the cases analyzed.

Figure 3: Proposal for Stages in Knowledge Management Based on the Hospitals Studied

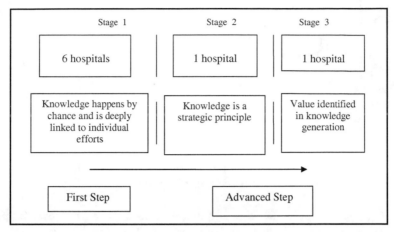

Table 1: Main Characteristics of the Three Stages of Knowledge Management in the Hospital Industry

Stage / Characteristics	First Stage	Intermediate Stage	Advanced Stage
Knowledge Acquisition	Knowledge is not seen as a strategic resource. Initiatives are sporadic, without focus.	More individual initiatives than organization-oriented ones.	Knowledge acquisition is clearly related to the strategic goals of the organization. Knowledge acquisition is an organizational effort.
Knowledge Dissemination	This is the main emphasis, specially related to measurement systems. Dissemination is developed essentially in informal ways.	Improvement in the dissemination ways, which include formal and informal approaches, wide participation of professionals from different technical areas and hierarchical levels. Greater emphasis on dissemination of knowledge acquired externally to the organization.	Information and knowledge exchange are considered fundamental to the organization. Groups organize themselves in order to create formal and informal ways for knowledge dissemination. External and internal knowledge is the benchmarking source for internal process improvement.
Knowledge Application	There is no formal control and evaluation related to the results of knowledge application. Existing capabilities and future needs are not clear.	First formal controls related to measurement systems. First efforts for capability identification and evaluation.	Existing capabilities are clear to organization members. Future capabilities are related to strategic plans and knowledge acquisition.

Competency Creation Based on Organizational Knowledge

Knowledge acquisition that creates competencies at a hospital can be considered as presenting two approaches: a proactive one and a reactive one. The first type — identified only at one hospital — seeks knowledge and competency creation according to its previously defined strategies.

Hospital E identified opportunities and trends in the healthcare environment and in the hospital industry through national and international benchmarking. It also seeks to acquire knowledge and competencies continually. Based on the external information, it has worked internally at identifying the external knowledge needed for the development of new services. The whole hospital is going through changes in order to adjust itself to the model proposed by the medical areas. From employee selection and training to administrative processes, all actions are according to the previously established strategic planning.

On the other hand, knowledge acquisition and creation of new competencies happens almost by chance in the reactive approach. This approach is present in most hospitals analyzed. In this case, the reported practice is that professionals, especially physicians, present proposals to the administration according to their professional interests. Depending also on the hospital's interests as well as the institutional goals, new services are accepted and implemented. There are no detailed previous studies. Additionally, in hospitals with a reactive approach there are no initiatives by managers to seek new knowledge and competencies. Rather, they adjust to suggestions from the medical area that take place individually.

Linking organizational knowledge and competency creation, it is possible to describe the cases studied as follows:

Cases Belonging to Stage 1

- The internal environment is not fitted to the continuous creation of new competencies in hospitals A and D. Indicators are restricted to working groups and there are teams that define guidelines and organizational processes. These guidelines and processes are only disseminated to the remaining employees and associates after they are first defined by the teams. Those two hospitals have the most centralized processes. Among the cases studied, they have the least developed knowledge dissemination, and competency creation is limited to certain groups.
- There are regular formal meetings to communicate the hospital's measurements and goals to all employees at hospital G. Competency generation is not much favored by such exchange, since the meetings play only an informative role.
- Indicators are available to all employees and associates through an intranet at hospitals B, C and F. In such cases, there is already some adjustment of the internal environment to competency development, since everyone has access to information and is able to directly contribute to the development and establishment of functional goals.

Case Belonging to Stage 2

- Knowledge dissemination is a strategic principle and the internal environment presents some conditions for creating new competencies at hospital H. Access to the measurements is still limited to specific working groups. Nevertheless, there are organized forms of knowledge dissemination through lectures, courses, seminars and symposiums. Informal and different ways of knowledge dissemination are also encouraged.

Case Belonging to Stage 3

- Competency generation follows the strategy established by the institutions at hospital E, which is at a more advanced stage of knowledge management. This policy orients the search for competencies in the market or their development internally, according to institutional interests. Internal measurements are available to all employees and associates. Ways of knowledge dissemination are freely established by working groups according to their needs.

The reports above point out that even hospitals in early stages of knowledge management may present different traits regarding their internal environment, favoring competency creation or not. However, the internal environment increasingly adjusts to the ongoing creation of new competencies, after the moment in which knowledge starts to be regarded as a strategic resource. The needs identified in the external environment and the internal creation of ways for knowledge dissemination orients competency creation.

COMPARING THE BEST PRACTICE WITH THE OTHER CASES

Hospital E was the one at the most advanced stage of strategic knowledge management within the cases analyzed. It combines formal and informal strategic processes and knowledge is managed as a strategic resource. Knowledge acquisition has a strategic approach; knowledge dissemination is wide, involving the different functional areas and hierarchical levels; and knowledge application is managed using clear performance measurements and seeking capability creation in their internal processes.

That happens because of:
- Information: the hospital collects it through information technology, concentrates it on just one system and makes it available to all employees.
- Internal environment: the hospital has created an internal learning environment in such way that people and working groups are able to identify the best way for carrying out information and knowledge exchange. Some ways are encouraged and formalized, but others are created by the associates themselves in order to help the process of knowledge dissemination. Externally, there is an awareness of the competition currently experienced by the hospital industry and willingness to be up-to-date through information and benchmarking. The hospital acknowledges competencies in the medical area, being the only one with a clear focus on the continuous improvement of services and management.
- Knowledge management: through access to national and international information and benchmarking, the hospital has identified opportunities and trends and it seeks

to acquire the needed knowledge externally. It identifies value in knowledge management, encouraging dissemination and internal application of that knowledge externally acquired. It acknowledges and publicizes internal knowledge, keeping it aligned to the previous planning.

Hospital E, being a 272-bed private institution, might have some initial advantages related to the dynamism of its management, considering the theoretical premises of this study. Even given that, this hospital still presents gaps regarding knowledge management. One aspect is its strategic process, preferentially centered on traditional strategic planning. On the other hand, public and university hospitals with more beds do not always have worse practices. Hospital C, a public hospital, carried out its strategic process also in an unstructured way, as well as hospital F, which widely communicates information through an intranet to all its employees.

Hospital G was the hospital in the least advanced knowledge management stage. In that healthcare institution, there is no established policy for a measurement system; dissemination methods are defined only by managers; information is concentrated in restricted working groups; and, there are no current practices for managing through managerial measurements. It would be fair to question if those aspects are related to the fact that the hospital is located in a small town away from the state capital, possibly with lower access to and less contact with more dynamic, competitive environments. Therefore, external dissemination of knowledge, easier for hospitals located in large urban centers, can be a means for improving existing practices. Thus, the cases studied can suggest that more isolated hospitals present disadvantages regarding knowledge exchange. For hospitals geographically isolated, participation in seminars, symposiums, and congresses might not be a priority regarding other activities due to the fact that they have no direct contact with reference institutions.

LESSONS LEARNED AND MANAGERIAL IMPLICATIONS

The following aspects might be considered for improving knowledge management in hospital organizations, following the main points examined in the cases included in this study.

Regarding knowledge acquisition:
- To seek information from distinct sources, both internally and externally;
- To allow access to information/indicators to all employees and associates through information technologies (computers, systems, e-mail, etc.) and other informal means;
- To decentralize information, making it available to several areas in order to allow multi-professional participation in process development and problem solving.

Regarding knowledge dissemination:
- To encourage working groups to create their own ways for information exchange: through presence or virtual meetings; formal and informal meetings; seminars, among others.

- To create conditions for the collective definition of the strategic organization's objectives.

Regarding knowledge application:
- To identify existing and potential competencies within the organization, according to previous planning and the organization's objectives;
- To reinforce existing competencies and to develop new ones that adjust to the demands of the external environment.

Regarding knowledge management as a whole:
- To seek organizational knowledge (acquisition - dissemination - application) as the guiding factor in many activities and not only as a strategic objective or an imposition from the organization's management;
- To identify ways for measuring the application and utilization of shared and acquired knowledge;
- To approach knowledge as an effectively important resource for the organization and to seek ways to acknowledge its creation and reward it.

CONCLUSIONS

This study aimed at presenting an initial view of strategic knowledge management in the hospital industry. The major part of the cases analyzed showed that knowledge management has great gaps to be bridged in the future by these healthcare organizations. In spite of this, the hospital at the most advanced stage of knowledge management presented practices close to the most competitive companies from more traditional industries. That points out to a clear strategic orientation in knowledge management, linking its practices and actions to the hospital strategy. In short, the cases analyzed corroborated some of the main theoretical references in knowledge management as well, such as Grant (1996) and Davenport and Prusak (1998).

Considering the fact that knowledge management is basically built on three stages — acquisition, dissemination and utilization of knowledge — it is important that a hospital's processes offer conditions that are ripe for people involved to create, share, make available, and influence knowledge at the organization in support of business strategies.

Within such an approach, it was possible to verify that the majority of the hospitals studied emphasize internal dissemination of knowledge. Such a fact reinforces the importance of cross-functional integration between the several functional areas in the hospital. The most frequently mentioned ways of knowledge dissemination were meetings and intranets.

Within a proposition of three stages for knowledge management, six hospitals were considered to be in the early stage. In this case, knowledge searching is strongly oriented by individual interests. In an intermediary stage, there is already an initial intention to manage knowledge being a strategic guideline, even though the preferential focus still resides on internal dissemination of knowledge in this stage. One case was identified at the most advanced stage. This hospital seeks strategically to acquire, disseminate, and apply knowledge, according to what was previously planned.

Finally, the results suggest that the characteristics of the hospitals studied — such as being public or private — had little influence on the stage of knowledge management which the hospital belongs to. The exception might be the geographic location. More isolation would lead to less contact with other reference institutions or hospitals, both in administrative and medical aspects.

We may mention as a limitation of this study the use of a single interviewer. The best orientation would be to take multiple views. In this case, we face some resistance, especially from the medical area.

Future research may investigate the following aspect related to this article:

* how these stages can be identified in other healthcare organizations, such as laboratories, public services, among others;
* the role of Information Technology in the strategic management of knowledge;
* quantitative studies in order to validate the first findings from this study.

REFERENCES

Begun, J. & Heawole, K. B. (1999). Strategic cycling: Shaking complacency in health care strategic planning. *Journal of Healthcare Management*, 44(5), 339-352.

Bruton, G., Oviatt, B. & Bruton, L. K. (1995). Strategic planning in hospitals: Review and proposal. *Healthcare Management Review*, 20(3), 16-25.

Campos, J. Q. & Campos, J. Q. (1982). *O hospital e sua humanização*. São Paulo: LTr.

Carapinheiro, G. (1998). *Saberes e poderes no hospital*. Porto: Edições Afrontamento.

Cunha, A. K. M. & Sordi, D. R. (2001). *A estratégia e a competição na área hospitalar: A contribuição do SIPAGEH*. Retrieved from the World Wide Web: http://www.sipageh.unisinos.br.

Davenport, T. H. & Prusak, L. (1998). *Working Knowledge*. Boston, MA: Harvard Business School Press.

Drain, M. & Godkin, L.A. (1996). Portfolio approach to strategic hospital analysis: Exposition and explanation. *Health Care Management Review*, 21(4), 68-74.

Drucker, P. (1999). Knowledge-worker productivity: The biggest challenge. *California Management Review*, 41(2), 79-95.

Gonçalves, E. L. (1983). *O hospital e a visão administrativa contemporânea*. São Paulo, Pioneira.

Grant, R. M. (1996). Prospering in dynamic-competitive environments: Organizational capability as knowledge integration. *Organization Science*, 7(4), 375-387.

Hamel, G. & Prahalad, C. K. (1990). The core competence of the corporation. *Harvard Business Review*, 68(3), 75-84.

Inamdar, N., Kaplan, R. S., Bower, M. & Reynolds, K. (2002). Applying the balanced scorecard in healthcare provider organizations. *Journal of Healthcare Management*, 47(3), 179-196.

Lafferty Jr., W. J. (2003). The development of a customer excellence master plan. *Journal of Healthcare Management*, 48(1), 62-71.

Landini, M. Z. S. & Damiani, J. H. S. (2000). *Gestão do conhecimento: Um estudo exploratório no Projeto Veículo Lançador de Satélites*. Retrieved from the World Wide Web: http://www.informal.com.br/artigos/a19102000.htm.

Lebrasseur, R., Whissell, R. & Ojha, A. (2002). Organizational learning, transformational leadership and implementation of continuous quality improvement in Canadian hospitals. *Australian Journal of Management*, 27(2), 141-162.

Leonard-Barton, D. (1992). The Factory as a Learning Laboratory. *Sloan Management Review*, 34(1), 23-38.

Leonard-Barton, D. (1994). *Wellsprings of Knowledge*. Boston: Harvard Business School Press.

Lipparini, A., Cazzola, F. & Pistarelli, P. (2000). Como sustentar o crescimento com base nos recursos e nas competências distintivas: A experiência da Illycaffè. *Revista de Administração de Empresas. São Paulo*, 40(2), 16-25.

Mintzberg, H., Ahlstrand, B. & Lampel, J. (1998). *Strategy Safari: A Guided Tour Through the Wilds of Strategic Management*. New York: The Free Press.

Mirshawka, V. (1994). *Hospital fui bem atendido: A hora e a vez do Brasil*. São Paulo: Makron Books.

Nevis, E. C., Dibella, A. J. & Gould, J. M. (1995). Understanding organizations as learning systems. *Sloan Management Review*, 36(2), 73-85.

Nonaka, I. (1995). A dynamic theory of organizational knowledge creation. *Organization Science*, 5(1), 14-37.

Paiva, E. L., Roth, A. V. & Fensterseifer, J. E. (1998). Knowledge Management and the Process of Manufacturing Strategy Formulation. *Proceedings of Production and Operations Management Society Conference*.

Popovich, K. & Popovich, M. (2000). Use of Q methodology for hospital strategic planning: a case study. *Journal of Healthcare Management*, 45(6), 405-414.

Probst, G., Raub, S. & Romhardt, K. (2000). *Managing Knowledge*. Chichester, UK: John Wiley and Sons.

Quinn, J. B. (1980). *Strategy for Change — Logical Incrementalism*. Homewood, IL: Richard Irwin.

Quintana, P., Roschke, M. A. & Ribeiro, E. C. (1994). Educación permanente, processo de trabajo y calidad de servicio em salud. In Q. J. Haddad et al. (Eds.), *Educación permanente e personal de salud*. Washington: OPS.

Ribeiro, H. P. (1993). *O hospital: História e crise*. São Paulo: Cortez.

Scott, G. (2001). Customer satisfaction: Six strategies for continuous improvement. *Journal of Healthcare Management*, 46(2), 82-85.

Toffler, A. (1994). *Powershift: As mudanças do poder*. Rio de Janeiro: Record.

Zahra, E. & Das, S. R. (1993). Building competitive advantage on manufacturing resources. *Long Range Planning*, 26(2), 90-101.

APPENDIX

Hospital Founder's SIPAGEH Averages – Year Of 2001

Hospital / Indicator	A	B	C	D	E	F	G	H
Customer -Satisfaction Public	59,5	NA	76,5	NA	NA	66,15	27,59	75,31
Customer -Satisfaction Private	62,84	NA	75,5	74,2	74,9	52,29	53,05	NA
Turnover	1,37	1,04	0,76	1,88	1,72	1,32	1,31	2,09
Absence rates	3,05	8,15	2,71	1,34	1,69	2,03	6,32	1,99
Frequency of work accidents	23,85	38,6	24,5	29,9	8,5	66,07	0	23,51
Bed occupation	80,75	88,3	89,5	81	85,5	86,35	65,57	87
Training Hours per Employee	0,53	0,31	2,58	4,8	4,84	6,53	5,14	2,39
Caesarian	NI	34,1	28,6	71	76,5	29,68	57,55	51,76
Average stay General	9,56	9,8	9,6	5,5	4,87	7,2	5,02	4,5
Average Stay Obstetric	NA	NA	3,05	3	NA	3	NA	NA
Avarege Stay Pediatric	NA	NA	13,9	NA	NA	5,8	NA	NA
Mortality General	4,9	6,7	4,9	2,2	2,16	4,2	2,5	2,09
Mortality Obstetric	NA	NA	0	0	NA	0	NA	NA
Mortality Pediatric	NA	NA	4,5	NA	NA	0,9	NA	NA
Liquid Margin	-1,71	-9,77	-2,45	9,55	-1,5	2,46	2,79	11,63
Infection Blood Stream	1	NA	0	2,05	NA	0,88	12,54	0
Infection related to Central Venous Catheter								
Hospital Infection in Clean Surgeries	NA	NA	1,8	2,05	NA	NA	2,11	NA

Chapter XXIII

Secure Knowledge Management for Healthcare Organizations

Darren Mundy, University of Hull, UK

David W. Chadwick, University of Salford, UK

ABSTRACT

As the healthcare industry enters the era of knowledge management it must place security at the foundation of the transition. Risks are pervasive to every aspect of information and knowledge management. Without secure practices that seek to avoid or mitigate the effects of these risks, how can healthcare organisations ensure that knowledge is captured, stored, distributed, used, destroyed and restored securely? In an age where risks and security threats are ever-increasing, secure knowledge management is an essential business practice. The cost of security breaches in a healthcare context can range from the unauthorized access of confidential information to the potential loss or unauthorized modification of patient information leading to patient injury. In this chapter the authors highlight different approaches to minimising these risks, based on the concepts of authentication, authorization, data integrity, availability and confidentiality. Security mechanisms have to be in-depth, rather like the layers of an onion, and security procedures have to be dynamic, due to the continually changing environment. For example, in the past, cryptographic algorithms that were proven to be safe, e.g., 56 bit key DES, have succumbed to advanced computer

*power or more sophisticated attacks, and have had to be replaced with more powerful
alternatives. The authors present a model for ensuring dynamic secure knowledge
management and demonstrate through the use of case studies, that if each of the security
layers are covered, then we can be reasonably sure of the strength of our system's
security.*

THE CONTEXT FOR SECURE
KNOWLEDGE MANAGEMENT

Knowledge is intangible, expensive to obtain, easy to lose and invaluable to
organizational success. An organization's knowledge can also be easy to view, steal,
manipulate and delete. In the physical world knowledge is protected by structures such
as non-disclosure agreements, filing cabinets and shredding machines. In the digital
world the same kind of mechanisms are required to ensure our knowledge is well
protected.

Security threats to organizational data are increasing exponentially both within
organizational boundaries and externally. According to the respected CSI/FBI Computer
Crime and Security Survey 2002 (Power, 2002), the largest majority of attacks on computer
networks are internal. In this chapter initially we present a conceptual model for ensuring
secure knowledge management in healthcare. Then we introduce key security technologies which can be used to implement components of the model, as well as providing
background information on how these components have traditionally been implemented
within IT systems. Finally we provide case studies of recent implementations that
illustrate use of the model. We believe this will convince the reader that security is a
necessity in the implementation of Knowledge Management Systems (KMS).

ENSURING SECURE KNOWLEDGE
MANAGEMENT IN HEALTHCARE

A model for ensuring secure knowledge management in healthcare is shown in
Figure 1.

- *authentication:* (1) Security measure designed to establish the validity of a
  transmission, message, or originator; (2) a means of verifying an individual's
  eligibility to receive specific categories of information (NIS, 1992) (see "Authentication Mechanisms");
- *authorization:* (1) The rights granted to a user to access, read, modify, insert, or
  delete certain data, or to execute certain programs; (2) access rights granted to a
  user, program, or process (NIS, 1992) (see "Authorization Mechanisms");
- *data security (privacy):* (The) protection of data from unauthorized (accidental or
  intentional) modification, destruction, or disclosure (NIS, 1992);
- *data integrity:* 1. (The) condition that exists when data is unchanged from its
  source and has not been accidentally or maliciously modified, altered, or destroyed
  (NIS, 1992) (see "Data Security and Integrity during Transfer");

Figure 1: Model for Secure Knowledge Management

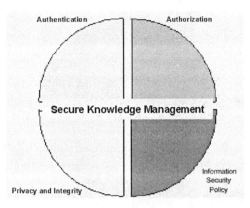

- *information security policy:* organizational guidelines, rules, regulations and procedures that are used to protect an organisation's information (see "Security Policy").

Each of the four components is essential and mutually supportive. Authentication without authorization would mean that only valid users could gain access, but could execute any operations they wish to within the KMS. For example, in a patient records system, secretaries (who might be authorized to update a patient's name and address only) could execute a command to access health details for all patients or change diagnoses. Conversely, authorization without authentication would mean that anyone could masquerade as anyone else and thus gain his or her access rights. Information security policy provides the risk management, the appropriate controls, the recovery procedures, and the auditing procedures, etc. Without an information security policy there would be no apparent requirement for secure practices, and security would either be ignored or implemented in an ad-hoc manner, with the result that some controls could be too rigid and others completely missing. Finally, a system without privacy and integrity would be untrustworthy, so the knowledge contained within the system would be virtually worthless. For example, in a knowledge base containing details about clinical procedures, erroneous changes could be made to the information without detection, possibly leading to fatal consequences for patients.   This model will be examined in greater depth in the next few sections, which provide information about mechanisms for implementing each segment of the model. Following these sections case material will be provided demonstrating the model in action.

AUTHENTICATION MECHANISMS
Authentication

How can you be sure that the user requesting access to your KMS is who they say they are? Traditionally, weak authentication systems, typically based on a username and/ or password, have been a key source of unauthorized access to networks and computer systems. From a healthcare KMS perspective, authentication mechanisms provide a means to ensure that external parties that we do not wish to access the KMS cannot gain access without acquiring an authentication token. If we choose a strong authentication mechanism, then it should make it extremely difficult, if not impossible, for these parties to gain access to our KMS. Particular risks of poor authentication in healthcare would include potential unauthorized access to a KMS containing information, for example, on patient conditions, quality of patient care or hospital procedures. All attacks potentially could result in decreased patient care and liability or negligence cases.

In the US and other countries, government regulations such as the Health Insurance Portability and Accountability Act (HIPAA) mandating the privacy of patient identifiable information require that access only be granted to those parties authorized to view the information. Strong authentication of users seeking access to a KMS containing patient-related material will be essential in achieving compliance with these kinds of regulations.

Present Practices: Passwords and their Frailties

Traditionally, authentication to networks and computer systems has been provided by the use of usernames and passwords. In early password authentication schemes, users would simply log on using their username and password and the computer system would do a simple lookup that the password given matched the password stored for the user. However, password files could frequently be obtained from the system itself and then posted for all to see. So developers were required to secure the scheme by taking the password and passing it through a programming routine called a onetime hashing algorithm. The hashing algorithm mathematically reduces the data into a small (typically 128 or 160 bits), indecipherable series of bits. The hashed password can then be stored in the system instead of the clear text password. When the user logs into the system, the password they input is hashed and the new hash and the stored hash are compared to see if they match.

Password hashing is now commonplace, but hashed passwords are still vulnerable to dictionary attacks. This is where the attacker runs all the words in a dictionary through the hashing algorithm, and compares the generated hashes with the stored hashed values. Bad as this might seem, a potentially far greater threat than poorly protected password storage is the threat of human weaknesses. Users are prone to picking poor passwords, writing passwords down, and giving their passwords out, etc. Management steps should be taken to educate users and strengthen password usage. Simple information security policy statements, such as passwords must be eight characters or more in length and must contain a mixture of capital letters, lowercase letters and digits, provide improvements to the basic system and usually render the passwords impervious to dictionary attacks. User education can also lead to a movement away from bad habits such as leaving passwords on post-it stickers and giving passwords out to other people.

However, even with the various protection mechanisms mentioned above, passwords are still relatively weak. To be effective they rely on secrecy and strict policy management. In health environments where perhaps access to PCs is not strictly controlled, especially on wards where patients or other parties could gain unauthorized access to the PC, passwords are not an effective authentication mechanism. To gain effective authentication other mechanisms can be used both in conjunction with and as replacements for passwords.

Key Technology Focus: Biometrics

Biometrics allow users to authenticate themselves using personal characteristics that are less easily stolen or copied. On a user there are certain uniquely identifying attributes that can be used to determine identity, e.g., fingerprints, retinal scans, facial imaging, voice recognition, hand readers, etc. Biometric authentication comprises three phases. Firstly, a template of the user's biometric feature is recorded by the system. A biometric device reads the user's biometric feature several times and stores the average of the readings in the system. Several readings are needed because biometrics vary according to temperature, humidity, blood pressure, etc. Then when the user wishes to authenticate to the system, a biometric device records the user's biometric feature (phase two). Finally, the reading is compared with the stored template using some predefined matching algorithm (phase three). Unfortunately, due to the imprecise nature of the matching, biometric authentication is prone to false positives and false negatives. False positives are when an attacker is wrongly identified as being the user, and false negatives are when the user is not recognised by the system.

Biometrics technology has been piloted in a number of organizations (e.g., Essex Police and Securicor (UK), Washington Hospital Centre (DC)) and full-scale implementations are already in place in a number of business sectors (e.g., Nigerian electoral process, and the City of Glendale (CA)). In future KMS, biometric authentication will increasingly become the authentication mechanism of choice.

Key Technology Focus: Public Key Cryptography, Public Key Infrastructure (PKI) and Digital Signatures

The concept of Public Key Cryptography was introduced to the academic community in 1976 by two researchers called Whitfield Diffie and Martin Hellman (Diffie & Hellman, 1976). Public Key Cryptography was initially applied to encryption (covered in "Key Technology Focus: Data Encryption," basically encryption means to disguise data and decryption means to retrieve the data that was previously disguised), but it also solved the problem of authentication. The basic idea of Public Key Cryptography is to have two different security tokens, called the *public* and *private* keys, which work together as a pair. They can be used to perform mathematical operations on data, either digital signing/verification or data encryption/decryption. The *public key* is viewable to all users whilst the *private key* remains a secret to the entity to whom the keys have been given. If data is encrypted with the *private key*, it can only be decrypted with the *public key*, and vice versa. It is not possible to both encrypt and decrypt the data with the same key, nor is it usually possible to determine one key from the other. When data is encrypted with the *private key* of a user, this allows the data to be authenticated as coming from that user. When data is encrypted with the *public key* of a user, this allows the data to be made confidential for that user.

However, public key cryptography is slower to execute than conventional cryptography, which uses a single key. For this reason, when data authentication is required, the data is first condensed using a hashing algorithm. The hash value is called a *message digest*. The *private key* of the user is then used to encrypt the *message digest*. The encrypted digest is known as the *digital signature* of the data. The *digital signature*, along with the original data, are then sent to the recipient. On receipt the receiver takes the *digital signature* and decrypts it using the signer's *public key*, to reveal the message digest created by the signer. The recipient then creates his own message digest from the data sent by the signer and compares the two. If the two *message digests* match then the recipient can be sure that the data was sent by the signer and it has not been changed en route.

However, this presupposes that the recipient is in possession of the genuine public key of the signer. Whilst it would be possible for all users to personally meet and exchange their public keys with each other, this is not a scalable solution. Consequently, we need a reliable and trustworthy way of distributing public keys. A trusted third party, called a Certification Authority (CA), is used to digitally sign the public keys of users, to ensure that they cannot be tampered with. A CA would be contained within and managed by a hierarchical authority, for example the Department of Health and Human Services or a hospital's Human Resources department. The CA signs a message containing the name of the user and their public key, and its own name, and these certified public key messages are called Public Key Certificates (PKCs).

Should a user's private key become compromised (e.g., stolen), then we have a requirement to communicate this knowledge to other users. This is generally done using a particular construct called a Certificate Revocation List (CRL). A CRL contains a list of all the public key certificates no longer considered to be valid because the private key has been compromised or revoked, and the CRL is signed and dated by the CA.

A Public Key Infrastructure is seen as, *"the set of hardware, software, people, policies and procedures needed to create, manage, store, distribute, and revoke PKCs based on public-key cryptography"* (Arsenault and Taylor, 2002). Recently mechanisms for digitally signing the popular eXtensible Markup Language (XML) documents have been introduced (Eastlake et al., 2002). Within a healthcare KMS, users would generate XML documents. The content of these documents would then be digitally signed with the user's private key. When any user wishes to retrieve the document, they can then check the verification of the XML Signature using the public key of the signing user.

Key Technology Focus: Smartcards

Modern smart cards contain a computer embedded chip and user-specific data, which can be used to provide authentication when placed in a smart card reading device. The user-specific data can be anything linked to the user, such as a private key or a digital fingerprint. Traditionally this user-specific data would have been stored as a software token on a PC, making it liable to theft or deletion. Smart cards provide increased security because the user specific data is never allowed to leave the smart card. All processing operations are carried out via the on-board chip so the user-specific data can never be copied. Usually the data is further protected via the use of a password.

Previously high costs and unreliability (Chadwick, 1999) have been a significant factor in the slow adoption of smart card technology. Costs have significantly decreased recently and reliability has improved, so the adoption of smart cards becomes a viable option to the other authentication alternatives.

AUTHORIZATION MECHANISMS

Authorization

Authorization provides assurance that the users accessing the KMS have permission to do so. When authorization is combined with a suitable authentication scheme, we can be sure that the users accessing the system are who they say they are and are authorized to access the resource. Different access control models have been developed to ensure that only authorized users can access resources. From a healthcare KMS perspective, we wish to ensure that users are, for example: authorized to access the system, authorized to generate new knowledge within the system, and authorized to make changes within the system.

Discretionary Access Control (DAC)

Discretionary Access Control (DAC) can be viewed as owner-based administration of access rights. In DAC the owner of an object has discretionary authority over which other users can access the object. For example, Alex has just set up his own KMS and he grants access to Kate and Lee, but denies access to Spencer. There are various types of DAC including a strict DAC where Kate and Lee would not be able to grant access to other users, and a liberal DAC where delegation is allowed either with a strict limitation on the number of delegation levels or with no restriction (i.e., Kate could grant access to Sophie who could grant to Johnny, etc.). The DAC approach has some limitations, the most notable being how the owner can delegate his discretionary power to other people.

Mandatory Access Control (MAC)

Mandatory Access Control (MAC) can be thought of in terms of security labels given to objects and users. Each object is given a label called a security classification and each user is given a label called a security clearance, which includes a classification list. This list identifies which type of classified object a user has access to. A typical hierarchical classification scheme used by the military is *unmarked*, *unclassified*, *restricted*, *confidential*, *secret*, and *top secret*. A MAC policy using such a hierarchical scheme would typically be "read down and write up," which would help stop information leakage. A user with clearance of *restricted* could read from objects with classifications of *unmarked* to *restricted* but only write to classifications of *restricted* to *top secret*. The same user could log in as unmarked to enable them to write to levels up to *restricted*.

Role Based Access Control (RBAC)

In the basic Role Based Access Control (RBAC) model, permissions are granted to roles, then these roles are assigned to users who, therefore, acquire the roles' access permissions. Roles typically represent organisational roles such as secretary, consultant, etc. Roles confer both access rights to resources and the right to assign roles to users. For example, a physician may have read access to a KMS but not have the access right to alter data within it. A KMS security officer may have the right to assign people to roles, but no access rights to the resources itself. A role and its permissions tend to change infrequently over time whereas the users associated with the role will change more regularly. This basic premise makes associating permissions with roles easier than associating permissions with users. Users can change roles and new users can be allocated roles. As needs change, roles can be granted new permissions or permissions can be removed. The main advantages of RBAC are in maintenance and scalability.

Key Technology Focus: Privilege Management Infrastructure (PMI)

Privilege Management Infrastructure is a new development in the world of authorization. A PMI is to authorization what a PKI is to authentication. In a PMI a user is allocated digitally signed privileges, called attribute certificates, and these attribute certificates can be presented to a resource in order to gain access to it. The resource is governed by an authorization policy that says which privileges users must have in order to gain access and under which conditions.

Attribute certificates are allocated to users by attribute authorities (analogous to certification authorities in a PKI). They are digitally signed by the attribute authority, and because of this they can be stored in a public repository or held by the user on their PC. In order to gain access to a resource, the user must first be authenticated by the resource to prove that he has the right to assert the privileges contained within his attribute certificates. This authentication could be by any means, e.g., Kerberos, or a digital signature and Public Key Certificate. After successful authentication, the attribute certificates containing the user's privileges are verified and checked against the authorization policy. If the policy states that the privileges are sufficient then the user is granted access, else access is denied. A number of different PMI solutions are available including PERMIS and AKENTI.

DATA SECURITY AND INTEGRITY DURING TRANSFER

Data Security and Integrity

A healthcare KMS without data security and data integrity should be thought of as being untrustworthy. The information held within the system could have been altered, modified or had key sections removed. Even more importantly a KMS without data security may have leaked sensitive information to unauthorized parties. One of the key stages at which information leakage can occur is during data transfer over the network, Intranet or Internet. From a healthcare KMS perspective, looking at regulations such as HIPAA, poorly configured data security could result in unauthorized users gaining access to patient information and noncompliance. Without data integrity, staff will not be able to use a healthcare KMS effectively, as the information it provides will be unreliable.

Key Technology Focus: Data Encryption

In data encryption understandable data (*plain text*) is transformed using an *encryption algorithm* into incomprehensible data (*cipher text*) under control of a *key*. When the previous *plain text* is required the *encryption algorithm*, the *key* and the *cipher text* are used in conjunction to retrieve it. The *cipher text* looks like a random bit stream and there is no way of establishing the *plain text* from the *cipher text* without the *key*. The *key* is usually a randomly generated bit string consisting of 64-256 bits (the longer the key, the stronger the encryption). Various *symmetric encryption algorithms* exist with the most popular being CAST (Adams, 1997), RC2 (Rivest, 1998) and Triple DES (ANSI, 1985).

Encryption provides protection of the information within a KMS from unauthorized viewing as long as the text is *cipher text* and the attacker does not have access to the *key*. There are two forms of encryption that can be used, single key (*symmetric*) or dual key (*asymmetric* or *public key*). In single key encryption both parties use the same key for encryption and decryption. Dual key encryption follows the same principles described in the Public Key Infrastructure section. Therefore, encryption comes with the disadvantages of key management (who should generate keys, how to distribute keys, what to do if keys are lost) and a decrease in system performance due to the encryption/decryption process. Also encryption does not actually provide any assurance that the data has not been altered in transit and only some assurance that the data came from the person it is stated to have come from.

Secure Data Transfer Technologies, e.g., Secure Sockets Layer (SSL)

SSL is a security protocol, which can be used to provide a secure channel between two machines (server and client) across an insecure network such as the Internet. The protocol has provisions for the protection of data in transit, using Message Authentication Codes (MACs) (Krawczyk, 1997), and strong authentication of the server using X.509 public key certificates. It can also provide authentication of the client and encryption of the data whilst in transit. An SSL connection consists of two phases; the handshake and data transfer phases. The handshake phase authenticates the server and optionally the client, and also establishes the shared secret that will subsequently be used in the MACs and optional encryption mechanism that will be used to protect the data. Once the handshake phase is completed the data is split up and transmitted in protected packets.

There are a large number of SSL implementations available, ranging from the free and high quality Open SLL implementation (www.openssl.org) to vendor toolkits from organisation such as RSA (www.rsasecurity.com) and IAIK (www.iaik.at). Other mechanisms exist which provide secure data transfer including Transport Layer Security (TLS) (Dierks & Allen, 1999), which is essentially an improved version of SSL, S/Mime (Dusse et al., 1998) to secure email transactions and Secure Shell (SSH) (Ylonen et al., 2000) often used for configuration management. In a healthcare KMS, SSL would be used to provide a protected channel for users to access information from the KMS.

Key Technology Focus: Firewalls

A firewall is a system designed to prevent unauthorized access to and from your private network. The firewall consists of a number of components:

- The Internet Use security policy for the organization. This stipulates at an organizational level the expected security required when connecting to the Internet. (For example, all external access must be through a strong authentication system.)
- The mapping of the policy onto designs and procedures to be observed when connecting to the Internet. (For example, SSL client authentication may be required.)
- The firewall hardware and/or software used to protect the network

Each of the components is required. Without a policy the firewall cannot be correctly configured, as the technical staff will not know which traffic to let in and which to exclude. Without enforcing the procedures then many aspects of the policy may simply be ignored, such as inspecting the logs on a daily basis. Firewalls can be complex. A couple of the techniques used are shown below.

- Packet Filtering. Filters network data packets based on their Internet Protocol (IP) and UDP/TCP source and destination addresses.
- Stateful Packet Inspection. Inspects data packets as they are arriving and filters on a specific set of security rules.

Firewalls help prevent attacks against insecure services, can secure external access to required network services and provide a cost advantage over securing each host on an organizational network. However, firewalls are not without their disadvantages. Like any computer system without regular updates/patches, intruders can gain access to the healthcare network. They may also make it difficult for legitimate users to be able to access required network services. Hackers can also often circumvent firewalls by using "backdoors" into the healthcare network, provided for example by modems situated behind the firewall. However, the biggest disadvantage of firewalls is they provide no protection against the internal hacker. Given that hospitals are public places, this can pose a serious problem. By placing a second firewall directly in front of the healthcare KMS server, this can ensure that requests to that server are authenticated and only passed through on certain ports, thereby restricting the attacker's options.

Key Technology Focus: Wireless Data Transfer

Wireless technology, based on the IEEE 802.11 standard, is increasingly being adopted, especially in areas such as healthcare where the benefits of mobility are great. Unfortunately 802.11 offers only a basic level of security (open or shared-key authentication and static wired equivalent privacy (WEP) keys). But worse still, many wireless LANs are installed with no security at all or are left in default out-of-the-box configurations, thus allowing all comers to gain access to the network. Wireless LANs should always be configured with 128-bit WEP as a minimum, but even this can be compromised by the determined hacker, so wireless technology should not be used for mission critical KM applications unless the basic security is enhanced with technologies such as TLS, VPNs, IPSEC or 802.1X/EAP.

Wireless Access Points are used to set up wireless networks and connect the wireless network to the physical hard-wired network. We can compare a Wireless Access Point directly to an internal modem on the organizational network (i.e., it is a "backdoor"). The addition of wireless to the healthcare network must not come at the cost of reduced security. Therefore, we must think about the key elements in securing this new technology.

- access and authentication – Open authentication involves configuring the correct service set ID (SSID) to the client. This is no more than a shared password, which, without WEP, is transferred in the clear over the airwaves, so anyone with a wireless receiver can capture it and thus gain access. By using WEP (see below), the SSID is encrypted prior to transfer, thus making it difficult for hackers to decipher the SSID. Shared-key authentication on the other hand simply uses the shared WEP key for authentication. The access point sends the client a challenge and the client must then encrypt this with the shared key and return it to the access point to gain access;
- data privacy (provided by using WEP encryption and shared symmetric keys);
- network location and access point security (physically placing the Wireless Access Point outside the healthcare organisations firewall may limit any damage).

Notwithstanding the security concerns above, the benefits of using wireless technology within KMSs are numerous. Specialists can record procedures in places where there might be limited "wired" access and doctors can be permanently online whilst doing their ward rounds.

SECURITY POLICY
Secure Data Management: Storage, Backup and Disposal

An information security policy is the key to secure data management. Without policies in place governing the storage, backup and disposal of information, no attention will be given to the procedures that need to be in place to enforce the policy. A security system is only as strong as its weakest link and the actual computer/storage device on which a KMS is situated can be an easy target if the attacker can gain physical access to it. Therefore, in circumstances where a machine stores confidential information or business critical information its physical security must be assured. Access restrictions to the room holding the machine must be in place and strictly enforced. Furthermore, the machine itself must be protected by secure authentication and authorization mechanisms.

Backup tapes must be treated with the same amount of physical security as the systems they are used to restore. This is because the information stored within your KMS is also stored on the backup medium. If a backup medium is stolen then it is reasonable to expect that your system has been compromised. Thus backup media should be physically secured by either storing them in a locked room or safe. In addition to physical security, the backup medium may also be logically protected either by using data encryption and/or an authentication mechanism to activate the restore process.

Secure disposal of storage media also needs to be an information security policy requirement. There have been instances where confidential data has been left on computers that have been passed on to other organizations. Even worse, computers can be left still set up to access your network or KMS. Simply deleting information on computers is not enough to erase the data from the hard drive. The data either has to be securely deleted using a commercial "secure delete" application or the media destroyed. Without secure deletion procedures the healthcare organization and its systems are not only at potential risk from release of confidential information but also at risk from backdoors into the system.

Key Business Focus: Business Continuity Planning/ Disaster Recovery

KMSs are invaluable resources. Losing the knowledge stored within such systems would invariably affect patient care and business continuation. In extreme cases the loss of an IT system can lead to the liquidation of an organisation. In the health community the loss of such a system could have results such as inefficient patient service, inaccurate diagnosis and loss of specialist practices. In extreme cases it could lead to the loss of human life (e.g., if important patient records are lost and diagnoses are lost or inappropriate drugs are prescribed).

The first step in the contingency process is to look at the business impact of losing the particular KMS combined with a risk and threat analysis. This will help to highlight areas of significant risk, which will need to be covered in detail by the contingency plan or mitigated by another measure. An analysis of the risks and threats facing the KMS will lead us in the second step to the development of a comprehensive contingency and recovery plan, plus risk-mitigating actions. The recovery plan will highlight procedures for ensuring business continuity should any of the risks and threats be realised. The third step will be to test out the recovery plan. A recovery plan which does not work is of little use in an emergency. If backup links and servers have been installed, then time needs to be set aside to test that an operational service can be brought back into use with them. If a third party backup service provider is being used, they will usually allow you time each year to test that their system can run an operational service for you.

The final step in the contingency process is the continual audit, review and update of the contingency plan and risk mitigating actions over the lifetime of the KMS. In other words, this is a continual process that never ends, so as to ensure that the recovery plan remains up-to-date and workable. Further, new risks are continually arising and these have to be taken into account and new mitigating actions devised. It is essential to ensure that key personnel know the recovery plan or know where to obtain it. If, for example, a change has been made in IT personnel between the last audit and the new one then the audit would record if the new personnel knew about the contingency plan.

CASE STUDY: PMI IMPLEMENTATION (AUTHORIZATION SEGMENT OF MODEL)

In this section we present an example of how a PMI implementation can be used to provide strong authorization in our recently developed Electronic Prescription Processing (EPP) Application Programming Interface (API). In the EPP API we have integrated the PERMIS PMI API (Chadwick & Otenko, 2002) so as to control who is authorized to execute commands such as prescribe and dispense prescriptions and also to ascertain patients' rights to exemption from charges (Chadwick & Mundy, 2003). In a KMS one could envisage using PERMIS to control rights to access the system, modify the data, etc.

The overseer of the UK National Health Service, which for all intents and purposes is the Secretary of State for Health in the UK Government, would generate and electronically sign a PERMIS policy stipulating who can carry out which actions in the Prescription Processing System. For example, the policy might state that the General Medical Council is trusted to allocate the role of Doctor to qualified Doctors, and that anyone with the role of Doctor is allowed to prescribe. Therefore, a signatory member of the General Medical Council indirectly gives all General Practitioners in the UK NHS the right to prescribe when they are issued with a Doctor role privilege certificate. When the GP is generating a prescription their prescription program will use the EPP API, and the latter will call the PERMIS decision engine to determine if the GP is authorised to prescribe according to the rules laid down in the policy. As long as the prescriber has the role of Doctor, they will have been granted permission to prescribe and they will be allowed access to the operation to generate an electronic prescription. Similar mechanisms exist for dispensers within the prescription processing system and for determining the exemption qualification of patients.

In a KMS we could reasonably expect the system administrator or systems manager to be the policy owner. The system manager could define roles such as reader, editor, administrator, and grant appropriate permissions to each of the roles. Each of the staff would be allocated one or more role attribute certificates according to their job functions. If for example an editor wished to modify information in the KMS then they would request access, the PERMIS decision engine would be consulted, their role attribute certificates would be retrieved and access granted or denied according to the policy.

CASE STUDY: SECURE DISTRIBUTION OF PATIENT DIABETES INFORMATION

Hospitals in the UK keep a large number of patient information databases recording information about patients with chronic diseases, for both research purposes and clinical health purposes. Most of the information is only available internally to the secondary carers, and no access is provided to other healthcare professionals who may also be involved in the patient's care. The sharing of information between primary and secondary carers will provide a more efficient disease control system and enhanced patient care through a combination of a reduction in the number of duplicate investigations, more accurate information being available to all, and a speeding up of the business processes.

As an example of secure knowledge management, we ran a project to provide primary healthcare professionals with secure Internet access to a hospital Diabetes Information System (DIS). The DIS was implemented in 1992 and provides a complete record of all registered diabetic patients in the local hospital area.

Figure 2: Distributed Diabetes Information System Security Infrastructure

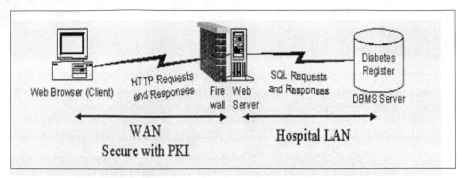

The DIS is situated on the secure hospital Intranet and to provide Internet access to the system we required a strong security infrastructure (*Figure 2*). This is because the Internet is a highly insecure network and not suitable for the transfer of unprotected, confidential patient information. The backbone behind our secure solution was a Public Key Infrastructure (PKI). The PKI provides the required prerequisites of strong authentication and data privacy through the use of strong encryption from accessing the hospitals internal trusted network.

Requests for patient data are transmitted from the primary carer's PC via the Hyper Text Transmission Protocol (HTTP) using a standard web browser. The HTTP requests are encrypted and digitally signed prior to transmission, using PKI software installed on the user's PC, thus forming a private channel to the hospital firewall from the PC.

The messages are decrypted and the digital signatures checked on the firewall, and then transferred to a web server on the hospital Local Area Network (LAN). Scripts on the web server convert the HTTP requests into Structured Query Language (SQL) requests for information from the DIS. The DIS processes the requests and sends SQL responses back to the web server. The patient information is then routed back to the client PC and displayed as web pages in Hyper Text Markup Language (HTML) format. All information transferred over the private channel is encrypted and digitally signed using either the user's private signing key (for requests) or the hospital's private signing key (for responses). If the user's digital signature is successfully authenticated, that person is allowed access through the firewall and into the DIS. If the hospital's digital signature is successfully authenticated, the patient information is displayed (otherwise it is discarded).

This example shows that secure distribution of knowledge is possible across the Internet, using new security mechanisms with legacy databases. A full description of this is provided in Young et al. (2001). Looking at how the segments of our model for secure KMS have been filled in this example; we have used PKI services to secure the channel between the client and the server thereby protecting the privacy and integrity of the transaction. Authentication is provided by means of the user's digital signature. Authorization is provided through ACLs within the DIS. Security policy is in place at the hospital with strict rules for who can gain access through the firewall, and who can access patient data. A firewall is positioned in front of the hospital network to prevent undesirable users.

SUMMARY

This chapter has provided an introduction to the wide range of different security techniques that can be used to secure knowledge management applications, none of which on their own can be seen as a panacea to all of your security requirements. Simply put, a combination of authentication, authorization, privacy, transmission security and good information security policies and practices are needed to help to ensure a more secure knowledge management environment.

Returning to our model, we have demonstrated through the case studies that if each of the segments is covered, then we can be reasonably sure of the strength of our system's security. We believe the implementation of PKI or the use of third party certification services will become widespread, not only in healthcare environments but also in the general business world. PKI services for authentication, data security and integrity coupled with PMI for authorization and firewalls for restricted access, all underpinned by an enforceable information security policy and procedures, combine together to provide a sound basis for secure KMSs.

REFERENCES

Adams, C. (1997). The CAST-128 Encryption Algorithm, *RFC2144*.

ANSI. (1985). American National Standard for Financial Institution Key Management (wholesale). *ANSI X9.17*.

Arsenault, A. & Turner, S. (2002). Internet X.509 Public Key Infrastructure: Roadmap. *PKIX Working Group Internet Draft*.

Chadwick, D. W. (1999). Smart Cards aren't always the Smart Choice. *IEEE Computer*, *32*(12), 142-143.

Chadwick, D. W. & Mundy, D. P. (2003). Policy Based Electronic Transmission of Prescriptions. *IEEE 4th International Workshop on Policies for Distributed Systems and Networks*, Como, Italy.

Chadwick, D. W. & Otenko, A. (2002). The PERMIS X.509 Role Based Privilege Management Infrastructure. *Seventh ACM Symposium On Access Control Models And Technologies,* (pp. 135-140).

Dierks, T. & Allen, C. (1999). The TLS Protocol Version 1.0. *RFC2246*.

Diffie, W. & Hellman, M. E. (1976). New directions in cryptography. *IEEE Transactions on Information Theory*, *22*(6), 644-654.

Dusse et al. (1998). S/Mime Version 2, Message Specification, *RFC2311*.

Eastlake, D., Reagle, D. & Solo, D. (2002). (Extensible Markup Language) XML-Signature Syntax and Processing. *RFC 3275*.

Krawczyk, H., Bellare, M. & Canetti (1997). HMAC: Keyed-Hashing for Message Authentication. *RFC2104*.

NIS. (1992). National Information Systems Security Glossary. *NSTISSI, 4009*.

Power, R. (2002). *CSI/FBI Computer Crime and Security Survey, Computer Security Issues and Trends, Computer Security Institute. VIII, 1*.

Rivest, R. A. (1998). Description of the RC2(r) Encryption Algorithm. *RFC2268*.

Ylonen, T., Saarinen, M., Rinne, T. & Lehtinen, S. (2000). SSH Transport Layer Security. *SECSH Working Group Internet Draft*.

Young, A. J., Chadwick, D. W. & New, J. (2001). Providing secure remote access to legacy applications. *IEE Computing and Control Engineering Journal, 12*(4), 148-156.

Chapter XXIV

Managing Knowledge to Improve Healthcare Quality in Banner Health

Twila Burdick, Banner Health, USA

John Hensing, Banner Health, USA

Bradford Kirkman-Liff, Arizona State University, USA

Pamela Nenaber, Banner Health, USA

Howard Silverman, Banner Health, USA

Maire Simington, Banner Health, USA

ABSTRACT

In 2001 Banner Health launched Care Management and Organizational Performance as a system-wide, collaborative and team-based effort to improve the performance consistency of the organization's core product: patient care. Functional Teams are composed of recognized knowledgeable clinical leaders who were viewed by peers as being experts with profound knowledge. Functional Teams have created more than 36 Work Groups that cut across organizational boundaries.

INTRODUCTION

The mission of Banner Health is to make a difference in people's lives through excellent patient care. Banner Health's core product is, in fact, patient care, and patients and other customers have increasing expectations of the healthcare they receive.

Delivering an excellent product and service is of paramount importance. One way to gauge the quality of the product is to measure its performance. Performance (clinical, financial, service) within every healthcare organization varies and can be described as "normally" distributed: some bad, some good, but most in the middle. Meeting changing demands requires ongoing improvement and different improvement approaches are required for different situations: bad performance or outcomes need to be reviewed and understood so that they can be avoided in the future. Outstanding performance or outcomes need a similar review to determine how such results can be consistently achieved. Performance in the middle can be improved by reducing variation (narrowing the area under the bell curve) and by improving processes (moving the curve). The Care Management and Organizational Performance Department at Banner Health is built on this premise. The mission of Care Management is to support the Banner Health mission by providing oversight and improvement of clinical care and patient safety that is coordinated across the system.

Banner Health is a new healthcare organization, formed as the result of a merger of Lutheran Health Systems and Samaritan Health System in September 1999 (see *Figure 1*). Banner Health is one of the nation's largest, nonprofit healthcare organizations in the US, with 19 hospitals, six long-term care centers and an array of other services, including family clinics, home care services and home medical equipment. Banner Health operates in nine Western and Midwestern states, with 21,500 employees, 2,569 acute care and 1,037 long-term care and rehabilitation beds. In addition to basic emergency and medical services, Banner Health medical centers offer a variety of specialized services, including heart care, cancer treatment, delivery of high-order multiple births, organ transplants, bone marrow transplants, rehabilitation services, and behavioral health services. Banner Health is nationally recognized for research in spinal cord injuries and Alzheimer's disease.

Improving quality of care has been a critical issue for healthcare institutions for decades. The Joint Commission for the Accreditation of Healthcare Organizations (JCAHO) has always had a focus on healthcare quality, and in recent years continuous process improvement has become a requirement for accreditation (JCAHO, 2003). The Institute of Medicine in recent years has issued a number of reports on the need to improve healthcare quality (Donaldson, 2000; Kohn et al., 2000; Adams & Corrigan, 2001; Hurtado et al., 2001). Following the approaches of TQM, CQI and Six Sigma, these efforts include measurement, analysis, prioritization, and process improvement, including implantation of proven practices (Besterfield et al., 2003; Endres, 2000; Evans & Lindsay, 2002; Barney et al., 2003; McLaughlin & Kaluzny, 1994; Wan & Connell, 2003). A number of journals (IJQHC, JCJQS, QSHC, IJHCQA, JQCP)[1] present numerous peer-reviewed case studies of various quality improvement and quality assurance activities in specific institutions, and a number of literature reviews examining this field have appeared (Counte & Meurer, 2001; Maguerez et al., 2001). In recent years several experts have recognized that current quality improvement and evidence-based practice efforts are not sufficient to significantly improve the outcomes of care (Haynes & Andrew, 1998; Plochg & Klazinga, 2002; Grol, 2000). While the potential for gains from using knowledge management in this area has been recognized, (Stefanelli, 2002; Burns, 2001; Malone, 2001; Zazzara, 2001; Horak, 2001; Stefanelli, 2001) detailed reports on the use of knowledge management concepts to support quality improvement efforts are difficult to

Figure 1: Location of Banner Health Facilities

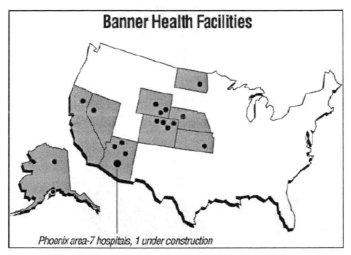

identify. In this chapter we contribute to closing the "theory-application gap" by describing the evolution of one organization's approach to quality improvement through the use of knowledge management approaches.

In 2001, Banner Health launched Care Management and Organizational Performance as a way to improve the performance consistency of the organization's core product: patient care. *Figure 2* presents a schematic of the Care Management vision. The center of the vision is the patient. A team surrounds the patient to provide care, including physicians and other caregivers: nurses, therapists, technicians and a variety of other roles. There are also specialized professionals in care coordination and utilization management who play important parts in care delivery. Lastly, an organization's leadership plays an important role as members of the team. The team's work process is surrounded by appropriate enabling technology, including information systems. The Care Management process is driven by external pressures for greater quality, safety, efficiency, and satisfaction, which require a focus on the processes of care delivery. The efforts are data-driven and include measurement, analysis, prioritization, and process improvement, including implementation of proven practices. The intent is to reduce variation and to shift those processes that have the greatest impact on outcomes to higher levels of quality. Outcomes are measured using a Balanced Scorecard, and include patient satisfaction, patient safety, clinical outcomes and other clinical measures, as well as organizational financial strength and innovation. Evidence-based decision support forms the foundation of clinical processes and in turn supports further improvement.

The Banner Healthcare Management vision evolved to include recognition of the importance of measurement, benchmarking and enabling technology. This is further explained in the model in *Figure 3*, described in part with a sports analogy. Every successful team coach has to plan the game prior to the start, manage the game during execution, and has to know the final statistics and score. The Banner Healthcare

Figure 2: Care Management Vision

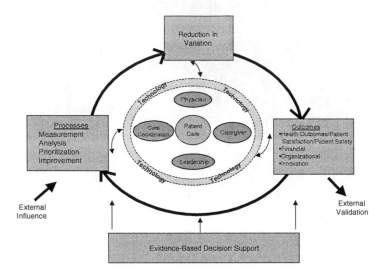

Management approach is a system-wide effort that starts with a prospective process of measurement, analysis, prioritization, and improvement of specific components of care delivery (*"Planning the Game"*). These are the traditional approaches of Continual Quality Improvement implemented by most healthcare organizations. The effectiveness of these activities is assessed by a number of metrics on performance and variation. Feedback from these metrics is provided in order to achieve a reduction in process variation and an improvement in performance (*"Managing the Game"*). The focus on these metrics is on system-wide reduction in process variation, achieved though reduction in variation in each institution and department. The effect of reduced variation is also measured system-wide, in metrics that retrospectively measure improved outcomes (*"Keeping Score"*). The "Keeping Score" function provides data that goes back to the "Planning the Game" cycle for further improvement.

Underlying these three efforts are three related activities. First, there is a continual effort to standardize policies, protocols and guidelines across the Banner Health facilities. In the past each institution had its own Continuous Quality Improvement efforts, which resulted in reduced variation and improved performance at each facility. However, the learning and knowledge gained by each institution through its own efforts was not shared in a systematic manner across all of the facilities. Care Management was intended to reduce "reinventing the wheel" across the system. Second, there is an ongoing effort to implement processes that diffuse the standardized policies and protocols. Standardized protocols are of little value if they are not implemented. New methods to promote system-wide implementation have been developed. Third, a variety of outcome tools are used to measure patient health status, patient satisfaction, patient

Figure 3: Expanded Care Management Conceptualization

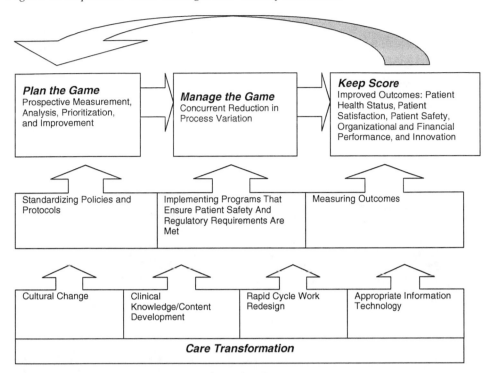

safety, organizational and financial performance, and innovation across all facilities against internal and external benchmarks as appropriate. Section II of the paper describes in detail how Care Management functions in these areas.

To support the mission of Care Management, a "joint sponsorship" between two departments: Information Technology and Care Management began working on a data architecture that would become the clinical information technology foundation for Banner Health. The effort evolved into a group known as CLINIC, the Clinical Informatics Implementation Council, because the effort was to produce such an important change in the organization. Known as Care Transformation, this effort would support the three activities of standardizing policies and protocols, program implementation and outcome measurement. Care Transformation is an organizational initiative that combines elements of appropriate clinical knowledge and content, technology; rapid cycle work redesign and cultural change, as seen in *Figure 4*. Clinical knowledge and content is developed to reduce variation and improve patient care quality and safety. Rapid cycle work redesign examines the detailed workflows within the institutions and redesigns workflows and jobs to embed standardized policies, protocol and developed clinical knowledge/content within the clinical information systems. Information technology would also be further designed so that the same clinical knowledge and content is incorporated into care rules: algorithms that would compare clinical orders and events to standards and alert the clinicians to potential problems. Such systems have existed for several years to identify potential adverse drug interactions: the intent of Care Transformation would be to broaden the use of rules to cover a variety of non-pharmacology issues.

Figure 4: Care Transformation

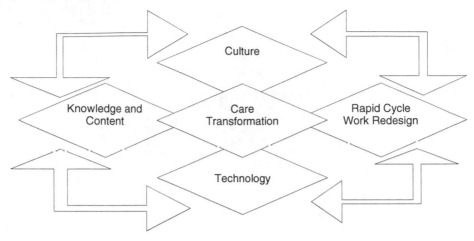

Care Transformation is the synthesis of rapid cycle work redesign and information technology along with cultural change and the development and use of clinical knowledge and content. Care Transformation is an organizational initiative across all stakeholders in the patient care experience to achieve an optimal health outcome.

STRUCTURE

Care Management is system-wide, collaborative and team-based. An initial assessment of functional areas to be included within Care Management was conducted through extensive interviews with managers within Banner Health. These examinations of function led to the identification of teams and team leaders (*Table 1*). The 12 functions reflect the "universe of care management" in descriptive terms rather than as departmental names. Other professionals in other institutions could easily have a different partitioning of the underlying functions. To provide system-wide representation, leadership and decision-making for Care Management, the Care Management Council was formed. The Council creates organizational policy, establishes priorities for Care Management activities, and provides a forum for the sharing of ideas and resolution of issues. This Council, led by the Chief Medical Officer, is composed of Care Management System Directors, leaders of Care Management teams as well as representatives of important organizational areas such as Operations, Information Technology, Finance, and Risk Management. The Functional Teams are composed of recognized knowledgeable clinical leaders throughout Banner Health who were viewed by peers as being experts with profound knowledge concerning these functional areas. Where appropriate, teams are co-chaired by a physician leader and an administrative leader. These teams cut across all traditional organizational unit boundaries. The focus is on the processes that affect patients regardless of where they are in a facility and which facility they are in. On an annual basis, the Care Management Council conducts a planning process to determine the major strategies required to achieve the desired outcomes and the Functional Team

Table 1: Inventory of Care Management Functional Areas

Function	Focus	Methods	Processes/ Examples
Patient Safety Consultation	Identify and eliminate sources of system failures to improve patient safety	Analyze processes for safe and effective clinical practices.	- Incident analysis and intervention - Sentinel event root cause analysis - Peer review facilitation - Physician profiling - Recommend formation of process improvement teams
Care Coordination	Meet the needs of individual patients and families during the episode of care.	Assure delivery of appropriate and timely care.	- Patient screening - Multi-disciplinary coordination of care - Evidence-based care delivery - Treatment and service coordination - Discharge and transfer planning - Patient and family counseling - Community resource referrals
Utilization Management	Optimize reimbursement and meet payer requirements	Manage appropriate level of care and resource utilization.	- Pre admission clinical and financial screening and placement - Verification of prior authorization - Determine appropriate level of care - Concurrent review and intervention - Continued Stay authorization - Prompt for complete and accurate clinical documentation - Denial and appeal management
Population Health Management	Reduce inappropriate variation and continuously improve clinical care and outcomes	Develop and/or implement best practices for specific patient populations.	- High volume/ risk/cost population identification - Literature review for best practices - Current practice review - Improvement strategy development and implementation - Development and implementation of standards of care, protocols, guidelines - Patient education
Regulatory/ Accreditation Consultation	Maintain licensure	Provide consultation for continuous survey readiness	- Standards review and dissemination - Accreditation standards monitoring - Survey preparation and consultation - External "auditor" liaison - Plans of correction development and monitoring
Clinical Data Management and Decision Support	Provide evidence for decision making	Provide data acquisition, analysis, and reporting	- Outcomes analysis - Database administration - Evaluation - Benchmarking - Physician practice pattern profiles - Computerized concurrent clinical decision support
Organizational Performance Measurement And Analysis	Determine process performance and capability	Select and analyze relevant performance measures	- Productivity measurement and reporting - External comparative performance - "Balanced" scorecard development - Goal setting - Critical success factor identification - Variation analysis (e.g., Statistical Process Control)
Performance Improvement	Meet and exceed changing requirements of patients and other customers	Evaluating and improving processes	- Customer focus groups - Process analysis - Process modeling (e.g., simulation) - Process design and redesign - Facilitation of multidisciplinary teams - Project management technique application
Customer Satisfaction Measurement	Recognize customer perceptions	Acquire and report customer satisfaction	- Ongoing Patient satisfaction survey processes - Ad hoc satisfaction measurement - Interpretation of survey scores - Customer focus group methodologies
Clinical Innovation	Implement new clinical care delivery methods	Identify, pilot and evaluate innovation methods	- Web based clinical connectivity for physicians - Environmental and 'low tech' innovations such as Planetree - "Expert" computer decision support systems - Replication of innovative best practice in other settings - Evaluation and prioritization of innovative ideas
Continuing Medical Education	Links physicians to Care Management	Design and implement physician educational programs	- Medical Director orientation and training - Physician development seminars and courses - CME physician credit for participation in care redesign - Maintain national CME accreditation
Research	Sponsor investigation of new health care delivery	Provide consultation and facilitate opportunities for research	- Assure compliance - Facilitate grant writing - Oversee Institutional Review Board - Develop new health services programs - Performs health outcomes research

Table 2: Care Management Outcomes, Strategies and Functional Team Responsibilities for 2002

Outcome Description	Strategy Description	Functional Team Responsibility
Health Outcomes/Patient Satisfaction/Patient Safety *Attain superior clinical processes and outcomes at all Banner facilities, recognized both internally and externally*	Develop systematic Care Coordination and Population Health Management methodology using evidence-based guidelines for BHS.	A: CC/UM B: Pop Hlth
	Select nationally recognized clinical indicators.	A: Pop Hlth B: Clin Data
	Collaborate with externally based organizations (ex. Leapfrog, JCAHO) on Patient Safety.	A: Pt Safety
	Measure patient satisfaction.	A: Cust Sat
	Maintain accreditation and regulatory compliance.	A: Regulatory
Financial *Achieve improved margin per case and targeted operational efficiency measures*	Develop systematic Utilization Management methodology for BHS.	A: CC/UM
	Develop systematic Care Coordination and Population Health management methodology using evidence-based guidelines for BHS	A: CC/UM
	Optimize reimbursement methodologies for changing clinical practices.	A: CC/UM B: Pop Hlth C: Innovation
	Develop standard approach and reporting for systematic margin analysis.	A: CC/UM B: Clin Data
Organizational *Demonstrate the value and create widespread knowledge and use of the business of care management*	Develop organizational structure at system, regional and facility levels for Care Management and Organizational Performance.	A: CMOP
	Articulate decision-making structure, process and criteria at system and regional levels for Care Management and Organizational Performance.	A: CMOP
	Develop the framework and process for deployment of system policies and replication of best practices.	A: PI
	Interface with regional and facility operations and medical organizations.	A: CMOP B: Liaisons
	Develop outcome reporting and analysis framework, incorporating financial return on improvement actions, for Care Management & Organizational Performance.	A: Clin Data B: Perf Meas
	Develop communication and education framework and process for CMOP	A: CMOP B: CME
	Determine appropriate data systems for Care Management and Organizational Performance.	A: Clin Data B: Perf Meas
	Develop BHS Care Management and Organizational Performance budgets.	A: CMOP
	Develop BHS Quality Plan.	A: Perf Imp
	Develop BHS reporting framework, format and methodologies for performance measurement and analysis. (Balanced scorecard)	A: Perf Meas B: Clin Data
	Establish process for BHS governance oversight of quality (Organizational Performance).	A: CMOP
	Identify ethical issues for consideration by BHS Care Management and Quality Committee.	A: CMOP
	Develop physician support in care redesign through national CME accreditation.	A: CME
Innovation *Incorporate innovation into patient care delivery*	Create skill development opportunities and tools for clinical innovation and promote clinical innovation throughout BHS.	A: Innovation
	Evaluate clinical innovations and identify pilot projects.	A: Innovation
	Coordinate clinical innovation with BHRI clinical trials and other research efforts and capabilities.	A: Innovation B: Research
	Seek external grant funding to support clinical innovation.	A: Innovation B: Research

responsibilities for those strategies. *Table 2* shows the overall plan for 2002. The 2002 plan's relatively higher weight given to organizational issues reflects the need to develop a clear organizational structure for Care Management. Relative to 2002, the 2003 plan has more efforts on health outcomes.

To accomplish this work, Functional Teams are empowered to create Work Groups that, like the team, cut across organizational boundaries based upon a charter drawn up by one of the Functional Teams. More than 36 Work Groups were established in the first two years of the project and there are more than 200 healthcare professionals who participate in the Functional Teams and Work Groups, with membership continuing to

Table 3: Examples of Work Groups, Missions and Actions

Workgroup	Mission	Actions
Adverse Drug Event Improvement Workgroup	To design and improve a medication use system (ordering, dispensing, and administering) for a specifically identified high-risk medication population that is safer as a result of a reduction in the rate of preventable Adverse Drug Events.	Reduce the incidence rate of preventable ADE's in a selected population.
		Coordinate the initiative for reduction of preventable ADE's.
		Recommend data needs, develop and define data collect method for ADE indicators.
		Review indicator data and recommend performance improvement actions
Surgical Site Identification Workgroup	Develop policies and procedures for surgical site identification	Survey current Surgical Site Identification policies and procedures to determine the presence and use of a Surgical Site identification policy at each BHS facility.
		Assess the policies for compliance with regulatory and standards of practice compliance
		Create a standardized policy for implementation across Banner Health
		Determine role of Patient Safety team in implementation of this policy

grow. Examples of the projects developed by several Work Groups can be seen in *Table 3*, addressing adverse drug events and surgical site identification. Each Work Group is chartered for a specific mission and has a planned set of actions developed by the Work Group members. These actions are reviewed and approved by the Functional Team that chartered the Work Group. Functional Teams are on-going, while Work Groups generally operate for six to nine months. The leader of the Work Group is a member of the Functional Team so the work of the Work Groups is connected. Coordination between Functional Team leaders is important in order to avoid duplicative work groups and to avoid overuse of key individuals.

The staff of the Care Management Department supports the work of the Functional Teams and Work Groups. The five major roles that support the Teams and Work Groups are System Directors, Clinical Data Analysts, Project Managers, Care Management Liaisons, and Administrative Assistants. The role of the Project Managers varies with each project. In some areas, the Project Manager provides support to the Functional Teams and the Work Groups. In others, they undertake a significant share of the work. The Care Management Liaisons are individuals identified in each region who work full-time for Care Management. In that role they work across all Functional Teams and Work Groups in terms of their activities in that region. The Banner Health intranet (which uses Microsoft SharePoint™ Portal Server 2001) is used as a means to disseminate information and reports to all Functional Teams, Work Groups and Banner Health employees. A screen shot is seen in *Figure 5*. The site provides a calendar for upcoming events, access to the initiative measures, separate sections for the Care Management Council, as well as each of the Functional Teams and most of the final Work Group products in the forms of toolkits and templates. This provides all members of Functional Teams and Work Groups with access to all plans, reports and documents in order to assure that overlap in Functional Team and Work Group activities is minimized through open coordination. Routine additions to the web site are made by Care Management staff.

Figure 5: Care Management Intranet Web Site

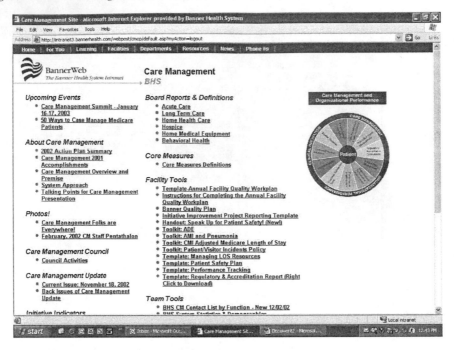

Process

The process by which knowledge is created, reviewed, and synthesized within the work groups is complex and varied from group to group, but a general description involves the six stages seen in *Figure 6*. The process starts with a discussion of individuals known to have expertise and knowledge related to the issue being examined by the Work Group. If the Functional Team members and Regional Liaisons do not know a specific person, they generally know who to ask within the institutions to help in the identification of experts. These identified people are asked to participate in the Work Group and are encouraged to identify others who in their view are more knowledgeable. The Work Group then meets face-to-face for representatives in central Arizona, with participants from other states joining by conference calls. The members discuss their experiences in their own institutions concerning the issue, conduct literature reviews and Internet searches, contribute standards and protocols from external, national organizations and meet with other Banner Health employees whose work relates to the issue. The experiences, knowledge, research and ideas from the group are consolidated into one or more written documents. These may be flow charts, spreadsheets, templates, or text documents such as policies or protocols. It is important to note that the processes of information and knowledge collection and document development may be iterated through several times, resulting in an increasingly refined set of work products. During this time, Work Group membership may change as the knowledge synthesis progresses, with new individuals with expertise and knowledge joining the Work Group and members who have contributed to their abilities leaving the Work Group.

Figure 6: Knowledge Creation, Review and Synthesis Process

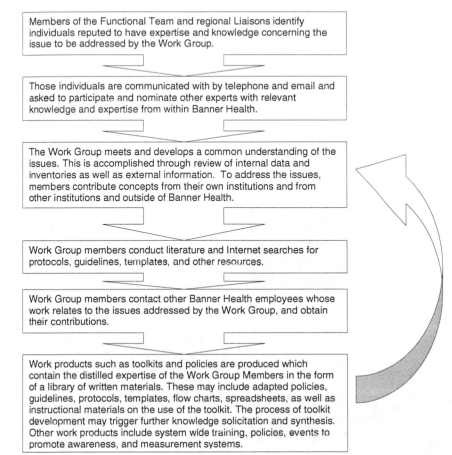

The development of toolkits, policies or other work products is seen as only the start of the activities of a Work Group. The major activity is the distribution, education and implementation of these materials in the various Banner Health facilities. This involves a five-stage process, which, relative to the toolkit development phase, is more structured and seen in *Figure 7*. The Functional Team and the Work Group together plan the final format of the materials and products, as well as the target audience, the feedback process, and the specific roles of various Care Management staff in the implementation. The specific details of model projects to implement the product of the Work Group are developed along with timelines, lists of those employees to be affected by the implementation, and other resources. The Care Management Council then approves this implementation design. If necessary, the Senior Management Group of Banner Health also approves the plan. Implementation involves a number of material distributions involving email of electronic documents, internal mail of paper documents, and presentations to managers and physicians. On-going data collection of metrics is used to assess the organizational and financial impact of each project. The details of the implementation plan vary significantly with the product and the particular issue being addressed.

Figure 7: Knowledge Distribution, Education and Implementation Process

Planning Phase – Conducted by the Functional Team and the Work Group:
> Define the form of the materials: a policy; a "Toolkit" of educational materials, forms, presentation scripts and slides; or other format
> Define the audience who will receive the materials
> Define the facility point person(s) and their responsibility relative to the work product implementation.
> Define the follow up and feedback required by the team i.e., brief feedback implementation process by facility
> Define the Project Managers role in the implementation process
> Define the role of the Regional Liaison in the project.
> Identify other staff and/or physicians who have roles and responsibilities

Design Phase – Primarily conducted by the Work Group with some assistance from the Functional Team
> Definitions of the objectives and expected outcomes and completion date
> Detailed description of project rationale
> Expectations of facilities relative to the implementation
> Individuals or departments affected by the implementation
> Location of materials including pertinent documents, communication plans, data sources, etc (Banner Health intranet, common drive location, etc).

Approval Phase
> Present to Care Management Council for approval and/or information
> Present information to or secure approval from Senior Management Group if necessary
> Communication back to Work Group and Functional Team

Implementation Phase
> Distribute materials for implementation
> Presentation to facility-based leadership
> Presentation to management groups at facilities and system departments as necessary
> Presentation to appropriate medical staff committees as needed
> Consider in depth discussion presentations with affected departments or services
> Contact facilities to confirm implementation and need for additional support

Evaluation
> Define evaluation process
> How / when will the impact of this project be measured
>> a. Operational impact
>> b. Financial Impact

After implementation, the Work Group or Functional Team monitors the various metrics selected for use with the implementation, and provides feedback to the Functional Team and Banner Health senior managers. Many of the facilities have process improvement events to showcase their improvement efforts. Recently such a system-wide event was held during Banner Health's Leadership Conference.

INTEREST IN AND FUTURE INTEGRATION OF FORMAL KNOWLEDGE MANAGEMENT

After concluding the first full year of designing, organizing and communicating about the intent of Care Management and Organizational Performance, the leadership of this group desired to take a prospective look at how best to replicate and assimilate the knowledge learned through the process of measuring, implementing and integrating its efforts. There was also a sense that the ideas and knowledge being both uncovered and created by these efforts were not diffusing rapidly enough throughout Banner Health. While dissemination was well planned, actual use may have been less than desired. The teams and work groups needed assistance in managing the sharing and reuse of knowledge. The leadership of Care Management began examining its efforts and wondered if there were other "best practices" for managing knowledge in other industries that could be useful for Banner's efforts. To this end, a relationship was forged with the W. P. Carey School of Business of Arizona State University to research these questions.

To assess the magnitude of the knowledge sharing and diffusion issues and to prioritize further knowledge management efforts, information was collected through three strategies. First, surveys of Functional Team leaders and users of the products produced by the Work Groups were conducted using the Banner intranet. Second, observers attended Functional Team and Work Group meetings and recorded comments and issues related to access to and organization of knowledge resources, difficulties with sharing knowledge, ideas, and problem solutions, and other related issues. Third, structured one-on-one interviews were held on the same issues with the co-leaders of the Functional Team and Work Groups. This triangulation approach led to a series of recommendations for specific knowledge management actions. Three of the preliminary recommendations are:

1. Development of an "Expertise Locator" tool as part of the Banner Health intranet. Banner Health includes a large number of health providers with expertise in rural healthcare, regulation in a large number of states, and individuals with experiences from a variety of pre-merger activities and initiatives. Banner Health culture is very supportive of "Not Reinventing the Wheel." At every meeting there is a constant focus on identifying those people who have expertise, knowledge and experiences — yet this identification process is time-consuming. An "Expertise Locator" as part of the Banner intranet would assist all organizational efforts in tapping into the valuable knowledge of the dispersed employees.

2. Development of additional mechanisms to capture the experiences of the recipients of the "Toolkit" in their use of the materials. Banner Health currently conducts forums to showcase performance improvement efforts with large audiences. The challenge is how to best capture this knowledge and how to assimilate this knowledge into employees' everyday work lives. One approach that appears to be useful, and would entail a continuation or transformation of the Work Groups, would be to establish "User Groups" as on-going forums to capture experiences with disseminating and encouraging the use of the approach and materials within each institution. Convening these on-going "User Groups" could be done via email, telephones, or chat rooms or discussion boards on the Internet. Membership of each User Group would consist of some members from the Work Group and some of members of the target audience who received the Work Group product.

3.   Better use of Internet-based tools to promote asynchronous communication and collaboration. The existing intranet web site was seen as somewhat difficult to navigate. Individuals would often send an email or call a Care Management Liaison in order to find where on the intranet a particular document could be located. The lack of an intranet-based discussion board also reduced Functional Team and Work Group effectiveness. To address these and related issues, Microsoft SharePoint™ Team Services will be implemented in 2003 for Care Management Functional Teams and Work Groups in order to order to provide a wider range of additional collaboration tools.

Banner Health is in the process of planning a major integration of their clinical information system architecture with Care Management and Care Transformation activities. This new architecture will incorporate external and internal knowledge resources into the minute-by-minute processes used in care delivery. It is important to distinguish this KM focus regarding "what-do-we-know-and-how-do-we-know-what-we-know-and-how-do-we-best-share-and-use-what-we-know" from the organization and delivery of clinical information (dictations, op reports, lab results, etc.) to the care providers. Portions of this architecture have already been implemented within some of the Banner Health facilities and one new facility that is being built is planned to be a "paper-light" hospital, with extensive use of electronic medical records with computerized physician order entry that would incorporate real-time, knowledge-based rules. The intent is to embed knowledge in the information technology to promote patient safety and quality in a continuous manner.

NEW QUESTIONS, NOT CONCLUSIONS

The process of integrating knowledge management into a multi-state healthcare system will be a continual process. Rather than state a series of end-point conclusions, among the "meta-knowledge" questions we are discussing and deliberating over are:

- How do we facilitate continued sharing of knowledge between "silos" within the organization?
- How do we synthesize knowledge from information when the volume of information increases rapidly?
- What methodologies work best for sharing various types of knowledge among different professions?
- How can we increase the signal:noise ratio in our knowledge acquisition and sharing efforts?
- What is the optimal role of technology in facilitating this sharing?
- What are the cultural, structural or other barriers facing us in this effort?

Banner Health sees knowledge management as one approach among many to improve the quality, safety, effectiveness and efficiency of the patient care processes. The focus of knowledge management — like all other activities — in Banner Health is on making a difference in people's lives through excellent patient care.

REFERENCES

Adams, K. & Corrigan, J. M. (eds.) (2001). *Priority Areas for National Action: Transforming Health Care Quality.* Washington, DC: National Academies Press.

Barney, M. & McCarty, T. (eds.) (2003). *The New Six Sigma: A Leader's Guide To Achieving Rapid Business Improvement And Sustainable Results.* Upper Saddle River, NJ: Prentice Hall.

Besterfield et al. (2003). *Total Quality Management* (third edition). Upper Saddle River, NJ: Prentice Hall.

Burns, S. (2001). Beyond Best Practices: Knowledge Management. *Healthcare Benchmarks,* 8(11), 129-31.

Counte, M. A. & Meurer, S. (2001). Issues in the Assessment of Continuous Quality Improvement Implementation in Health Care Organizations. *International Journal for Quality in Health Care, 13*(3), 197-207.

Donaldson, M. S. (ed.) (1999). *Measuring the Quality of Health Care.* Washington, DC: National Academies Press.

Endres, A. (2000). *Implementing Juran's Road Map For Quality Leadership: Benchmarks And Results.* New York: Wiley.

Evans, J. R. & Lindsay, W. M. (2002). *The Management and Control of Quality* (fifth edition). Cincinnati, OH: South-Western.

Grol, R. (2000). Between Evidence-Based Practice And Total Quality Management: The Implementation Of Cost-Effective Care. *International Journal for Quality in Health Care, 12*(4), 297-304.

Haynes, B. & Haines, A. (1998). Barriers and Bridges to Evidence Based Clinical Practice. *British Medical Journal, 317,* 273-276.

Horak, B. J. (2001). Dealing with Human Factors and Managing Change in Knowledge Management: A Phased Approach. *Topics in Health Information Management, 21*(3), 8-17.

Hurtado, M. P., Swift, E. K. & Corrigan, J. M. (eds.) (2001). *Envisioning The National Health Care Quality Report.* Washington, DC: National Academies Press.

IJHCQA. (n.d.). *International Journal Of Health Care Quality Assurance.* Bradford, UK: Emerald Publishing.

IJQHC. (n.d.). *International Journal for Quality in Health Care.* Oxford: Oxford University Press.

JCAHCO. (n.d.). Joint Commission for Accreditation of Health Care Organization. *Proposed Revisions to Performance Improvement for Hospitals.* Retrieved from the World Wide Web: http://www.jcaho.org/accredited+organizations/hospitals/standards/draft+standards/proposed+revisions+to+performance +improvement+for+hospitals.htm.

JCJQS. (n.d.). *The Joint Commission Journal on Quality and Safety.* Chicago: Joint Commission for Accreditation of Health Care Organization.

JQCP. (n.d.). Journal *of Quality In Clinical Practice.* Oxford: Blackwell Publishing.

Kohn, L. T., Corrigan, J. M. & Donaldson, M. S. (eds.) (2000). *To Err Is Human: Building a Safer Health System.* Washington, DC: National Academies Press.

Maguerez, G., Erbault, M., Terra, J. L., Maisonneuve, H. & Matillon, Y. (2001). Evaluation of 60 Continuous Quality Improvement Projects in French Hospitals. *International Journal for Quality in Health Care, 13*(2), 89-97.

Malone, S. M. (2001). Knowledge Management: White Knight or White Elephant? *Topics in Health Information Management*, 21(3), 33-43.

McLaughlin, C. P. & Kaluzny, A. D. (eds.) (1994). *Continuous Quality Improvement In Health Care: Theory, Implementation And Applications*. Gaithersburg, MD: Aspen Publishers.

QSHC. (n.d.). *Quality and Safety in Health Care*. London: BMJ Publishing.

Stefanelli, M. (2001). The socio-organizational age of artificial intelligence in medicine. *Artificial Intelligence in Medicine*, 23(1), 25-47.

Stefanelli, M. (2002). Knowledge Management to Support Performance-Based Medicine. *Methods of Information in Medicine*, 41(1), 36-43.

Plochg, T. & Klazinga, N. S. (2002). Community-Based Integrated Care: Myth or Must? *International Journal for Quality in Health Care*, 14(2), 91-101.

Wan, T. T. H. & Connell, A. M. (2003). *Monitoring the quality of health care: Issues and scientific approaches*. Boston, MA: Kluwer Academic.

Zazzara, P. (2001). Operationalizing Knowledge Management in Health Care. *Topics in Health Information Management*, 21(3), 1-7.

ENDNOTE

[1]   All issues are relevant.

About the Authors

Nilmini Wickramasinghe is an assistant professor in the Computer and Information Science Department at the James J. Nance College of Business Administration at Cleveland State University, Ohio (USA). She teaches IS at the undergraduate and graduate levels in the areas of knowledge management as well as e-commerce and m-commerce, IT for competitive advantage organizational impacts of technology and health care issues. In addition, Dr. Wickramasinghe teaches and presents regularly in many universities in Europe and Australia. She is currently carrying out research and is published in the areas of management of technology, in the field of health care as well as focusing on IS issues especially as they relate to knowledge work and e-business. Dr. Wickramasinghe is honored to be able to represent the US for the Healthcare Technology Management (HCTM) Association (URL*http://www.hctm.net/Conferences/2003/Conference_2003.html*).

Jatinder N.D. Gupta is currently an eminent scholar of management, Professor of Management Information Systems, and chairperson of the Department of Accounting and Information Systems in the College of Administrative Science at the University of Alabama in Huntsville, Alabama, USA. Most recently, he was a professor of Management, Information and Communication Sciences, and Industry and Technology at Ball State University, Muncie, Indiana (USA). He holds a PhD in Industrial Engineering (with specialization in Production Management and Information Systems) from Texas Tech University. A co-author of a textbook in operation research, Dr. Gupta serves on the editorial boards of several national and international journals. A recipient of the Outstanding Faculty and Outstanding Researcher awards from Ball State University, he has published numerous papers in such journals as the *Journal of Management Information Systems,* the *International Journal of Information Management, INFORMS Journal of Computing, Annals of Operations Research*, and *Mathematics of Operations Research*. More recently, he served as a co-editor of a special issue on *Neutral Networks in Business of Computers and Operation Research* and a book titled *Neutral Networks in Business: Techniques and Applications*. His current research interests include information and decision technologies, scheduling, planning, and control, organizational learning and effectiveness, systems education, and knowledge management. Dr. Gupta is a member of several academic and professional societies including the Production and Operations Management Society (POMS), the Decision Sciences Institute (DSI), and the Information Resources Management Association (IRMA).

Sushil K. Sharma is currently an assistant professor in the Department of Information Systems & Operations Management, at Ball State University, Muncie, Indiana (USA). He received his Ph.D. in Information Systems. Dr. Sharma has a unique distinction of having been conferred two doctoral degrees. Prior to joining Ball State, Dr. Sharma held the associate professor position at the Indian Institute of Management, Lucknow (India) and visiting research associate professor at the Department of Management Science, University of Waterloo, Canada. Co-author of two textbooks in IT (*Programming in C* and *Understanding Unix*), Dr. Sharma's research contributions have appeared in many peer-reviewed national and international journals, conferences and seminars' proceedings. Dr. Sharma's primary teaching and research interests are in e-commerce, networking environments, network security, ERP systems, database management systems, information systems analysis & design and knowledge management. Apart from teaching and guiding students for various innovative IS related topics, Dr. Sharma has wide experience of consulting in information systems and e-commerce area, network security and has served as an advisor and consultant to several government and private organizations including World Bank funded projects. Dr. Sharma has also conducted a number of executive development programs for the corporate world and government organizations on e-commerce, networking environments, and database related subjects.

* * *

Jae-Hyeon Ahn is an associate professor at KAIST (Korea Advanced Institute of Science and Technology) in Seoul, Korea. He received his B.S. and M.S. in Industrial Engineering both from Seoul National University, South Korea (1984 and 1986, respectively), and a PhD in Management Science & Engineering from Stanford University (1993). After graduation, he worked as a senior researcher at AT&T Bell Labs (1993-1998). His current research interests are focused on knowledge management, managerial decision-making, strategy analysis in telecommunications industry, and customer loyalty in e-business. He has published papers in *Management Science, Decision Support Systems, Medical Decision Making, IEEE on Vehicular Technology,* the *Journal of Information Technology,* and *European Journal of Operations Research.*

Nabeel A. Y. Al-Qirim is a lecturer of information systems, a module coordinator of e-BusinessIT and a researcher (path) in the School of Computer and Information Sciences, Faculty of Business, Auckland University of Technology, Auckland, New Zealand. He has a Cert. (Education), a bachelor's degree in Electrical Engineering, PostGradDipInfoSys. (Honors with distinction), MBA, and PhD. His research interests and publications are in IT, e/m-commerce and e/m-business in different countries and contexts: SCM, strategy (outsourcing, adoption, usage, policy), telemedicine, small businesses, NGOs and developing countries. He has many publications in leading conferences, books and journals, and he is a member of the editorial advising committee of IJCEC and JECO. He is the editor of the book titled *Electronic Business in Small to Medium-Sized Enterprises: Frameworks, Issues and Implication*s, and a co-editor of the book *e-Business,* *e-Government & Small and Medium-Size Enterprises: Opportunities & Challenges.* Before joining academia, he worked in the IT industry with companies such as IBM, Compaq, Data General, Group Bull, and Siemens Nixdorf for 12 years as a consultant for managing total IT solutions to different commercial and governmental entities.

Twila Burdick is the system director for Organizational Performance at Banner Health (USA), and is responsible for clinical data management, organizational performance measurement, including customer satisfaction data, and performance improvement. She previously served as Samaritan Health System's coordinator for Continuous Quality Improvement with responsibility for coordination of all activities related to the implementation of CQI, and as director of Management Engineering. Twila holds a BS in Secondary Education from Montana State University and an MBA from the University of Montana. She has had the opportunity to study extensively in the quality management field.

Tanya Castleman is a professor of Information Systems at Deakin University, Australia, and a member of the Centre for Business Research in the Deakin Business School, Melbourne. She was previously a member of the Center for Information Systems Research at Swinburne University of Technology. The main focus of her research is the organizational, social and community aspects of information and communication technologies, especially the Internet and e-commerce. Her research is practically oriented and she has conducted a broad range of research and consultancy projects. Tanya has published internationally on issues including: the adoption and implementation of e-commerce by small and medium enterprises, employment implications of e-commerce applications, the Internet and regional sustainability, ICT in health and human service delivery and government electronic service delivery.

David W. Chadwick is a professor of Information Systems Security at the University of Salford, UK. He holds a BS and PhD in Chemistry from Salford University. Professor Chadwick is an internationally recognized expert in X.500, the international standard for Directory Services, and LDAP, the Internet standard for directory access. He has published widely on this topic, including one major book, *Understanding X.500: The Directory* (*http://www.salford.ac.uk/its024/X500.htm*), one Internet RFC "RFC 2120 Managing the X.500 Root Naming Context" (*ftp://ftp.isi.edu/in-notes/rfc2120.txt*), and two co-authored guides which were sponsored by the DTI. He gives seminars (*http://www.salford.ac.uk/its024/seminars.htm*) at home and abroad on X.500 and LDAP. He is an active participant in the Internet LDAP standards work, and the author of several current LDAP Internet drafts. He is also the BSI representative to ISO/ITU-T X.500 standardization meetings, and was the international editor for the 1993 enhancements to Part 4 of the Standard. His research interests include PKI usability, trust management, and policy-based security.

Suk-Gwon Chang is a professor of MIS and Telecommunications at Hanyang University, Korea. He received his PhD in Management Science from KAIST (Korea Advanced Institute of Science and Technology). His research interests include telecommunications management, information systems strategy, Internet industry analysis, telecommunications and e-business collaboration, and knowledge management. He has published papers in computers & OR, IEEE transactions on communications, operations research, telecommunication systems, information economics & policy, decision support systems and telecommunication policy. He is now serving as an associate editor of *Telecommunication Systems*.

Paul S. Craft is director of the Medical Oncology Unit of Canberra Hospital in Australia. He has wide clinical research interests ranging from studies of health outcomes and quality of life in advanced cancer to basic research in breast and prostate cancer. He serves on a number of government committees including the Medical Services Advisory Committee of the Australian Department of Health.

Peter Croll started programming in 1970 prior to his BS in Computer Science. His industry experience involved designing reliable microprocessor control systems. At Sheffield University, his PhD focused on development methods for real-time parallel processing applications. His academic career transverses three continents: the UK, Singapore and Australia. He is a chartered engineer and a fellow of the BCS. His research maintains industry relevance and is widely published. As head of the School of IT and Computer Science, University of Wollongong, Professor Croll's current research interest is the reduction of risk using rigorous yet agile software engineering methods for safety-related applications, including e-health.

Ana Karina Marimon da Cunha is an assistant professor and executive coordinator of the Undergraduate Course of Hospital Management at the University of Vale do Rio dos Sinos – UNISINOS, Brazil. She received her MS in Business Administration from UNISINOS. Her research interests are related to health care management. She coordinates the SIPAGEH (Standardized Measurement Systems for Hospital Management) research project.

Graydon Davison joined the College of Law and Business at the University of Western Sydney in 2000, following careers in public and private sector management and in management consulting. Graydon holds a Master of Technology Management and is currently completing his PhD He teaches Organizational Behavior and Management and Decision Making. His PhD thesis, "Innovative Practice in the Process of Patient Management in Palliative Care," is a non-clinical view of the management of innovation in a complex, dynamic environment where the results of innovation are social advantage, care and well-being of people.

Pranay Desai is currently an information systems consultant with F5-System Integrators (Brisbane, Australia). He completed his Master of Information Systems and is also a certified Oracle developer. Mr. Desai is currently lecturing at Griffith University (Brisbane, Australia) in a number of subjects. These include business processes and models, application development, advanced programming, data communication and information system development. Mr. Desai has extensive practical experience in database development and business process analysis within organizations in India, where he was born, and Australia.

Kevin C. Desouza has served as a consultant to numerous corporations in the areas of knowledge management and strategic management of information. He has authored

Managing Knowledge with Artificial Intelligence (Quorum Books), and more than 30 refereed articles either published or forthcoming in journals such as the *Communications of the ACM, Information & Management, Industrial Management, Technology Forecasting and Social Change, Journal of Business Strategy, Human Resource Magazine, International Journal of Healthcare Technology and Management, Journal of Engineering and Technology Management, International Journal of Information Management, Government Information Quarterly, Journal of Contingencies and Crisis Management, IT Professional, Human Systems Management, Competitive Intelligence Review, Business Horizons, Competitive Intelligence Magazine, Across the Board, Emergence, Journal of Knowledge Management, Knowledge Process and Management, European Management Journal, Business Process Management Journal* and the likes. He is currently serving as a senior associate editor of the *Journal of Information Science and Technology*, and is a guest editor of the *International Journal of Healthcare Technology and Management*. His research interests include knowledge management, national security, and military intelligence. He is currently completing his doctoral work at the University of Illinois at Chicago.

Susan West Engelkemeyer is an associate professor of Management and director of the One Year M.B.A. Program at Babson College in Wellesley, Massachusetts. She served as the College's director of quality for 5 years. She also serves as a consultant for the American Association for Higher Education (AAHE) in Washington, DC, and was a senior examiner for the Malcolm Baldrige National Quality Award for 6 years. She has published in *Quality Management, Quality Progress, and Journal of Innovative Management,* and has authored several book chapters. Her current research is focused on systemic organizational change and assessment, key performance measures, and knowledge management. She holds an MBA from East Carolina University, and a PhD from Clemson University.

Adam Fadlalla is an associate professor of Computer and Information Science in the College of Business Administration at Cleveland State University, Cleveland, Ohio (USA). He holds an MBA in Finance and Decision Sciences from Miami University, Oxford, Ohio, an MS in Computer Science and a PhD in Computer Information Systems from the University of Cincinnati, Cincinnati, Ohio. His current research interests include decision support systems, artificial intelligence applications and knowledge discovery in databases. His research has been published in many journals, including *Computers and Operations Research, Omega, Interfaces, Journal of the American Medical Informatics Association*, and *Information Systems Management.*

Danielle Fowler is an assistant professor of Management Information Systems at the University of Baltimore, Maryland (USA). Fowler earned her PhD from Swinburne University of Technology (1998) and was on the staff of the School of Information Technology there before moving to the University of Baltimore in 2000. Her areas of specialization include requirement engineering, e-commerce and object orientation, on which she has published internationally. She is also a member on a number of international conference committees.

John Gammack is a professor in Information Systems at Griffith University (Australia) and the School's research director. Formerly he was director of the Centre for Electronic Commerce and Internet Studies at Murdoch University, Perth, Australia and head of the IT school. His primary research interests include modeling knowledge and decision in organizations, and the development of information systems related to this. He has approximately 150 publications in these and related areas. His currently funded research examines the (electronic) branding of cities, and various issues, particularly technological, relating to sustainable development in the Asia-Pacific region.

Vidyaranya B. Gargeya is an associate professor in the Department of Information Systems and Operations Management, Joseph M. Bryan School of Business and Economics, University of North Carolina at Greensboro, USA. He earned his PhD from Georgia State University. Dr. Gargeya's research interests include management of information technology services, services operations management, technology in services, total quality management, and service chain management.

Eliezer (Elie) Geisler is a professor and associate dean for research at the Stuart Graduate School of Business, Illinois Institute of Technology (USA). He holds a doctorate degree from the Kellogg School at Northwestern University. Dr. Geisler is the author of approximately 90 papers in the areas of technology and innovation management, the evaluation of R&D, science and technology, and the management of medical technology. He is the author of eight books, including: *The Metrics of Science and Technology* (2000) and *Creating Value with Science and Technology* (2001). Dr. Geisler was founder and editor of the Department of Information Technology for the *IEEE Transactions on Engineering Management*, and is associate editor of the *International Journal of Healthcare Technology and Management.* He consulted for major corporations and for many US federal departments, such as Defense, Commerce, EPA, Energy, and NASA. Dr. Geisler is director of IIT's Center for the Management of Medical Technology (CMMT). Dr. Geisler co-chairs the annual conference on the Hospital of the Future. His most recent books are: *Installing and Managing Workable Knowledge Management Systems* (Praeger, 2003, co-authored with Rubenstein) and *Technology, Healthcare and Management in the Hospital of the Future* (2003, with Krabbendam and Schuring). His forthcoming book is: *The Structure and Progress of Knowledge: Applications in Databases and Management Systems* (M.E. Sharpe, 2004).

William Golden is a member of the Centre for Innovation and Structural Change and a lecturer in Information Systems at NUI, Galway (Ireland). He has held this position since 1991. He completed his doctorate on B2B electronic commerce at the University of Warwick, UK. He has presented papers at both national and international conferences. He has co-authored a book, contributed chapters to other texts and published papers in the areas of e-commerce and IS in *Omega, The International Journal of Management Science, International Journal of Electronic Commerce, Journal of Agile Management Systems* and the *Journal of Decision Systems.*

W. A. Groothuis completed his education in information science, with specialization office automation and information analysis, and then began working as a consultant with Doctors without Borders. Selection and implementation of information systems, issues concerning the Internet and training of employees were elements of his work. In 1998, he joined the advisory group Healthcare of Cap Gemini Ernst & Young (CGEY). His main areas of attention were decision support technology, information systems, knowledge management and mobile communication. In 2003, he left the Netherlands to live with his wife and son in Sweden.

John A. Hensing is Senior Vice President of Care Management and Quality at Banner Health (USA). He joined the organization in 1995. His responsibilities include care management and organizational performance for the system, including medical management, care coordination and case management, management engineering and organizational performance improvement. He also oversees operations of the Banner Health Research Institute. He has practiced internal medicine in Tempe for 18 years and was awarded the Distinguished Internist of the Year Award in 1993. He is a fellow in the American College of Physicians and has served on multiple boards including The Samaritan Foundation, Samaritan Health System, HealthPartners of Arizona and the Arizona Medicare Demonstration Project 1999.

Amanda H. Hoffmeister is Director of Accounting at Cookeville Regional Medical Center in Cookeville, Tennessee (USA). She received her undergraduate degree in business and an MBA from Tennessee Technological University. While in the MBA program, she developed an interest in quality improvement issues, and in particular in patient safety and errors in health care, and how practices from other industries could help to prevent them. She is also a past Tennessee Quality Award examiner.

Martin Hughes is a lecturer in Information Systems at NUI, Galway (Ireland), a position he has held since 2000. He is currently pursuing a PhD on e-business at the University of Bath, UK. His research interests include knowledge management, inter-organizational systems and risk, and e-commerce and the small firm. His work has been published in book chapters, leading international IS conferences and in the *Journal of End User Computing, Journal of Electronic Commerce in Organizations, Journal of Small Business and Enterprise Development,* and the *Irish Marketing Review.*

T. Inoue is an assistant professor in the Department of Industrial and Management Systems Engineering, Waseda University. He transferred from graduate school in Musashi Institute of Technology to Graduate School of Sciences and Engineering, Waseda University to complete his doctoral dissertation on organizational climate and innovative action.

Bradford L. Kirkman-Liff has been a faculty member in the W. P. Carey School of Business, Arizona State University (USA) since 1981. His current research and teaching are in the areas of the global pharmaceutical and biotechnology industries, knowledge management and information technology strategies, and negotiation. His past research and teaching was in the areas of managed care, health insurance, and health reform in industrialized nations. He has been a World Health Organization fellow and has served as a consultant to governments (including the US Congressional Budget Office and the US General Accounting Office), hospitals, pharmaceutical and biotechnology businesses, and health insurers in the US, Canada, the UK, Belgium, Ireland and the Netherlands.

Darren Mundy is taking up the post of lecturer of Internet Computing at the University of Hull's Scarborough Campus, UK. Prior to this, he was a research assistant for 3 years in the Information Systems Security Research Group (*http://sec.isi.salford.ac.uk*) at the University of Salford, UK. He has been involved in a large variety of research projects including secure electronic prescription processing, secure electronic discharge notes and secure direct access to a diabetic database by opticians. He holds a First Class Honors Degree in Computer Science and Information Systems from the University of Salford, and is presently progressing toward a PhD in the field of Internet Security.

Sharon Muret-Wagstaff is an instructor in Pediatrics at Harvard Medical School and associate director of the Harvard Pediatric Health Services Research Fellowship Program (USA). Sharon also teaches quality and organization of health care in the Boston Combined Residency Program in Pediatrics, and she consults at other universities and health care organizations on building organizational infrastructure and capacity for research and performance excellence. Sharon was an examiner for the Malcolm Baldrige National Quality Award for 6 years. She holds an MS in Public Health and a PhD in Developmental Psychology from the University of Minnesota, and an MPA in Policy and Management from the Kennedy School of Government at Harvard University. She is certified as a Six Sigma Black Belt by the American Society for Quality.

R. Nat Natarajan is the W.E. Mayberry professor of Management at Tennessee Technological University (USA). He received his MS from the Kellogg Graduate School of Management, Northwestern University and his PhD in Business from the University of Kansas. He has published in journals such as the *International Journal of Production Economics, Decision Sciences, Total Quality Management* and in the *Encyclopedia of Production and Manufacturing Management.* He has made presentations and participated in numerous conferences and professional programs in the US and abroad. He has served as an examiner for the Baldrige National Quality Award and for the Tennessee Quality Award.

Pamela M. Nenaber is the system director for Care Management and has responsibility for the oversight, coordination and improvement of clinical care and patient safety for all facilities within Banner Health. Prior positions include operational and consultative experience in multiple settings, including not-for-profit hospitals, corporate multi-hospital systems and national for-profit home health. She received her BS degree with highest honors from Columbia University and earned a master's degree in Health Services Administration from Arizona State University.

Ely Laureano Paiva is an assistant professor and Executive Coordinator of the Graduate Program of Administration at Universidade do Vale do Rio dos Sinos – UNISINOS (Brazil). He received his PhD from Federal University of Rio Grande do Sul, Brazil. He was fellow researcher in the University of North Carolina at Chapel Hill. He publishes regularly in international and Brazilian journals. His research topics are related to operations management, including operations strategy, knowledge management and international operations.

Richard J. Puerzer is an assistant professor of Engineering at Hofstra University where he directs instruction in the Industrial Engineering and Engineering Management programs. He received his BS, MS, and PhD in Industrial Engineering from the University of Pittsburgh (1989, 1991, and 1997, respectively). His teaching includes courses in statistics, operations research, simulation, engineering economics, and engineering methods. His research interests include engineering assessment and the application of automatic identification tools in health care industries.

Harsha P. Reddy was born in India. She completed her bachelor's degree in Computer Science and Engineering from Sri Krishna Devaraya University, a reputable university in India. Believing that the broad overview gained during the undergraduate studies can be consummated only by the in-depth study that a graduate study will entail, she accepted a scholarship to undertake MS at Cleveland State University, Ohio (USA). She did an independent study in "Data Stream Management System" with Dr. Arndt, Cleveland State University. This research increased her interest in the areas of efficient data association and knowledge management, which is one of the prominent reasons for writing this chapter. She also worked as a Web programmer in the Cleveland Clinic Foundation, Cleveland, where she enhanced her skills in Web management. Currently, Reddy is working as an application developer in IntelliCorp, Solon, Ohio (USA), a nationwide provider of online criminal records, driving records and other public records. By applying her comprehensive theoretical knowledge in the real world, she could achieve a perfect blend of theoretical and practical knowledge. She is honored to be in National Dean's List for 2002. She is interested in obtaining a PhD in Computer Sciences and believes that this degree would enable her to combine a teaching career with advising business on software industry.

Albert H. Rubenstein is Founder and President of International Applied Science and Technology Associates (IASTA, Inc.) and professor emeritus at Northwestern University, where he established the program of Research on the Management of R&D/Innovation, the Engineering Management Program, and the Center for Information and Telecommunication Technology. His latest books are *Managing Technology in the Decentralized Firm* and *Installing and Managing Workable Knowledge Management System* (with Elie Geister). In addition, Rubenstein has consulted with more than 100 industrial firms and technology-based government agencies in the US and 12 other countries. He has more than 150 publications and two doctorates in engineering and management.

George C. Runger is a professor of Industrial Engineering at Arizona State University (USA). He is author of two books and many technical papers in the field of industrial statistics. He is a recipient of the Brumbaugh Award from the American Society for Quality Control. Among his professional interests are multivariate process monitoring and control and statistical methods for massive data sets. He is the co-director of the Modeling and Analysis of Semiconductor Manufacturing Laboratory at ASU. He holds degrees in industrial engineering and statistics.

M. Saito is a professor in the Graduate School and Department of Industrial and Management Systems Engineering, Waseda University, holding a doctorate from the Faculty of Medicine, University of Tokyo. Research interests are workplace redesign, human-centered system design in industries and process management in providing health care in hospital and in community.

Kuldeep Sandhu is a lecturer at Griffith University's School of Management and also director of Postgraduate Studies in Information Systems within the school. He teaches in the areas of applications development, computer simulation, distributed decision support systems, data communications and internships. He is also program director for the Graduate Certificate and advanced masters courses in IS, including the Master of Strategic Information Systems Management. He has extensive practical experience before joining the university and in research work. His current research interests are in e-development and design, business systems integration and the relationship between KM and IT.

H. Seki is an associate professor, Faculty of Distribution and Logistics Systems, Ryutsu Keizai University. After completing graduate school in Waseda University, he was assistant professor in Waseda University for 3 years and took position of Associate Professor in Ryutsu Keizai University. His major interests are mathematical statistics and organizational ergonomics.

Bruce Shadbolt is a senior lecturer with the Canberra Clinical School at the Canberra Hospital (Australia) affiliated with the University of Sydney's Faculty of Medicine and the Australian National University Medical School. He is Director of the Centre for Advances in Epidemiology & IT, and head of Medical Informatics at the National Health Sciences Centre. Dr. Shadbolt is a leading researcher in health outcomes studies and expert in clinical trial methodology.

Howard Silverman currently serves as Education Director for the Program in Integrative Medicine and Clinical Professor of Family and Community Medicine at the University of Arizona's College of Medicine (USA). He was formerly system director of Medical Informatics and Clinical Innovation at Banner Health (USA), where he had organizational responsibility for creating synergy between care transformation activities, clinical innovation and information technology. He graduated Phi Beta Kappa from Purdue University, majoring in mathematics and German. He earned his MS in Computer Science at MIT, where he specialized in artificial intelligence applications in medical decision making. He then attended Stanford University School of Medicine followed by a residency in family practice at Good Samaritan Medical Center in Phoenix, Arizona.

Maire Simington is the director of Care Management Services and is responsible for oversight of knowledge management, project management, publishing and liaison activity for care management. Prior to joining Banner Health (USA), she was the chair of Marketing/Communications at Mayo Clinic in Scottsdale and has worked in marketing and communication in multiple settings. She graduated Phi Beta Kappa from Hofstra University where she majored in English, and earned her PhD in English at Arizona State University. She also holds an MBA from the University of Phoenix.

Edward A. Smith received a bachelor's degree in Mathematics and a master's degree in Computer Science and Medical Informatics from the University of Utah prior to receiving his medical degree from the University of Arizona. After completing a residency in internal medicine at the University of Texas at San Antonio, he practiced in Mesa, Arizona for 16 years. Recently he decided to return to academia, completed an MPH degree at the Harvard School of Public Health and joined the faculty at Arizona State University. He is currently on the faculty at the University of Arizona College of Medicine and an investigator at the Translational Genomics Research Institute in Phoenix, Arizona.

Deborah I. Sorrell is employed as an Integration Analyst at High Point Regional Hospital and Health System and has more than 20 years' experience in the health care industry. Her expertise spans diverse areas such as diagnostic medicine, operations management, and IT. She has a Bachelor's degree in Medical Technology, a Master's in Business Administration, and Master of Science in Information Technology and Management.

Paul A. Swatman is a professor of Information Systems at Deakin Business School, Melbourne, Australia. Previously he has held positions as professor and Dean of Information Systems at the Stuttgart Institute of Management and Technology, Germany; professor and head of the School of Management Information Systems at Deakin University; and as Foundation Director of the Center for Information Systems Research at Swinburne University of Technology. He was visiting professor at numerous universities and research centers. His research interests include: methods for the acquisition/development of high-quality information systems, systems development as a problem solving activity and organizational and social change resulting from information and telecommunications technology innovation.

Murat Caner Testik is an assistant professor of Industrial Engineering at Cukurova University. He holds a PhD in Industrial Engineering from Arizona State University. His research interests are statistical quality control and data mining for quality improvement.

A.E. Wahle completed her education to be a nurse and, in 1993, chose to study Medical Information Sciences at the University of Amsterdam. She worked for a year and a half at the Academic Medical Centre (AMC) of Amsterdam as an information analyst. In 1998, she left to work with Cap Gemini Ernst & Young (CGEY). She is now senior consultant at an advisory group, specialized in health care. Her main areas of attention are information and knowledge management, combined with issues about quality and patient safety.

Rui Wang is system architect and key developer of the PHT system. Rui holds a graduate diploma in computing science and has many years of experience in software development. Her main IT interest is enterprise Web application development methodology and implementation.

Khin Than Win is a lecturer in the School of IT and Computer Science at the University of Wollongong. She is a medical doctor with a post graduate degree in Computer Information System. Her background of medicine and computer information systems has made her an efficient and enthusiastic researcher in health informatics. Her research interests are in issues related to electronic health record systems. She has published several peer review conference and journal papers in Health Informatics.

Heidemarie Winklhofer is a lecturer in Information Systems at Griffith University Brisbane, Australia. Prior to her appointment, she worked for 8 years in the IT industry in Canberra, Australia. She has presented papers at IS conferences in Australia and overseas. She is currently studying toward a PhD in IS. Her major research interests include project management, system development methodologies, organizational change and m-commerce.

Index

E

e-benefits 115
e-bonnectivity 114
e-health 51, 110
e-healthcare 50
e-hospital 50
e-hospital network 57
electronic data collection 208
electronic health record 92
electronic prescription system (EPS) 37
enterprise business processes 51
e-procurement 114
evidence-based medicine 125, 133
explicit knowledge 3, 17, 237

F

factual knowledge 33
fault tree analysis 105
firewalls 330

G

granularity problem 215
gross domestic product (GDP) 15

H

health and hospital services (HHS) 195
health care providers 194
health data users 93
health information systems 91
health insurance portability and account-
    ability Ac 58
health services system 207
healthcare 239
healthcare costs 150
healthcare enterprises 14
healthcare leaders 151
healthcare organization 1, 44, 50, 78, 286,
    321
healthcare quality 337
HIPAA 165
home based support (HBS) 211
hospital industry 14, 44, 65, 304
human services 208

I

ID cards 214
implicit knowledge 3
India 235
Indian companies 235
information age 110
information revolution 6
intellectual capital (IC) 45
intellectual nuggets 45
intelligent agents 7
intranet utilization patterns 229
intranets 222
iterative software development model 94

J

JCAHO 338

K

KM practices 231
KM systems 44
knowledge 223, 290
knowledge acquisition 306
knowledge application 306
knowledge assets 164
knowledge capture 20
knowledge creation 18, 306
knowledge databases 240
knowledge discovery 78
knowledge discovery in data bases (KDD)
    16
knowledge dissemination 306
knowledge elicitation 18
knowledge flows 238
knowledge management (KM) 1, 14, 45,
    91, 110, 165, 224, 235, 306, 349
knowledge management process model 14
knowledge mapping 7
knowledge of procedures 33
knowledge perspectives 207
knowledge productivity measurement 286
knowledge repositories 17
knowledge retrieval 16
knowledge sharing 243
knowledge storage media 2
knowledge transfer 17

T

tacit knowing 237
tacit knowledge 3, 17
tele-medicine 193, 197

U

unified medical vocabulary 23

V

vendor "solutions" 237
video conferencing (VC) 195
virtual work environment 238

W

waterfall model 94
Web browsers 8
wireless data transfer 330

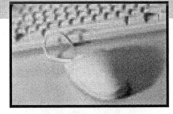
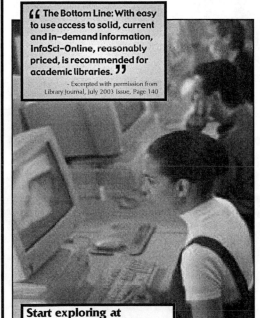

Books on Healthcare Information Systems

Effective Healthcare Information Systems

Adi Armoni, Ph.D., Tel Aviv University, Israel

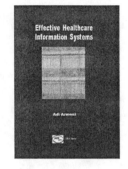

Health and medical informatics encompass a very broad field that is rapidly developing in both its research and operational aspects. The discipline has many dimensions, including social, legal, ethical and economic. This book, *Effective Healthcare Information Systems* puts a special emphasis on issues dealing with the most recent innovations such as telemedicine, Web-based medical Information and consulting systems, expert systems and artificial intelligence.

ISBN: 1-931777-01-2; eISBN: 1-931777-20-9; Copyright: 2002
Pages: 295 (s/c); Price: US $59.95

Strategies for Healthcare Information Systems

Robert Stegwee, Ph.D., University of Twente, The Netherlands
Ton Spil, University of Twente, The Netherlands

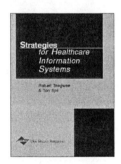

Information technologies of the past two decades have created significant fundamental changes in the delivery of healthcare services by healthcare provider organizations. *Strategies for Healthcare Information Systems* provides an overall coverage of different aspects of healthcare information systems strategies and challenges facing these organizations.

ISBN: 1-878289-89-6; Copyright: 2001; Pages: 232 (s/c); Price: US $74.95

Knowledge Media in Healthcare: Opportunities and Challenges

Edited by Rolf Grutter, Ph.D., University of St. Gallen, Switzerland

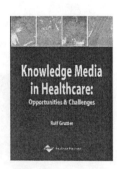

Because the field of healthcare reflects forms of both explicit and tacit knowledge such as evidence-based knowledge, clinical guidelines and the physician's experience, knowledge media have significant potential in this area. *Knowledge Media in Healthcare: Opportunities and Challenges* is an innovative new book which strives to show the positive impact that Knowledge Media and communication technology can have on human communication within the field of healthcare.

ISBN 1-930708-13-0; eISBN: 1-59140-006-6; Copyright: 2002; Pages: 296; Price: US$74.95

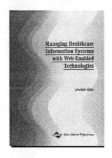
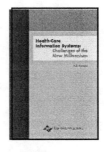

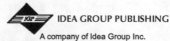